Online Nursing Education

A Collaborative Approach

Melissa Robinson, PhD, RN
Professor and Division Chair, Nursing Programs
University of Providence
Great Falls, MT

Henny Breen, PhD, RN
Professor of Nursing Program and
Service Learning Coordinator
RN-to-BSN Program
Linfield University, School of Nursing
Portland, OR

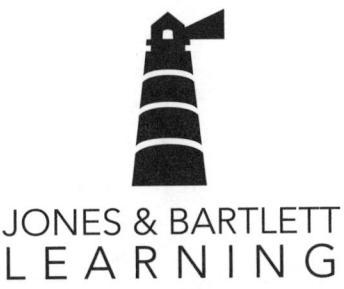

JONES & BARTLETT
LEARNING

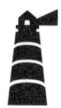

World Headquarters
Jones & Bartlett Learning
5 Wall Street
Burlington, MA 01803
978-443-5000
info@jblearning.com
www.jblearning.com

Jones & Bartlett Learning books and products are available through most bookstores and online booksellers. To contact Jones & Bartlett Learning directly, call 800-832-0034, fax 978-443-8000, or visit our website, www.jblearning.com.

Substantial discounts on bulk quantities of Jones & Bartlett Learning publications are available to corporations, professional associations, and other qualified organizations. For details and specific discount information, contact the special sales department at Jones & Bartlett Learning via the above contact information or send an email to specialsales@jblearning.com.

Production Credits

VP, Product Operations: Christine Emerton
Director of Product Management: Matthew Kane
Product Manager: Tina Chen
Content Specialist: Melina Leon-Haley
Project Manager: Kristen Rogers
Digital Project Specialist: Rachel DiMaggio
Director of Marketing: Andrea DeFronzo
Senior Marketing Manager: Lindsay White
VP, Manufacturing and Inventory Control: Therese Connell
Product Fulfillment Manager: Wendy Kilborn
Composition: S4Carlisle Publishing Services
Project Management: S4Carlisle Publishing Services
Cover Design: Michael O'Donnell
Text Design: Kristin E. Parker
Senior Media Development Editor: Troy Liston
Rights & Permissions Manager: John Rusk
Rights Specialist: James Fortney
Cover Image (Title Page, Part Opener, Chapter Opener): © Thinz/Shutterstock
Printing and Binding: Sheridan

Library of Congress Cataloging-in-Publication Data

Names: Robinson, Melissa, author. | Breen, Henny, author.
Title: Online nursing education : a collaborative approach / Melissa Robinson, Henny Breen.
Description: Burlington, Massachusetts : Jones & Bartlett Learning, [2022]
| Includes bibliographical references and index.
Identifiers: LCCN 2020028512 | ISBN 9781284181173 (paperback)
Subjects: MESH: Education, Nursing--methods | Education, Distance--methods
| Interdisciplinary Placement--methods | Curriculum--standards |
Students, Nursing
Classification: LCC RT73 | NLM WY 18 | DDC 610.73071/1--dc23
LC record available at https://lccn.loc.gov/2020028512

6048

Printed in the United States of America
24 23 22 21 20   10 9 8 7 6 5 4 3 2 1

Brief Contents

About the Authors   **xiv**

Acknowledgments   **xv**

Preface   **xvi**

CHAPTER 1	**Collaborative Model for Online Nursing Education** 1
CHAPTER 2	**Philosophical and Theoretical Approaches to Online Education** . . . 9
CHAPTER 3	**Online Nursing Students** 21
CHAPTER 4	**Successful Academic Progression and Online Nursing Students** 43
CHAPTER 5	**Leadership of Online Nursing Programs** 61
CHAPTER 6	**Quality Assurance in Online Nursing Programs** 71
CHAPTER 7	**Curriculum Development** 87
CHAPTER 8	**Online Course Design** 101
CHAPTER 9	**Online Teaching Strategies** 127
CHAPTER 10	**Learning Through Writing in Online Classrooms** 149
CHAPTER 11	**Experiential Learning in Online Nursing Programs** 163
CHAPTER 12	**Narrative Pedagogy** 193
CHAPTER 13	**Faculty Role in Academia** 211

CHAPTER 14   **The Influence of Generational Differences on Learning in the Online Classroom: Research Exemplar** 241

CHAPTER 15   **Assessing Online Collaborative Discourse** 259

CHAPTER 16   **Academic Partnerships: Social Determinants of Health Addressed Through Service Learning** 273

Index   **289**

Contents

About the Authors xiv

Acknowledgments xv

Preface xvi

**CHAPTER 1 Collaborative Model for Online
Nursing Education** **1**

Overview 1

Collaborative Approach to Online Nursing Education 1

Collaboration 3

Collaborative Model for Online Nursing Education 3

Guiding Principles 4

    Nurse Education Is an Advanced Specialty of Nursing Practice 4

    Online Nursing Education Is a Subspecialty of Nursing Education 5

    Online Nursing Education Should Be Integrated Within the Institution 5

    Technology Is Secondary to Education Theory and Best Practice 6

Summary 6

References 7

**CHAPTER 2 Philosophical and Theoretical
Approaches to Online Education** **9**

Overview 9

Philosophical Approach to Education 10

    Constructivist Learning Theories 10

    Collaborativist Learning Theory 12

    Experiential Learning Theory 13

    Transformative Learning Theory 14

Adult Learning Theory 15

Narrative Pedagogy 15

Summary 18

Best-Practice Recommendations for Online Teaching 18

References 19

CHAPTER 3 Online Nursing Students 21

Overview 21
Enrollment Trends in Higher Education 21
Educational Pathways to Nursing 22
Demand for Higher Levels of Nursing Education 23
Characteristics of Online Nursing Students 24
     Cultural, Ethnic, and Gender Diversity 24
     English as a Second Language 26
     Generational Diversity 28
     Learning Styles and Preferences 29
     Personality Traits 30
     Student Motivation 31
Humanistic Education 32
Student–Faculty Relationships 34
Promoting a Sense of Belonging 35
     Respect 35
Social Presence: Teacher Immediacy 35
     Synchronous Meeting Times 36
     Individual Phone Calls 36
     Student Support During a Crisis 37
Best-Practice Recommendations for Online Teaching 38
References 38

CHAPTER 4 Successful Academic Progression and Online Nursing Students 43

Overview 43
Background 43
Motivation for Higher Levels of Nursing Education 44
Barriers to Degree Advancement for Nurses 44
Student Persistence 45
Holistic Academic Progression for Nurses:
    An Interprofessional Model 45
Program Description 47
Interprofessional Team 47
     Outreach Coordinator 48
     Admissions Counselor 48
     Academic Advisor 49
     Program Director and Online Faculty 50
Community Partnerships 52
Program Evaluation: The Interprofessional Model 53

Measurements of Student Persistence 54
Student Survey: Feedback From Students on
    Academic Advising 54
Community Partner Survey. 56
Outcomes of Program Evaluation. 56
Best-Practice Recommendations for Online Programs. 57
Acknowledgment. 58
References 58

**CHAPTER 5 Leadership of Online Nursing
Programs. 61**

Overview. 61
Background 61
Acceptance of Online Education 62
Dedicated Program Leadership 63
    Collaborative Leadership Model 63
    Coordinator of Online Programs. 64
    Service-Learning Coordinator 67
    Course Lead 67
Summary 69
Best-Practice Recommendations for Online Programs. 69
References 70

**CHAPTER 6 Quality Assurance in Online
Nursing Programs. 71**

Overview. 71
Background 71
Institutional Support for Quality Online Education 72
Quality in Online Programs. 73
Assessment and Evaluation of Online Learning 74
    Course Evaluation 74
    Student Persistence Rates 75
Academic Program Review. 76
Quality Assurance Specific to the Online Nursing Program. 76
Preparation for Online Teaching. 76
Best Practices for Online Teaching 76
Peer Appraisal 79
Online Course Expectations 79
Student Feedback 79
Summary 83

Best-Practice Recommendations for Online Programs 83

References 83

CHAPTER 7 **Curriculum Development** **87**

Overview 87

Healthcare and Societal Issues Affecting Nursing Education 87

Program Development 88

Alignment 88

Curriculum Design 91

    Concept-Based Curriculum 91

    Alignment Design 95

    Integrated Design 95

Integration of Models as Applied
to an Online RN-to-BSN Curriculum 96

Assessment of Learning 96

Progression of Learning Through the Semesters 96

Best-Practice Recommendations for Online Teaching 98

References 98

CHAPTER 8 **Online Course Design** **101**

Overview 101

Best Practices for Online Course Design 101

    The Learner Is at the Center of the Course Design 102

    Collaborative Learning 102

    Develop a Clear and Consistent Structure 102

    Collaborate on Course Design 103

    Collaborative and Individual Reflection 103

Process of Online Course Design 103

Collaborative Design and Development Process 105

Design and Development 105

    Learning Outcomes 105

    Assessment 108

    Integration of Assessment and Learning Activities 111

    Assessments and Grading Rubrics 114

Structure and Sequencing of the Course 121

Learning Modules 121

Learning Materials 122

Leveling and Scaffolding 124

Evaluation 125

Best-Practice Recommendations for Online Teaching 125

References 126

CHAPTER 9 Online Teaching Strategies 127

Overview 127

Faculty Preparation for Teaching Online 127

Learner-Centered Teaching 128

Concept-Based and Competency-Based Teaching 129

The Faculty Role in Constructivist Teaching 129

Scaffolded Teaching 129

Active Learning and Teaching 130

Develop a Community of Learners 132

Community of Inquiry 132

Social Presence 133

Cognitive Presence 134

Teaching Presence 134

The Learner in the Community of Inquiry Model 135

Teaching Strategies to Demonstrate Presence
and Engagement 136

Online Collaborative Activities 137

Group Work 138

Asynchronous Discussions 138

Facilitating Reflective, Critical, and Analytical Thinking 139

Socratic Method 141

Facilitation Challenges 142

Grading and Feedback 142

Instructional Resources 142

Feedback Banks 143

Group Feedback 143

Personalization 143

Grading and Timeliness 145

Summary 146

Best-Practice Recommendations for Online Teaching 146

References 147

CHAPTER 10 Learning Through Writing in
Online Classrooms 149

Overview 149

Information Literacy 150

Collaboration Between Librarians and Nursing Faculty 150

Embedded Librarians 150

Research Guides and Tutorials 151

Student-Centered Learning 151

Writing Across the Curriculum in Nursing Education 152

Institutional-Level Policies 154

Technical Aspects of Writing for the Discipline 154

Mechanics 155
Academic Integrity 156

Types of Writing Students Do in Online Nursing Programs 159

Best-Practice Recommendations for Online Programs 159

References 160

CHAPTER 11 Experiential Learning in Online Nursing Programs **163**

Overview 163

Experiential Learning Overview 163

Simulation 164

Simulations as Experiential Learning 164
Synchronous Versus Asynchronous Simulation 166

Experiential Learning Cycle by Kolb and Kolb 166

Learning Is an Endlessly Recurring Cycle, Not a Linear Process 166
Experiencing Is Necessary for Learning 168
The Brain Is Built for Experiential Learning 169
The Dialectic Poles of the Learning Cycle Are What
    Motivates Learning 170

Adapting the Model for Online Nursing Education 170

Semester 1 172
Semester 2 172
Semester 3 172

Other Experiential Learning Strategies 172

Arts and Literature Activity 172
Interviews 177
Small-Group Work Using a Case Study 177
Service Learning 178

Summary 179

Best-Practice Recommendations for Online Teaching 180

References 180

Appendix

Experiential Learning: Using Virtual Simulation
    in an Online RN-to-BSN Program 182

CHAPTER 12 Narrative Pedagogy **193**

Overview 193

Narrative Pedagogy 193

Interpretative Approach 194

The Concernful Practices of Schooling Learning Teaching 195

    Gathering: Welcoming and Calling Forth 195

    Interpreting: Unlearning and Becoming 196

    Inviting: Waiting and Letting Be 196

    Listening: Knowing and Connecting. 197

The Use of Narrative Pedagogy in Online Classrooms 197

    Virtual Communities 198

    Art Forms: Literature, Cinema, Podcasts, Music 198

    Experiential Storytelling. 204

Summary 208

Best-Practice Recommendations for Online Teaching. 209

References 209

CHAPTER 13 Faculty Role in Academia **211**

Overview. 211

Nurses in Academia 211

Demand for Faculty in Nursing. 212

Readiness for Online Teaching 212

Preparation and Competency for Online Teaching 212

Competent Online Teaching 213

    Online Adjunct Faculty 213

    Orientation. 214

    Mentorship. 214

Professional Development 215

    Certified Nurse Educator 218

    Certified Online Instructor (COI). 219

    Quality Matters. 220

Scholarship in Nursing Education 220

Boyer's Model of Scholarship 221

    Scholarship of Teaching 221

    Scholarship of Application 221

    Scholarship of Discovery 221

    Scholarship of Integration. 221

Faculty Promotion and Tenure 222

Our Journey to the Scholarship of Teaching and Learning. 224

Growth in Teaching 224

    Reflection on Teaching 224

    Reflection on Teaching Philosophy 225

Exchanging Knowledge About Teaching and Learning. 227

    Formal Mentorship Program. 227

Growth in the Scholarship of Teaching. 229

Collaborative Scholarship 230

Summary 232

Best-Practice Recommendations for Online Programs 232

References 233

Appendix A
Faculty Mentor Position Summary 235

Appendix B
Faculty Orientation and Mentorship Checklist. 237

**CHAPTER 14 The Influence of Generational
Differences on Learning in the Online Classroom:
Research Exemplar 241**

Overview 241

Generational Diversity in Nursing Education. 241

Study Methodology. 242

Finding 1: Increased Nursing Knowledge 242

Finding 2: Expanded Perspectives 243

Finding 3: Leadership Development. 245

   Mentorship. 247

Finding 4: Enhanced Communication Skills 250

Finding 5: Personal Growth. 252

Finding 6: Improved Technology Skills. 253

Implications for Nursing Education Practice and Research. 254

Recommendations for Future Research 255

Strategies That Support a Generationally Diverse Online Classroom . . . 256

References 256

CHAPTER 15 Assessing Online Collaborative Discourse. . .259

Overview 259

Collaborative Learning 259

Literature Review. 260

Online Collaborative Learning Theory 261

   Phase One: Idea Generating 261

   Phase Two: Idea Organizing 261

   Phase Three: Intellectual Convergence 261

Method and Design 261

   Setting and Participants 262

   Data Collection, Coding, and Analysis 262

   Ethical Considerations 264

Findings 264
    Week One (Entire Class). 264
    Week Two: Group Forums 267
Discussion 268
Conclusion/Recommendations. 270
    Online Instruction 270
    Evaluation 271
    Further Research. 271
References 272

**CHAPTER 16 Academic Partnerships: Social
Determinants of Health Addressed Through
Service Learning 273**

Overview 273
Background 273
Literature Review. 274
Methodology. 275
Data Sources and Analysis 276
Findings: Students. 278
    Vulnerable Populations. 280
    Challenges in Access to Care. 281
    Leadership Skills—Communication, Collaboration, and Advocacy. 281
    Improved Awareness of Community Resources. 281
    Impact on Nursing Practice 282
Findings: Community Organizations 282
    Access to Health Education. 282
    Involvement of Clients in Health-Promotion Activities 285
    Increased Quality of Care and Services 285
    Increased Trust and Confidence in the Organization. 286
Discussion 286
Acknowledgments 287
Funding. 287
References 287

Index 289

About the Authors

Melissa Robinson, PhD, RN, is a professor of nursing and division chair at the University of Providence. She has been a registered nurse since 1991, with experience in hospice and palliative care nursing, community and tribal health, and nursing leadership. She has taught in online nursing education since 2006, initially in an adjunct role in the online registered nurse–bachelor of science (RN-to-BSN) program at Salish Kootenai College, then as a professor of nursing at Linfield University, School of Nursing from 2008 to 2020. She is a certified hospice and palliative care nurse, a certified online instructor, and has served as a master reviewer for Quality Matters. She has authored a number of peer-reviewed journal articles and regularly presents at local, state, and national conferences on issues related to nursing education, including best practices in online education, online teaching strategies, and population health. She is currently serving as the lead editor for the 7th edition of *Family Health Care Nursing: Theory, Practice, and Research.*

Henny Breen, PhD, RN, is a professor of nursing in the RN-to-BSN program at Linfield University, School of Nursing since 2011. She started nursing as a diploma graduate 45 years ago in Ontario, Canada, and moved to Hawaii 20 years later. Her nursing experience includes mental health in a variety of roles, including staff nurse, community health, private practice, and as a clinical nurse specialist in a women and children's hospital. She has also worked in quality management, nursing management, and as a supervisor for a high-risk pregnancy disease management program. Nursing education became her full-time nursing practice 16 years ago in Kaneohe, Hawaii, teaching for a BSN program at Hawaii Pacific University. She has 13 years of online teaching experience, and for the past 9 years has focused most of her teaching practice online with postlicensure nursing students after moving to Portland, Oregon. She currently lives in Boise, Idaho. She is a certified nurse educator and a certified online instructor. She has authored a number of peer-reviewed articles and chapters for various texts and regularly delivers peer-reviewed presentations at national and international conferences related to online education and service learning.

Acknowledgments

"If your actions inspire others to dream more, learn more, do more and become more, you are a leader."

—John Quincy Adams

We would like to acknowledge that our work would not be possible without the colleagues and mentors who have shared their knowledge and support with us over the years. The success of our online students is significantly affected by our interprofessional team, and we are sincerely grateful to them.

For their dedication to student success and their contributions to developing the interprofessional model, we would like to recognize Jessica Mole, Joanne Swenson, Reese Hiller, and Anna Harrington-Chaudhary.

For their contributions to creating high-quality learning experiences for online nursing students, we would like to acknowledge the distance librarians on our team, including Carol McCulley and Brandon Wilkinson.

We would also like to sincerely thank our online students. Supporting your growth and development in nursing has been an honor and a privilege. As nurse leaders of the future, you have inspired us and humbled us, and we are forever grateful to you.

Henny Breen
Melissa Robinson

Preface

We are excited to share with you the absolute joy of teaching nursing education online. We both have experience teaching prelicensure and postlicensure nursing students and thoroughly enjoy how online teaching offers us the opportunity to intimately engage with each student in a way that is not possible in the traditional classroom. Although this book has an emphasis on registered nurses with a diploma or associate degree who are furthering their education, we wish to provide practical and theoretical evidence for how the online learning environment can be used to enhance learning in a deep and meaningful way, regardless of the educational level. Online teaching has provided us with opportunities to make a difference in the personal and professional lives of nurses, which has fueled our desire to achieve the best possible outcomes for students.

Teaching exclusively online within a private, liberal arts institution that includes traditional, residential, and online campuses has presented challenges in gaining recognition as a rigorous, high-quality degree program within the institution. We have been inspired to develop the online nursing program through the implementation of policies, professional development of faculty, and best practices that support high-quality teaching and better outcomes for students backed by evaluation studies and qualitative research.

Based on our own experiences in nursing practice and higher education, we have been committed to ensuring that graduates from a variety of backgrounds have access to opportunities that build their confidence and help them grow personally and professionally while advancing their education. It has been our goal to create learning experiences that give online nursing students the ability to realize their full potential for leadership in a variety of settings.

In thinking about how to structure this book, it was important to us that each chapter would stand alone so that readers could pick and choose the parts of the book that were most interesting and relevant to them. However, we found that there is a great deal of interdependence among the different topics addressed, which only serves to reinforce our collaborative model for online nursing education. It was our desire to expand on what is currently in the literature about online teaching and online program delivery to include the importance of a collaborative interprofessional team that is focused on the successful academic progression of students.

This book reflects the work of a deeply reflective and collaborative process between us. In the beginning, we met to develop an outline and brainstormed what should be included in each chapter and assigned a lead to each chapter. The first name on each chapter is the lead who did the beginning research for the chapter and began the writing process. From there, each chapter went back and forth between us by email, through video conferencing, and/or in person until we were both satisfied.

It is our shared love for the profession of nursing and our deep commitment to mentoring nurses who will grow as leaders, influencers, and lifelong learners that inspired us to share what we have learned through our academic practice as educators.

Henny Breen
Melissa Robinson

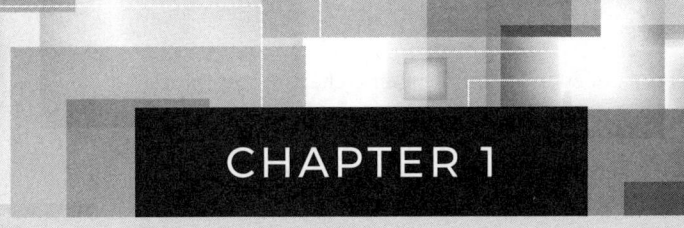

CHAPTER 1

Collaborative Model for Online Nursing Education

Henny Breen and Melissa Robinson

"When I have experienced 'Excellence' in my own life, it has come about as a result of collaborative effort with another. It is evident in the relationship of a supportive employer, spouse, or group of individuals, or a patient where we are striving to accomplish a goal."

(Online registered nurse–bachelor of science in nursing student)

Overview

It is our belief that collaboration is at the heart of any successful online program. This chapter introduces our collaborative model, which is integrated throughout the book. It is based on the following four principles: (1) Nurse education is an advanced specialty of nursing practice, (2) online nursing education is a subspecialty of nursing education, (3) online nursing education should be integrated within the institution, and (4) technology is secondary to education theory and best practices. This chapter also introduces the content of this book.

Collaborative Approach to Online Nursing Education

Our approach to online nursing education grew out of our experience as nurse educators, teaching and conducting research in online education. As full-time faculty members with a workload dedicated entirely to the online nursing program in our institution, we have intentionally developed our teaching practice as a specialty within nursing education. Together, we have over two decades of online teaching experience, specifically in postlicensure education, and have gained experience with the expectations of faculty members related to teaching effectiveness, professional achievement and scholarship, and service to the institution and community.

Our professional development and contributions to nursing scholarship, including our doctoral research, have been focused in the areas of online pedagogy and postlicensure nursing education. We have attended local, national, and international conferences that have allowed us to learn from experts in online education and from leaders within our discipline. To further extend our knowledge and share our experiences, we have disseminated our work widely in professional presentations that emphasize our research findings, innovative teaching strategies, factors involved in the leadership of an online program, strategies that support successful academic progression for online students, and more, which we discuss throughout this book.

When we became colleagues and started teaching in the same program, we recognized how similar our experiences in higher education had been. Earlier in our careers and after practicing as registered nurses (RNs) for approximately a decade, we had both advanced to the bachelor of science in nursing (BSN) degree by attending an RN-to-BSN program. We are both first-generation bachelor's degree students who were naïve to the academic world. We became excited about the new learning and expanded opportunities, which then motivated us to earn our master's degrees while continuing to work in hospitals and community settings and raising a family. After transitioning to full-time teaching, we began the journey to earning our doctorate degrees. We have experienced the challenges of needing to meet in realtime in a classroom and welcomed the opportunity to learn online so that we could continue with our other obligations. It is from our shared background as students and educators that we wrote this text and developed a collaborative model for online education to illustrate the value of collaboration in the development and delivery of an online nursing program.

We perceive online learning as the perfect platform not only to meet the needs of students with diverse schedules and responsibilities but also to provide a safe environment for deep personal reflection. The online learning environment based on social constructivism provides students with the opportunity to think deeply about complex concepts and topics and integrate new understanding in their nursing practice. Nurses today need a broader knowledge base that requires them to be familiar with a range of diverse topics, such as ethical decision making; proficiency in creative problem solving and decision making; critical thinking; and leadership that comes from being grounded in theory, evidence, and experience.

We believe our students, regardless of the mind-set they come into the educational process with, will grow and become even more excited about the work they do when they feel respected for their knowledge and experience and can build on that. We have found that even the most resistant nurses, such as those who verbalize that they are advancing their education for the purposes of job security only, experience changes. They often become very engaged in the learning process—some even report being transformed or "changed forever"—when a social constructivist approach is used. In fact, many even decide to continue on to earn a graduate degree. We believe it is our job to ignite or reawaken the passion that lies within every student who chose to become a nurse and advance their education beyond the diploma or degree that began their entry into nursing as an RN.

Collaboration

Collaboration is an important concept to the nursing profession and is often simply perceived as working together as a member of a patient care team. However, collaboration is much more; it is multifaceted and complex. It is conceptualized as both a dynamic process among two or more people and as an outcome in which there is a synthesis or merging of different perspectives in understanding complex problems and coming to a solution. The American Nurses Association (ANA) *Scope and Standards of Practice* (2015) provides a definition that speaks to complexity, defining collaboration as follows:

> A professional healthcare partnership grounded in reciprocal and respectful recognition and acceptance of: each partner's unique expertise, power, and sphere of influence and responsibilities; the commonality of goals; the mutual safeguarding of the legitimate interest of each part; and the advantages of such a relationship. (p. 86)

It requires the ability to know where and how to leverage influence in working with others. True collaboration needs to be based on mutual trust, respect, open discussion, and shared decision making. There is no room for withholding of information, power grabbing, and personal agendas. The focus needs to be on a shared goal, which in our case is educating students.

Collaborative Model for Online Nursing Education

The success of an online program lies in the ability to collaborate with all stakeholders within the program, the institution, and the community. More specifically, the success of online students and of online programs, overall, relies on effective collaboration to develop the curriculum, recruit and admit students, support the academic success of students, advertise and promote the program, develop partnerships with employers, and so on. It is only through collaboration that all these essential components can be integrated in a way that promotes success. From this premise, we developed our collaborative model depicted in **Figure 1-1** and shared our experiences in this text.

It is important to understand that all parts are related to each other in order to fully implement a successful online program. Collaboration is central to the model because the collaborative process is integrated throughout. For example, collaboration occurs among different team members, such as administrators, advisors, recruiters, and faculty, to name a few. Collaboration also occurs with community leaders to identify workforce learning needs and with students to ensure their learning needs are met. Further, collaborative learning forms the basis of our theoretical approach to teaching. Our model came from our reflections about what was needed to have a successful online nursing program within a liberal arts institution. As a result, four beliefs emerged that we identify as guiding principles.

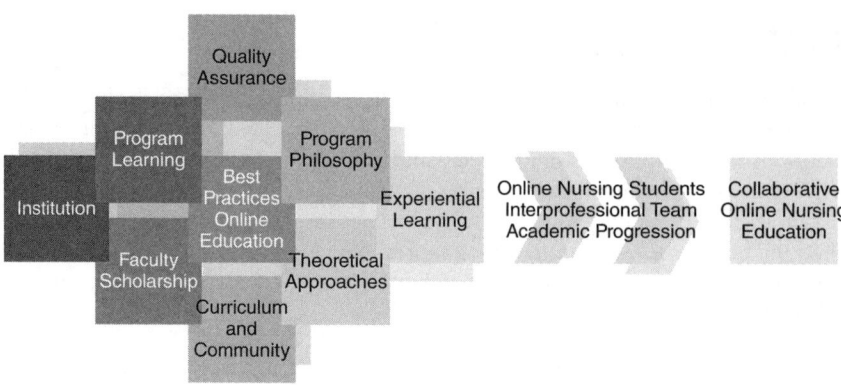

Figure 1-1 Collaborative model for online nursing education

Guiding Principles

The following four principles guide our teaching and leadership in the online nursing program. They also make up the primary components of the collaborative model for online nursing education that we share in this text:

1. Nurse education is an advanced specialty of nursing practice.
2. Online nursing education is a subspecialty of nursing education.
3. Online nursing education should be integrated within the institution.
4. Technology is secondary to education theory and best practices.

Nurse Education Is an Advanced Specialty of Nursing Practice

There has been a long-standing debate about whether nursing education should be considered an advanced practice role, with strong arguments on both sides. This issue was debated by Emerson Ea and Maryann Alexander (2011) in an opinion piece in *The Journal for Nurse Practitioners* and the question posed by the editor, Donald Gardenier. Although nurse educators have advanced knowledge and function at an advanced level, they are not considered advanced practice nurses by licensure or regulation. Both the American Association of Colleges of Nursing (AACN) and the National League for Nursing (NLN) support nursing education as an advanced practice in that advanced practice includes indirect care (Ea & Alexander, 2011).

The NLN supports the position that nurse educators are an advanced specialty role through the Academic Nurse Educator Certification Program, which has eight core competencies, as listed on their website. These competencies promote excellence in the advanced specialty role of the academic nurse educator (NLN, 2020). Faculty can demonstrate they have met the competencies through an initial exam and provide evidence demonstrating ongoing competency every 5 years in order to maintain their certification as a certified nurse educator (CNE). However, it is not regulated or licensed, as is required for certified nurse practitioners, nurse anesthetists, and nurse midwives (Ea & Alexander, 2011). Further, not all faculty are required to have the CNE certification or even required to have expertise in pedagogy in order to teach.

However, Ea and Alexander (2011) make the point that state boards of nursing have rules related to ensuring faculty are qualified to teach, and to regulate them beyond this requirement would be burdensome to nursing by requiring additional fees for licensure and certification. They also state that it would be confusing to the public because other educators do not require a separate license or legal recognition. They claim it would not add any benefit in terms of public safety (Ea & Alexander, 2011). It is a conundrum to us that nurse educators who are responsible for ensuring that those they teach are able to function as RNs or advance practice nurses are not recognized as advanced practice nurses themselves and that they are not required to be educated in pedagogy. At the same time, we recognize that this is a much larger issue with implications beyond nursing. Should nurse educators be required to be certified by the NLN as some nursing schools are requiring? Is this a movement much like the movement to require a BSN to practice nursing? We leave it to readers to think about this and come to their own decision.

Online Nursing Education Is a Subspecialty of Nursing Education

Online nursing education is a subspecialty of nursing education because it requires specialized knowledge and skill. Quality online curriculum development and teaching build on pedagogy for traditional classroom teaching. However, faculty require additional training and support for online education to ensure that learning outcomes are met. In our institution, we require all full-time faculty who teach nursing online to be certified in online teaching. Adjunct faculty are closely mentored by full-time online nursing faculty to ensure a quality learning experience for the student. Having full-time faculty dedicated to online teaching fosters ongoing development in this subspecialty of nursing education.

We have been writing this text during the 2019 novel coronavirus (COVID-19) pandemic, in which institutions of higher learning across the country had to quickly move teaching online to ensure public health safety. This is a time of renewed conflicting opinions about online education. To this day, online education continues to carry the stigma that online learning is of lower quality than face-to-face learning, despite research demonstrating otherwise. The term *emergency remote teaching* has been proposed (Hodges, Moore, Lockee, Trust, & Bond, 2020). It is important to recognize the difference between remote *teaching* and online *teaching and learning* that has been studied for years to ensure quality online course design, teaching, and learning, which is the premise of this text. Remote teaching attempts to mimic the face-to-face classroom through synchronous class meetings via video conferencing with platforms such as Zoom and narrated lectures placed online.

Online Nursing Education Should Be Integrated Within the Institution

Our focus is on liberal arts institutions with professional programs as opposed to larger institutions with massive online programs. Much like the addition of professional programs, online programs are often perceived as a way to bring in revenue and as taking away from the mission of a pure liberal arts education. Chief academic officers continue to report that the acceptance of online learning by faculty has not improved. Only 29.1% of chief academic officers surveyed believed their faculty accepted the value and legitimacy of online education; this rate is lower than the rate recorded in 2004 (Allen, Seaman, Pouline, & Taylor Straut, 2016). At the same time, there is declining enrollment in liberal arts majors as more and more students gravitate toward career-directed programs, like nursing, that will secure them an income upon graduation (Ferrall, 2008).

Online programs for advanced nursing education have increased to meet the needs of nurses working in the profession. These circumstances have led to an ongoing struggle within our institution and many others to accept the legitimacy of online education, which is discussed in the chapter on leadership. There is an ongoing need to work with faculty and administrators within institutions to promote the value of online education.

Technology Is Secondary to Education Theory and Best Practice

It is our belief that the modality of delivering education is secondary to education theory and best practices. Therefore, decisions about what technology to use are based on how it can best support the educational experience of the student population. This premise is discussed throughout the text.

Summary

This text is a cumulation of our life's work specific to online education. It is about our experience in an online nursing education program positioned within a small liberal arts college. We start with our philosophy and theoretical approaches to online education in Chapter 2. In Chapter 3, we discuss the demographics and characteristics of online nursing students and what they need to promote and support their success. In Chapter 4, we share an interprofessional model that was developed by our interprofessional team to support online students from the initial point of contact with the institution through successful completion of the degree. Community partnerships, which are critical to a nursing program's success, are also addressed. Leadership of online programs, quality, and outcomes at the program level are addressed in the next two chapters.

Starting in Chapter 7, we move to more direct teaching-related matters, starting with curriculum development and moving to online course design in Chapter 8 and teaching strategies in Chapter 9. In Chapters 10–12, we highlight some unique learning opportunities for online students: learning through writing, experiential learning, and narrative pedagogy. In Chapter 13, we share our experience as online faculty moving through the ranks of academia. We propose that collaboration in teaching and scholarship can be an effective way to improve productivity and enhance faculty satisfaction. The final three chapters are examples of our research that illustrate some of the points we make in this book. The collaborative approach (or model) provides a framework for ensuring that the online educational program is one in which the student perceives the online learning community as a rich, engaging experience.

References

Allen, I. E., Seaman, J., Pouline, R., & Taylor Straut, T. (2016). *Online report card: Tracking online education in the United States.* http://onlinelearningsurvey.com/reports/onlinereportcard.pdf

American Nurses Association. (2015). *Nursing: Scope and standards of practice* (3rd ed.). Author.

Ea, E., & Anderson, M. (2011). Is nursing education considered an advanced practice role? *The Journal for Nurse Practitioners, 7*(5), 370–371.

Ferrall, V. E. (2008). *Can liberal arts colleges be saved?* https://www.insidehighered.com/views/2008/02/11/can-liberal-arts-colleges-be-saved

Hodges, C., Moore, S., Lockee, B., Trust, T., & Bond, A. (2020). The difference between emergency remote teaching and online learning. *EDUCAUSE Review.* https://er.educause.edu/articles/2020/3/the-difference-between-emergency-remote-teaching-and-online-learning

National League for Nursing. (2020). *Nurse educator core competency.* http://www.nln.org/professional-development-programs/competencies-for-nursing-education/nurse-educator-core-competency

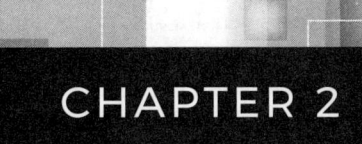

CHAPTER 2

Philosophical and Theoretical Approaches to Online Education

Henny Breen and Melissa Robinson

"The most important single factor influencing learning is what the learner already knows. Ascertain this, and teach him [or her] accordingly."

(**Ausubel**, 1968, p. 1)

Overview

The purpose of this chapter is to discuss the philosophical beliefs held by the authors regarding how adults learn and the theoretical approaches to nursing education that we believe are essential to high-quality teaching and learning in the online classroom. It has been our experience as online learners and educators that discussions about online education are often technology driven as opposed to being driven by educational theory and best practices in education.

Curriculum development in nursing education programs requires that faculty members consider a variety of factors, including the mission and goals of the program, learning outcomes, content areas, teaching strategies, levels of learning for specific student populations, and more. Because learning theories explain how learning occurs, a conceptual or theoretical foundation for learning provides a consistent rationale for decision making within the curriculum (Harasim, 2017; Saylor, 2011). Collaborative curriculum development and approaches to teaching in online programs require ongoing discussion among faculty about their beliefs and perspectives for how learning occurs, given that the theories "we employ (even unknowingly) shape how we design and implement our practice" (Harasim, 2017, p. 5).

It is our commitment to provide a theoretical foundation for online nursing education that emerges from our philosophy of constructivism. The theories that guide our practice include cognitive constructivist theory, social constructivist theory, collaborativist learning theory (previously known as *collaborative online learning theory*), transformative learning theory, experiential learning theory, and adult learning theory. Although narrative pedagogy is considered a strategy or an approach to nursing education and not a theory, it is within the realm of constructivist learning theory. Narrative pedagogy is a research-based pedagogy developed within the discipline of nursing that arose out of the common *lived experiences* of students, teachers, and clinicians in nursing education (Nehls, 1995). We felt it was important to address it in this chapter, given how influential this strategy is to our teaching practice, especially when it comes to difficult topics. This chapter provides foundational knowledge about these theories, which will be applied in subsequent chapters.

Philosophical Approach to Education

Our philosophical approach to education is based on constructivism, a concept that is derived from the work of several fields, including psychology, philosophy, anthropology, and education (Legg, Adelman, Mueller, & Levitt, 2009). Constructivism has two philosophical roots, ontology and epistemology. Ontology is concerned with "the nature of being," whereas epistemology refers to "the origin, foundation, limits, and validity of knowledge" (Oxford, 1997, p. 37). Within radical constructivism, the ontological stance is that reality exists in ideas, and no conclusive claims can be made about reality because people construct their own understanding of reality (Oxford, 1997; von Glasersfeld, 1984, 2005). This sharply differs from the positivist beliefs of most scientists, who work to discover truth as they increase their knowledge (von Glasersfeld, 1984).

The constructivist epistemological stance is that reality or truth cannot be revealed through instruction independent of human perception because knowledge about the world is only obtained through the interaction with experience (Windschitl, 2002). Although *constructivism* as a philosophy refers to the nature or epistemology of learning, *constructivist learning theory* refers to how people learn (Harasim, 2017). Constructivism was built on the premise that the development of knowledge is different for all learners based on their unique, individual experiences and how individuals interact in their environment. Constructivist philosophies appreciate multiple socially constructed realities and perspectives (Guba & Lincoln, 1994). Constructivist learning theory suggests that learning is an active process in which learners make meaning of new information and construct new knowledge through experience and reflection upon that experience (Harasim, 2017). The two major categories of constructivist pedagogy are cognitive constructivism, which suggests that meaningful learning is rooted in personal experience (Brown, Collins, & Duguid, 1989), and social or cultural constructivism, which views knowledge as being shaped by an individual's social and cultural influences (Vygotsky, 1978/1997). This is an important distinction because cognitivism is understood as an individual pursuit of knowledge, whereas social constructivism is a pursuit of knowledge through social interaction.

Constructivist Learning Theories

Whereas our philosophy of learning in the online classroom provides a foundation for understanding our epistemological approach to learning, learning theory provides an explanation of why and how learning occurs. A solid understanding of a variety of educational theories as applied to the online classroom is critical for effective online teaching in nursing education. Truly, the value of theory is the insight that it provides for understanding how learning occurs and the teaching strategies that evolve out of that understanding (Cusatis Phillips, 2018). The following sections describe the learning theories that guide our teaching practice in the online classroom.

Cognitive Constructivism

Cognitive learning theory was derived from Jean Piaget's (1896–1980) biological approach to learning (Harasim, 2017). Piaget believed that learning is an extensive cognitive activity that has many phases, based on the developmental level of the individual. He believed that humans pass through the same stages of cognitive development at around the same age while they make sense of new knowledge by applying it to what they already know and making modifications to their thinking as needed (Harasim, 2017). Cognitive theory arose from neurophysiological and psychological research that led to knowledge about how the brain processes information and retrieves knowledge from memory (Bruner, Goodnow, & Austin, 1986).

Based on aspects of cognitive theory and constructivism, cognitive constructivist learning theory addresses meaningful learning (Garrison, 1993). Cognitive theories are applied to learning experiences through problem solving, analysis, and memorization activities. There is a focus on memorizing information and retrieving that information. By combining a constructivist approach and cognitive learning, individuals also have the opportunity to develop their own interpretations while they build their cognitive skills and knowledge. Cognitive constructivist theory supports learning as an active, complex, and interconnected process during which an individual assimilates and integrates new knowledge (Divesta & Rieber, 1987). Further, it provides a strong foundation for understanding how adults modify their thinking as they make sense of new knowledge based on previous experiences.

Social Constructivism

The social constructivist theory of cognitive development emphasizes the social context rather than the stages of development, as in Piaget's theory. Biological development does not occur in isolation because social and cultural factors influence learning. These social interactions were the focus of Vygotsky's work because he believed that higher individual cognitive development occurred in these interactions (Vygotsky 1978/1997).

Vygotsky's research focused on social constructivism and learning that occurs through collaborative learning experiences, as a result of social interaction and within a cultural context. His theories emphasized interaction as a primary element of effective learning in the classroom. Social interactions in a classroom, combined with a personal critical thinking process, comprise social constructivist learning theory (Powell & Kalina, 2009). Vygotsky also believed that learning is an interpersonal process involving active learning experiences that engage the individual, instructor, and peers in the process. Based on adults' rich life and work experiences, the social, situated nature of constructivist learning is uniquely valid for adults (Ruey, 2010). Social constructivist theory applies the general philosophical approach of constructivism to a social learning environment in which individuals construct knowledge through their interactions with others. Thus, the social constructivist theory of cognitive development emphasizes the social context rather than the stages of development emphasized in cognitive constructivist theory. The zone of proximal development is a key principle derived from social constructivist theory.

Zone of Proximal Development. Vygotsky (1978/1997) believed that individuals could learn beyond their developmental level. As a result of this belief, he developed the concept of the zone of proximal development (ZPD), which theorizes that learning takes place when learners solve problems beyond their actual developmental level but within their potential development under the guidance of a more knowledgeable person. The ZPD considers "not only the cycles and maturation processes that have already been completed but also those processes that are currently in a state of formation, that are just beginning to mature and develop" (Vygotsky, 1978/1997, p. 33). In other words, the ZPD considers not only the actual biological developmental level, as in Piaget's theory, but also the potential development. Another important distinction in this theory is that the actual developmental level is determined independently through problem-solving skills, for example, whereas problem-solving skills at the potential developmental level are achieved in collaboration with more capable peers or under the guidance of an adult, who could be an instructor or mentor (Vygotsky, 1978/1997).

Collaborativist Learning Theory

Collaborativist learning theory is about knowledge building based in an online group. This theory, previously known as *online collaborative theory*, evolved over more than three decades based on an inductive approach to theory building (Harasim, 2017). Before describing the theory, it is important to understand that collaboration is conceptualized as both a dynamic process in which the group moves through different developmental stages and as an outcome in which there is a synthesis or merging of different perspectives in understanding complex problems and coming to a solution (Gardner, 2005). Collaborative learning advances active and reflective learning and encourages teamwork, which provides opportunities for students to become accountable for their own and others' work (Billings & Halstead, 2016). Collaborative activities are important to guide teaching and learning because these are attributes required of practicing nurses. Nurses must be able to collaborate with other nurses and professionals. To maximize the impact of the learning experience, it is important for faculty to be able to differentiate between cooperation and collaboration in curriculum development and teaching.

A concept analysis found that the terms *collaboration* and *cooperation* are often used interchangeably, with some delineation found in the literature (Breen, 2013). Some researchers, such as Tutty and Klein (2008), place collaboration and cooperation on either end of a continuum, whereas others identify cooperative learning as a division of labor and collaboration as co-labor (Harasim, 2017). As a result of the concept analysis, *virtual collaboration* was defined as "an interdependent and democratic online group process grounded in constructivist pedagogy in which students debate and reflect on shared knowledge, to construct new understanding of relevant information" (Breen, 2013, p. 267).

Collaborativist learning theory defines *learning* as intellectual convergence (Harasim, 2017). A good understanding of the process of collaboration is needed.

Three processes or phases comprise Collaborativist Learning Theory, which leads from divergent thinking to intellectual convergence (Harasim, 2017):

> *Idea generating.* This phase refers to divergent thinking within a group and may involve brainstorming, talking, or writing it out. Information is generated as ideas are shared through a democratic process in which different perspectives are provided from group members' personal observations and experiences.

> *Idea organizing.* Group members begin to acknowledge and recognize different perspectives. Conceptual change demonstrates intellectual progress as group members begin to identify how the different perspectives relate or do not relate to one another and the topic, and there is a beginning movement toward convergence.

> *Intellectual convergence.* Convergent thinking reflects a shared understanding, which includes agreeing to disagree. It may result in a mutual contribution to the construction of a knowledge product, such as a group project.

Experiential Learning Theory

Experiential learning theory is built on six propositions shared by multiple scholars who gave experience a central role in their theories of human learning and development. They include Jean Piaget (cognitive constructivism), Lev Vygotsky (social constructivism), John Dewey (experiential education), and David Kolb (experiential learning). The six propositions discussed by Kolb (1984, 2013) include:

1. *Learning Is Best Conceived as a Process, Not in Terms of Outcomes.* "Learning is an emergent process whose outcomes represent only historical record, not knowledge of the future" (Kolb, 1984, p. 26). What this means is that the emphasis needs to be on engaging students in learning and providing feedback as they continue to construct new knowledge so that skill is developed in the acquisition of knowledge.
2. *Learning Is a Continuous Process Grounded in Experience.* Learning involves re-learning, in that beliefs and ideas about a concept or subject are examined in light of new knowledge. Piaget referred to this proposition as *constructivism* because new knowledge is constructed when students begin to realize how new information conflicts with their prior beliefs and experiences. In this interplay between expectations and experience, learning occurs.
3. *The Process of Learning Requires the Resolution of Conflict Between Dialectically Opposed Modes of Adaptation to the World.* The learning process is driven by conflict, differences, and disagreement resolved through iterations involving reflection, action, feeling, and thinking. New knowledge, skills, or attitudes are achieved through confrontation among these four modes of learning, known as *concrete experience* (CE), *abstract conceptualization* (AC), *reflective observation* (RO), and *active experimentation* (AE) in Kolb's theory of experiential learning.
4. *Learning Is a Holistic Process of Adaptation to the World.* Learning involves the whole person rather than merely cognition. It involves the integration of thinking, feeling, perceiving, and behaving. It is a holistic process of adaptation to the world, moving from the scientific method to problem solving, decision making, and creativity.

5. *Learning Involves Transactions Between the Person and the Environment.* John Dewey (1859–1952), an American philosopher, psychologist, and educational reformer, believed, as do many constructivist theorists, that learners construct new knowledge based on previous knowledge and experience. He emphasized the unique and individualized nature of interaction in the learning environment (Boettcher & Conrad, 2010). Kolb (1984) felt that the term *interaction* did not speak adequately to the complexity of the relationship between objective and subjective experience and proposed that the word *transaction* was more appropriate. Learning results from ongoing transactions between the student and the environment as new experiences assimilate into existing concepts and existing concepts accommodate to new experience. The concept of mutually determined transactions between the student and the learning environment is central to experiential learning.

6. *Learning Is the Process of Creating Knowledge.* Experiential learning theory is viewed as the transactions made between social knowledge and personal knowledge. Social knowledge is co-constructed in a sociohistorical context, whereas personal knowledge is the subjective experience of the student. Therefore, experiential learning theory is clearly based on constructivist theory in which social knowledge is created and re-created in the personal knowledge of the student (Kolb & Kolb, 2013). The social interactions were the focus of Vygotsky's (1896–1934) work.

Kolb (1984) summarized the six propositions by offering a definition of learning that emphasizes several critical aspects of learning from the experiential perspective. "Learning is the process whereby knowledge is created through the transformation of experience" (p. 38). Kolb's (1984) theory of experiential learning helps explain how experience is transformed into learning through a holistic perspective that combines experience, perception, cognition, and behavior.

Transformative Learning Theory

Transformative learning theory is based on cognitive constructivism. Mezirow (1996), a pioneer in transformative learning, asserted that "learning is understood as the process of using a prior interpretation to construe a new or revised interpretation of the meaning of one's experience in order to guide future action" (p. 162). He believed learning can be transformative if it involves thinking critically and reflectively about one's experiences, beliefs, values, feelings, self-concept, and prior learning. Transformative learning is much more than changing one's opinion. It involves major changes in one's worldviews (Merriam, Caffarella, & Baumgartner, 2007). Transformative learning offers substantial relevance for adults because they are often in a position of needing to make responsible, informed decisions based on their own interpretations and judgment, as opposed to relying on others as they did as children (Saylor, 2011; Taylor, 2008). A change in worldview requires a profound or unexpected disorienting event to occur during the educational experience that challenges students to examine prior beliefs and ways of thinking. Critical reflection is prompted, which can lead to new insights, thinking, or awareness (Morris & Faulk, 2007). Some strategies that have demonstrated positive outcomes for promoting transformative learning in nursing include narrative learning, service learning, and collaborative learning, which are listed in **Table 2-1**. These are discussed in more detail in subsequent chapters.

Adult Learning Theory

Understanding adult learning theory is an important adjunct to understanding and applying constructivist learning theories for teaching online nursing students. Although Malcolm Knowles did not coin the term *andragogy*, it became synonymous with Knowles's adult learning theory. He defined *andragogy* as "the art and science of helping adults learn" (Knowles, 1978, p. 43). He focused his theory on adults and their life experiences. Knowles (1978) identified six principles of andragogy for adults that address the motivational aspects of adult learning:

- Adults need to know the reason for learning something.
- Experience provides the basis for learning activities.
- Adults need to be responsible for their decisions on education and should be involved in the planning and evaluation of their instruction.
- Adults are most interested in learning subjects having immediate relevance to their work and/or personal lives.
- Adult learning is problem-centered rather than content oriented. (p. 40)

Knowles based his theory of adult learning on the assumption that adults are increasingly self-directed and have experiences that provide for a rich learning environment (Manning, 2007). Nursing students are adult learners, and most online courses are taught to postlicensure students with professional and life experiences. Therefore, we see ourselves as colleagues in the online learning environment with a responsibility to provide meaningful learning experiences that are relevant to the life and work experiences of students.

Narrative Pedagogy

Narrative pedagogy is a teaching strategy in which teachers, students, and clinicians share experiences that are examined and debated (Billings & Halstead, 2016). The narrative approach has been used consistently by nurse educators, given the rich experience they have from their clinical experiences, which, when shared, illuminate the concepts they are teaching. More recently, narratives have become recognized as a way to develop insight into patients' lived experiences. Narrative learning is based on transformative learning theory (Clark, 2010) and principles of adult learning (Knowles, 1978) that prioritize life experiences as a major resource for learning.

Fitzpatrick (2017) maintained that narrative nursing is focused on the use of reflective practice in order to improve nursing interventions as understanding increases through examining the actions and processes inherent in narrative stories. When used purposefully to meet the educational needs of students, narratives can prepare learners for nursing practice that often includes dealing with difficult and stressful situations (Walsh & van Soeren, 2012).

Given the current understanding of constructivism and experiential learning, Fenwick (2004) expanded on narrative learning to consider the cultural context. Nursing students come to a shared understanding of what real stories mean for patients and can challenge "conventional wisdom, exposing assumptions and analyzing multiple perspectives" (Walsh & van Soeren, 2012, p. 45). This can lead to deep learning. Woodhouse (2007) differentiates storytelling from narrative. A story is the telling of a sequence of events, whereas a narrative is the way it is being told. This is very important for students to understand because the narrative can be altered by manipulating the context. Understanding the context is critical to understanding the narrative. It can change how it is perceived by the learner and the meaning assigned to it.

Ironside (2014) noted that teachers might not attend to the importance of waiting and silence in their courses. This is an important skill to master to allow for deep thinking as students process shared experiences. The deep thinking that comes from using this strategy is ideal in asynchronous online classrooms because students and teachers have the time to process written narratives. Thus, narrative pedagogy in which both faculty and students share their life experiences can result in transformative learning opportunities.

Table 2-1 Application of Theory to Online Teaching Practice

Theory	Learning Process	Teaching Strategies and Methods
Cognitive constructivism	■ Consider developmental level of learner ■ Incorporate previous knowledge and experiences to construct new knowledge ■ Retrieve knowledge from memory ■ Problem solving ■ Individual reflection ■ Enhances critical thinking	■ Journal writing ■ Interviews ■ Case studies ■ Tests, quizzes ■ Memorization activities
Social constructivism	■ Social context rather than stages of development ■ Cultural factors influence learning ■ Learning is an interpersonal process that requires engagement of students and faculty ■ Learning occurs through collaboration or social interaction ■ Improves critical thinking and clinical reasoning ■ Constructing knowledge requires interacting with others	■ Group discussions ■ Group activities
Zone of proximal development	■ Learn beyond development level under the guidance of a more knowledgeable person ■ Zone relies on the influence of more knowledgeable peers, such as instructors, mentors, or more experienced students	■ Group discussions ■ Activities that engage students in work that promotes diverse and varied experiences

Theory	Learning Process	Teaching Strategies and Methods
	■ Considers the student's potential for development	■ Role modeling ■ Mentorship activities
Collaborativist learning theory	■ Is specific to online learning ■ Knowledge construction ■ Advances active and reflective learning ■ Encourages teamwork ■ Merging of different perspectives ■ Understanding complex problems ■ Solution oriented	■ Group discussions ■ Instructor-led activities ■ Student-led activities
	■ Accountability for their own work and work of others ■ Differentiate between cooperative and collaborative work ■ Interdependent and democratic process ■ Moves students from divergent thinking to intellectual convergence	
Experiential and transformative learning theory	■ Prior interpretation is revised to guide future action ■ Assumptions are challenged ■ Beliefs, values, and self-concept are reconsidered ■ More than opinion ■ Major changes in one's worldview ■ Requires profound or disorienting event ■ New insights and awareness	■ Narrative learning ■ Service learning ■ Collaborative learning ■ Critical reflection ■ Clinical experiences
Adult learning theory	■ Adult learning is the art and science of helping adults learn ■ Focus is on adults and their life experiences ■ Motivated by subjects that are relevant to their work or personal lives ■ Problem centered rather than content oriented	■ Learning activities recognize previous experiences (life, education, work) ■ Self-assessment of learning ■ Provide choices for assignments that are relevant to students' learning needs and interest

(continues)

Table 2-1 Application of Theory to Online Teaching Practice   *(continued)*

Theory	Learning Process	Teaching Strategies and Methods
Narrative pedagogy	■ A teaching/learning strategy ■ Students and faculty share experiences that are examined and debated ■ Shared experiences are interpreted, and assumptions are challenged ■ Meaningful sharing leads to deep learning	■ Art, film, literature ■ Storytelling ■ Case studies based on real experiences ■ Problem-based learning ■ Group discussion ■ Unfolding case studies

Summary

In this chapter, we have shared our philosophy for how adults learn in the online classroom. We have also addressed the primary theoretical approaches that guide our online teaching practice. Constructivism as a philosophy is a worldview in which reality exists in ideas and people construct their own understanding of their experiences. Several theories arose out of constructivism. The important thing to remember about these theories is that knowledge is advanced through individual reflection on new knowledge and current experiences in order for students to challenge their assumptions and develop their own interpretations. Further, new knowledge is advanced through collaborative experiences in which learners share experiences and debate new knowledge. Learning can be transformative, and nursing practice improves when educators understand theory and apply it to their practice. Nurses work with patients at their most vulnerable moments and work within an increasingly complex healthcare environment, requiring educational practices that advance critical thinking and clinical reasoning skills. The principles of adult learning provide a guide for educators who want to create a learning environment in which nursing students are respected as adult learners.

Table 2-1 highlights the key points of the theories discussed in this chapter. Descriptions of the ways that students learn and some suggested strategies and methods for online teaching are provided. More detailed discussion of the application of theory to the practice of online teaching is included in the chapters on curriculum and teaching.

Best-Practice Recommendations for Online Teaching

- Collaborate with faculty colleagues to develop a philosophical approach to how learning occurs in your online program.
- Use learning theory and evidence to guide pedagogical decisions about teaching methods.

References

Ausubel, D. P. (1968). *Educational psychology: A cognitive view*. Holt, Rinehart and Winston.

Billings, D. M., & Halstead, J. A. (2016). *Teaching in nursing: A guide for faculty* (3rd ed.). Saunders-Elsevier.

Breen, H. (2013). Virtual collaboration in the online education setting: A concept analysis. *Nursing Forum, 48*(4), 262–270. http://doi.org/10.1111/nuf.12034

Brown, J. S., Collins, A., & Duguid, P. (1989). Situated cognition and the culture of learning. *Educational Researcher, 18*(1), 32–42.

Bruner, J., Goodnow, J. J., & Austin, G. (1986). *A study of thinking*. Transaction.

Clark, C. M. (2010). Narrative learning: Its contours and its possibilities. *New Directions for Adult and Continuing Education, 126*, 3–11. http://doi.org/10.1002/ace.367

Cusatis Phillips, B. (2018). Learning theories. In M. H. Oermann, J. C. DeGagne, & B. Cusatis Phillips (Eds.), *Teaching in nursing and role of the educator* (pp. 29–44). Springer.

Divesta, F. J., & Rieber, L. P. (1987). Characteristics of cognitive engineering: The next generation of instructional system. *Educational Communications and Technology Journal, 35*, 213–230.

Fenwick, T. J. (2004). *Learning through experience: Troubling orthodoxies and intersecting questions*. Krieger.

Fitzpatrick, J. J. (2017). Narrative nursing: Applications in practice, education, and research [Editorial]. *Applied Nursing Research, 37*(10), 67. http://dx.doi.org/10.1016/j.apnr.2017.08.005

Gardner, D. (2005). Ten lessons in collaboration. *Online Journal of Issues in Nursing, 10*(1). http://ojin.nursingworld.org/mainmenucategories/anamarketplace/anaperiodicals/ojin/tableofcontents/volume102005/no1jan05/tpc26_116008.html

Garrison, D. R. (1993). A cognitive constructivist view of distance education: An analysis of teaching-learning assumptions. *Distance Education, 14*(2), 199–211. http://doi.org/10.1080/0158791930140204

Guba, E. G., & Lincoln, Y. S. (1994). Competing paradigms in qualitative research. In N. Denzin & S. Lincoln (Eds.), *Handbook of qualitative research* (pp. 105–117). Sage.

Harasim, L. (2017). *Learning theory and online technologies* (2nd ed.). New York, NY: Routledge.

Ironside, P. M. (2014). Enabling narrative pedagogy: Inviting, waiting, and letting be. *Nursing Education Perspectives, 35*(4), 212–218. http://doi.org/10.5480/13-1125.1

Knowles, M. (1978). Andragogy: Adult learning theory in perspective. *Community College Review, 5*(3), 9–20. http://doi.org/10.1177/009155217800500302

Kolb, A., & Kolb, D. A. (2103). *The Kolb Learning Style Inventory 4.0: A comprehensive guide to the theory, psychometrics, research on validity and educational applications*. https://learningfromexperience.com/research-library/the-kolb-learning-style-inventory-4-0/

Kolb, D. A. (1984). *Experiential learning: Experience as the source of learning and development*. Upper Prentice-Hall.

Legg, T. J., Adelman, D., Mueller, D., & Levitt, C. (2009). Constructivist strategies in online distance education in nursing. *Journal of Nursing Education, 48*(2), 64–69. http://10.3928/01484834-20090201-08

Manning, G. (2007). Self-directed learning: A key component of adult learning theory. *Journal of the Washington Institute of China Studies, 2*(2), 104–115.

Merriam, S., Caffarella, R., & Baumgartner, L. (2007). *Learning in adulthood: A comprehensive guide*. Jossey-Bass.

Mezirow, J. (1996). Contemporary paradigms of learning. *Adult Education Quarterly, 46*, 158–172.

Morris, A., & Faulk, D. (2007). Perspective transformation: Enhancing the development of professionalism in RN-to-BSN students. *Journal of Nursing Education, 46*(10), 445–451. http://doi.org/10.2202/1548-923X.2052

Nehls, N. (1995). Narrative pedagogy: Rethinking nursing education. *Journal of Nursing Education, 34*(5), 204–210.

Oxford, R. L. (1997). Constructivism: Shape-shifting, substance, and teacher education applications. *Peabody Journal of Education, 72*(1), 35–66.

Powell, K. C., & Kalina, C. J. (2009). Cognitive and social constructivism: Developing tools for an effective classroom. *Education, 130*(2), 241–250.

Ruey, S. (2010). A case study of constructivist instructional strategies for adult online learning. *British Journal of Educational Technology*, *41*(5), 706–720.

Saylor, C. (2011). Learning theories applied to curriculum development. In S. Keating (Ed.), *Curriculum development and evaluation in nursing* (pp. 49–69). Springer.

Taylor, E. W. (2008). Transformative learning theory. *New Directions for Adult & Continuing Education*, *119*, 5–15. http://doi.org/10.1002/ace.301

Tutty, J., & Klein, J. (2008). Computer-mediated instruction: A comparison of online and face-to-face collaboration. *Educational Technology Research & Development*, *56*(2), 101–124. http://doi.org/10.1007/s11423-007-9050-9

von Glasersfeld, E. (1984). An introduction to radical constructivism. In P. Watzlawick (Ed.), *The invented reality* (pp. 17–40). Norton.

von Glasersfeld, E. (2005). Thirty years constructivism. *Constructivist Foundations*, *1*(1), 9–12.

Vygotsky, L. (1997). Interaction between learning and development. In M. Gauvain & M. Cole (Eds.), *Readings on the development of children* (Vol. 2, pp. 29–36). W. H. Freeman and Company. (Reprinted from *Mind and society*, pp. 79–91, by L. Vygotsky, 1978, Cambridge University Press.)

Walsh, M., & van Soren, M. (2012). Interprofessional learning and virtual communities: An opportunity. *Journal of Interprofessional Care*, *26*, 43–49.

Windschitl, M. (2002). Framing constructivism in practice as the negotiation of dilemmas: An analysis of the conceptual, pedagogical, cultural, and political challenges facing teachers. *Review of Educational Research*, *72*(2), 131–175.

Woodhouse, J. (2007). *Strategies for healthcare education: How to teach in the 21st century*. Radcliffe.

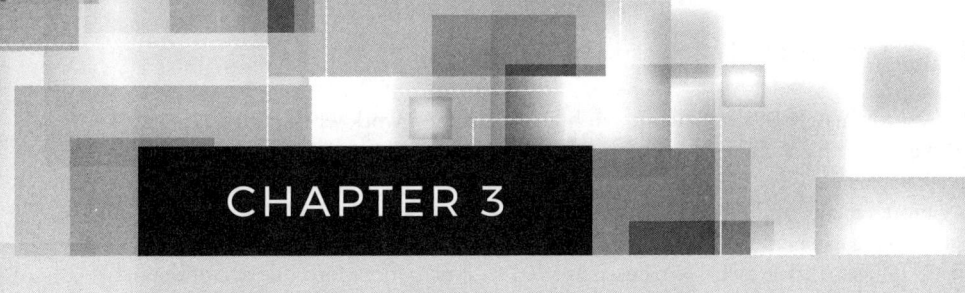

CHAPTER 3

Online Nursing Students

Melissa Robinson and Henny Breen

"Learning is facilitated in an environment that is caring and respectful, and where students believe they are safe to express their questions, ideas, or emerging thoughts."

(**Lewis, Rogers, & Naef**, 2006, p. 32)

Overview

It is our belief that a deep understanding of the unique characteristics of online nursing students is needed to truly achieve student-centeredness and high-quality online teaching. This chapter begins with a discussion of trends in higher education, pathways in nursing education, and the characteristics of online nursing students. Humanistic education is presented as an approach to online education that prioritizes caring, empathy, and the development of strong interpersonal relationships with online students that support their success in the online classroom.

Enrollment Trends in Higher Education

The demographics of higher education have changed dramatically in recent years. Enrollment in traditional face-to-face campus college and university programs has declined, and enrollment in distance-education programs has increased significantly. Between 2011 and 2016, enrollment in U.S. institutions dropped by 7.8%, which is attributed to the rising costs of education for students and families, students choosing to delay or not attend postsecondary education, and declining high school enrollment (Hershan & Lauderdale, 2018). Today, approximately 38% of undergraduate students are older than 25 years of age, and that number is predicted to grow dramatically through 2025 (Inside Track, 2019).

Approximately 85% of students in higher education work while taking classes, and many also have children and other family responsibilities (Inside Track, 2019; Jenzabar, 2019). Over the past two decades, the U.S. population has grown not only more racially and ethnically diverse but also more educated, partly as a result of a growing Hispanic population seeking higher education more than ever before (Espinosa, Turk, Taylor, & Chessman, 2019). First-generation college students, older adults, and women are among the groups increasingly represented in postsecondary degree programs. Additionally, in 2017, almost 40% of students in higher education reported having difficulty with depression in the previous year, and 61% reported overwhelming anxiety (Oster, 2019). Anxiety and depression are the two most common reasons that students seek mental health services (Penn State University, 2017). Many students are balancing full- or part-time jobs, family responsibilities, social or extracurricular activities, and coursework, which can be very stressful. Administrators and faculty in higher education are adapting to the changing needs of students in order to successfully recruit, retain, and support them.

At the same time, distance-education programs are becoming more widely accepted and serving the needs of students who are part of the shifting demographics. Enrollment in online courses has more than quadrupled in the last 15 years (Dusst & Winthrop, 2019). In 2018, the Education Department's National Center for Education Statistics (NCES) reported an overall drop of nearly 90,000 students between the fall of 2016 and the fall of 2017. The number of all students who took at least some of their courses online grew by 5.7%, or more than 350,000 students (NCES, 2019). During the same time frame, the number of students enrolled in exclusively online programs grew from 14.7% to 15.4%, or about 1 in 6 students (NCES, 2019). In nursing education, enrollment in baccalaureate, master's degree, and doctor of nursing practice (DNP) programs has been steady. Nursing ranks among the top three most popular online majors (Clinefelter & Aslanian, 2015). In 2016, more than 50% of registered nurse (RN)–bachelor of science in nursing (BSN) programs were offered completely online, with enrollment increasing every year in more than 600 of the 747 RN-to-BSN programs in the United States (American Association of Colleges of Nurses [AACN], 2017a).

Educational Pathways to Nursing

Nursing is unique in that there are multiple educational pathways to prepare nurses for entry-level practice as RNs. Prelicensure nursing students are able to take the licensure exam after completing any of a number of nursing educational programs, including a diploma in nursing, an associate degree in nursing, or a BSN degree in nursing. Accelerated second-degree baccalaureate programs have also become popular options for students who have a degree in another field (Keating, 2018). Postlicensure nursing education has become increasingly important as many employers have added BSN requirements to their hiring and promotion criteria, resulting in more RNs making the decision to enter RN-to-BSN programs, also referred to as *RN completion programs*. BSN and graduate programs at the master's level prepare nurses for advanced roles in case management, nursing leadership, nurse education, and clinical leadership. At the doctoral level, there are different tracks that include research-focused degrees (PhD) and practice-focused degrees (DNP). Each level of nursing education is supported by the AACN Essentials, which guide curriculum development, program planning, and accreditation.

Demand for Higher Levels of Nursing Education

Distance-education programs have had a positive impact on the nursing workforce by making higher education more accessible, flexible, and cost-effective for students across the country, including those balancing work and family responsibilities. By leveraging technology to develop online curricula, nursing education programs provide opportunities for students who may otherwise experience scheduling and geographical barriers. Online nursing education has been instrumental, particularly in rural communities, in providing access to specialized courses and degree programs that enhance the knowledge and skills of the nursing workforce (Wros, Wheeler, & Jones, 2014). The nursing workforce is expected to grow from 2.7 million in 2014 to 3.2 million in 2024, which is a 16% increase (AACN, 2017b). In addition, it is predicted that 649,100 replacement nurses will be needed to address the retirement of baby boomer nurses (AACN, 2017b). According to the Bureau of Labor Statistics publication *Employment Projections 2018–2028* (U.S. Department of Labor, Bureau of Labor Statistics, 2018), nurse practitioners and nurse faculty are projected to be among the top 30 fastest-growing occupations between 2018 and 2028.

As the demand for nurses educated at higher levels continues to grow, nurse leaders have started to question if the time has come to move to a graduate level of practice as the entry into practice. When nurses slowly advance their education through different levels, they often earn more credits "than their colleagues in medicine, education, engineering, religion and law" (Keating, 2018, p. 173). The experience is familiar for many nurses who started practicing with a diploma or associate degree in nursing and added additional levels of education over the past few decades. Recently, the number of RN-to-BSN graduates in the United States, compared with other BSN graduates, increased from 30.6% in 2010 to 47.4% in 2016 (AACN, 2017a). Once nurses have earned the BSN, they are well prepared to advance their education to fill roles in advanced practice, leadership, and academia.

In 2011, the Institute of Medicine, now known as the National Academy of Medicine, published the *Future of Nursing: Leading Change, Advancing Health*. The key messages that were developed to transform the nursing profession have had a direct impact on nursing education, including (1) nurses should practice to the full extent of their education and training, (2) nurses should achieve higher levels of education and training through an improved education system that promotes seamless academic progression, (3) nurses should be full partners with physicians and other health professionals in redesigning health care, and (4) effective workforce planning and policymaking require better data collection and improved information infrastructures (National Academy of Medicine, 2011). Postlicensure online nursing education programs are making it possible for nurses to move through the education system to earn higher levels of education, including graduate degrees. One of the aims discussed in the *Future of Nursing* report (National Academy of Medicine, 2011) included doubling the number of nurses with doctorate degrees by 2020. Although more progress is needed to reach that goal, nurses with doctorate degrees are essential to replenish the faculty pool, advance nursing science, contribute to the literature on quality and safety in patient care, and provide leadership in healthcare reform (National Academy of Medicine, 2011).

Characteristics of Online Nursing Students

We believe that to truly achieve student-centeredness and quality online teaching, a deep understanding of the unique characteristics of the online nursing student is needed. Students come to online nursing programs from a variety of backgrounds and with diverse perspectives, life and work experiences, goals, and needs. Historically, nurses have pursued continuing education and lifelong learning opportunities to stay current with healthcare changes, achieve higher levels of nursing education, or advance professionally. Faculty benefit from understanding the diverse characteristics of online students, which can affect their learning and their ability to succeed in online education, including their culture and ethnicity, generational cohort, learning styles and preferences, and degree of motivation (Cusatis Phillips, 2018). Some of the characteristics of online nursing students and strategies that faculty can implement to support them are addressed in the following sections.

Cultural, Ethnic, and Gender Diversity

The American Nurses Association (ANA) and the National League for Nursing (NLN) have addressed the importance of increasing diversity in all nursing programs in order to reflect the diversity in the community that is cared for by nurses. Diversity and quality health care are inextricably linked, creating a path to increased access and improved health in order to eliminate health disparities (NLN, 2016). To that end, the NLN is committed to the education of exemplary nurses who value and represent the richness of diversity and inclusion to help advance the health of the nation and the global community:

> Diversity signifies that each individual is unique and recognizes individual differences—race, ethnicity, gender, sexual orientation and gender identity, socio-economic status, age, physical abilities, religious beliefs, political beliefs, or other attributes. It encourages self-awareness and respect for all persons, embracing and celebrating the richness of each individual. It also encompasses organizational, institutional, and system-wide behaviors in nursing, nursing education, and health care. (NLN, 2016, p. 2)

The AACN (2019) has encouraged nurse leaders in academic and practice settings to prepare leaders representative of all racial and ethnic groups, advance cultural humility as a core competency for nursing students and practicing nurses, and collaborate on the recruitment and retention of nursing students and nurses of color. **Table 3-1** includes current data reflecting ethnic and gender diversity within educational and practice settings. In recent years, the nursing profession has moved from being predominantly White and female to having more representation of men and more nurses from diverse racial and ethnic backgrounds. Racial and ethnic diversity has increased from less than 15% of all nurses in 1995 to more than 20% in recent years (Villarruel, Washington, Lecher, & Carver, 2015), and the percentage of men in nursing has increased by 1.1% since 2015 (National Council of State

Table 3-1 Diversity Represented in Nursing Education and Practice Settings

Time Period	U.S. Nursing Education and Practice Demographics
2008–2017	Enrolled students from minority backgrounds; populations underrepresented in nursing: ■ 35% of students in entry-level baccalaureate programs ■ 34% of master's students in graduate programs ■ 32.5% of students in research-focused doctoral programs
2017	■ Racial and ethnic backgrounds in nursing (registered nurses [RNs]) represented: • 80.8% White/Caucasian • 6.2% African American • 7.5% Asian • 5.3% Hispanic • 0.4% American Indian/Alaska Native • 0.5% Native Hawaiian/Pacific Islander • 1.7% two or more races • 2.9% Other
2017	■ Men in nursing account for 9.1% of the RN workforce—an increase of 1.1% since 2015 ■ The highest representation of men is in nurse anesthetist positions (41%)

Data from Fang, D., Li, Y., Turinetti, M., & Trautman, D.E. (2018). *2017–2018 enrollment and graduations in baccalaureate and graduate programs in nursing.* American Association of Colleges of Nursing.

Boards of Nursing [NCSBN], 2017). Men in nursing are slightly more likely to be from a minority group (25%) than their female counterparts (20%), which underscores the need to continue to focus on both gender inclusion and racial and ethnic diversity in the profession (Auerbach, Buerhaus, Staiger, & Skinner, 2017). The diversity of the nursing workforce still lags far behind that of the general population. By 2043, it is estimated that the United States will become a majority–minority nation, which highlights the urgency to diversify nursing and other health professions (Villarruel et al., 2015).

To support the commitment to enhance the diversity of students in nursing education and nurses in practice, online nursing faculty must also be prepared for the opportunities and challenges of a diverse online classroom. One early challenge in an online course is that visual cues as to the gender and race of both faculty and students are absent, which can be overcome by asking students and faculty to post their pictures and share their background in an introduction (Rumay Alexander, 2016). It is important to consider that when faculty assume the role of facilitator of learning or seem to be an equal participant in the learning process, students from certain cultural backgrounds may be uncomfortable with the less formal role of the faculty member (Rumay Alexander, 2016).

On the other hand, online classrooms are ideally suited for open, structured discussions about the impact that cultural differences have on educational interactions, health outcomes, and social conditions. An important approach to supporting the diversity of every student in the online classroom is for faculty to openly acknowledge the differences and welcome students to reflect on their values, beliefs, or culture as they share their backgrounds and experience. Faculty can also model this by sharing their own backgrounds and making the value of the diversity known within the online classroom (Bednarz, Schim, & Doorenbos, 2010). This can be done by developing introductory activities or icebreakers to encourage students and faculty to get to know each other and begin to develop rapport. As the course progresses, faculty can integrate course assignments that also address the value and importance of diversity in the classroom, within the healthcare system, and in the global community. This may include individual reflection assignments, small-group work, or community-based activities. **Table 3-2** includes examples of online course activities that emphasize and support diversity in the online classroom.

English as a Second Language

The online classroom is a unique environment for English as a second language (ESL) students. There is limited literature to understand best practices for supporting ESL students in the online classroom. In a qualitative study that explored the lived experiences of 10 ESL students attending an online RN-to-BSN program, researchers used semistructured interviews to ask participants to talk about their experience with learning in the online classroom, to discuss their interactions with other nursing students and faculty, and to discuss whether they felt that language and culture affected their online course interactions (Sailsman, Rutherford, Tovin, & Cianelli, 2018). The following experiences reported by participants illustrate key opportunities for faculty awareness and support:

- Participants shared memories of fears and anxieties related to misunderstanding course expectations and lack of timely responses from peers and faculty.
- Time was considered a benefit of online learning because they could take their time with the course material without feeling rushed when language was a barrier.
- Participants believed that their level of comfort with online learning improved over time as they learned how to balance their workload and utilize available resources.
- Without verbal communication, their peers did not hear their accents and did not know they spoke ESL.
- When they enrolled in classes, they looked for "cultural affinity connections" by looking at the last names on the course roster so they could connect with these students.
- Participants benefited from online group activities because they could connect with peers on a more meaningful level.
- Writing assignments were described as difficult, overwhelming, and anxiety producing.
- Participants spent a considerable amount of time formulating their thoughts, translating concepts, creating proper sentence structure, and submitting a final paper or post that made them proud.
- Participants expressed gratitude for learning resources provided by the institution; they also appreciated having a neutral person to review their work and

Table 3-2 **Course Activities That Support Diversity in the Online Classroom**

Introductory Email From Faculty

Welcome, class!

I am excited that we are starting the semester. Whether you are new to online learning or you have taken multiple online courses, I want you each to know how important you are to our online learning community. Each of us comes to this community with our own unique background (familial, cultural, generational, and more) and has a variety of life and work experiences that will enrich our learning. As we get started in the course this week, you will notice that we will start with an introduction where you can share as much of your background as you feel comfortable with. As we move through the course, I will be asking you to share your own experiences to apply to the learning activities. You have an important foundation of education and experience to draw from as we collaborate to develop new knowledge and share ideas. I look forward to getting to know you!

Introductory Activities, Icebreakers

1. Please share your personal and professional background. Share as much as you feel comfortable with. Let us know your preferred name, nickname, or other details that will enhance our communication.
2. Please share one detail about your family heritage or cultural identity that you would like us to know.

Discussion Activities

1. What family stories have been passed down from your family of origin? Discuss two or three family rituals or traditions that are unique to your family's heritage. Are there any that relate to health and health practices?
2. What comes to mind when you think of the demographic diversity of your home community? What are your images of poverty in your community; what does it look like?
3. Discuss an encounter you had with a patient from a different culture that was highly satisfying. What was it about this encounter that made it satisfying?
4. Discuss an encounter with a patient of a different culture that was very disappointing to you. What do you think led to this unsatisfying encounter? What would you do differently if you were to have that encounter again?

Reflective Activities

1. Describe a time when you may have experienced or witnessed stereotyping, discrimination, or racism. How did you feel?
2. Discuss the challenges or opportunities of caring for an individual or family that has a different socioeconomic background than you do.
3. Discuss the challenges or opportunities of caring for an individual or family that has strong ties to a culture you are not familiar with.

give them feedback, and some students had family members review their writing ahead of time.

- Participants appreciated faculty members who asked about them and those who demonstrated kindness, professionalism, and caring (Sailsman et al., 2018).

Ultimately, ESL students expressed appreciation for online faculty members who took the time to get to know them on a personal level and for those who expressed genuine interest in their success with online learning. Although the Sailsman et al. study was conducted with a small sample of 10 participants, it resonated closely with our experience teaching ESL nursing students in the online classroom. The recommendations provided in this chapter include specific strategies for supporting ESL students as well as general best practices for online education.

Generational Diversity

The generational differences in today's online classrooms can enrich the learning experience for all students, but it can also present challenges. It is not uncommon to have students representing up to four generations in the same classroom, as well as represented in the nursing workforce, including baby boomers, GenXers, millennials, and Generation Z students. Generational differences reflect diverse experiences and perspectives. Each generational cohort has a common set of values, ideas, ethics, communication styles, and cultural influences that affects how cohort members interact with each other (Bednarz et al., 2010; Cusatis Phillips, 2018). The differences have added to the complexity of the learning needs of a diverse student population while also creating an opportunity to increase awareness of generational issues in the classroom.

It is not assumed that individuals have certain characteristics based solely on their generation or that age is a reflection of nursing practice experience, given the increase in older students entering the nursing profession. Rather, the generations are described in this chapter using broad generalizations found in the literature. The four generations typically represented in online classrooms in higher education include the following:

1. *Baby boomers* represent the largest group of nurses in the workforce; however, in recent years, many have prepared for retirement. Baby boomers have been characterized as appreciating recognition and respect, valuing education and personal growth, and enjoying opportunities for interpersonal communication to build rapport with peers (Stanley, 2010). They prefer a caring environment for learning, prefer face-to-face communication, and appreciate assignments that consider their previous life experiences and knowledge (Robinson, Scollan-Koliopoulos, Kamienski, & Burke, 2012).
2. *Generation X* students are characterized as being self-directed, career oriented, and seeking flexibility in work and educational opportunities. They often strive for a balance between their personal and professional lives and value diversity, travel, and technology, yet they are also career driven and view nursing as a profession full of opportunities (Irvine, 2010). They tend to be motivated by mastering clinical skills; achieving short-term, challenging goals; and interacting face to face and in groups (Lipscomb, 2010). They want practical information and opportunities to learn in a fun, engaging environment.
3. *Millennials* make up the majority of current undergraduate nursing students. They are considered a global generation that accepts multiculturalism, technology, and instant communication as a way of life (Pardue & Morgan, 2008). Millennials have grown up with strong ties to their families and demonstrate positive, friendly attitudes toward learning and work. Millennials are typically skilled at multitasking and enjoy group activities that involve technology. They

are interested in professional certification and continuing education and are very comfortable with online learning. Millennials are actively engaged in the learning process and expect to learn using technology and innovative learning strategies. They appreciate experiential learning, active questioning, group work, and multimedia. (Pardue & Morgan, 2008)

A better understanding of the generational diversity that is represented in higher education can lead to the development of effective pedagogical practices in nursing education and to healthier work environments for nurses. A description of a qualitative study examining the impact of generational differences on learning in the online classroom is found in Chapter 14. Two participant narratives are highlighted here to demonstrate the value of a generationally diverse online classroom:

> The exposure to multi-generations in the learning environment is a microcosm of the diversity of all the generations that I care for in my nursing practice. I welcome the diversity of opinion that can certainly differ from my personal philosophy. Through the diversity of opinion and perspective, I learn tolerance, and can reflect on new perspectives and outlooks. This can also extend into tolerance and understanding of the cultural diversity encountered in the healthcare environment. (online RN-to-BSN program graduate)

Another study participant spoke of the relative anonymity of the online classroom, which made her feel safe to share her beliefs and experiences. She felt the environment helped her learn in ways that were free from possible biases or judgments based on her age, body size, or physical appearance, and therefore, she felt she also grew in her acceptance of others:

> The diversity in opinion and perspective from varying [sic] generations was challenging and fun. It allows the student to free themselves [sic] from preconceived notions and biases that we all possess. Maybe just the awareness of our bias and prejudgment frees us and breaks down the barriers that restricts [sic] us from truly embracing the diversity we experience with our patients (impact on patient care). The acceptance of this diversity of opinions and perspectives allowed for my personal growth and awareness of the differences in the patients I encounter in my everyday nursing practice. This was a great practice in patience and acceptance and allowed me to be less quick to judge people in my personal and professional life. (online RN-to-BSN program graduate)

Table 3-3 includes recommendations for supporting a generationally diverse online classroom.

Learning Styles and Preferences

Learning styles and preferences have been discussed repeatedly in the literature as the manner in which a learner perceives, interacts with, and responds most effectively to the learning environment (Kolb & Kolb, 2005). The literature supports the elements of learning style as cognitive, affective, and physiological, which can be influenced by the learner's cultural background (Popkess & Frey, 2016). The learning experience

Table 3-3 **Recommendations for Supporting a Generationally Diverse Online Classroom**

- Begin class with an introduction so that students can share their backgrounds and experiences.
- Encourage students to share life and work experiences in collaborative discussions.
- Facilitate student–peer interaction as well as student–faculty interaction.
- Create generationally diverse groups to enhance peer engagement and learning.
- Provide opportunities to access course textbooks in a variety of formats, including e-books.
- Utilize a variety of media that support learning but do not overwhelm students.
- Develop an orientation that includes support for technology, and provide ongoing support for navigating the learning management system and other technology needs.
- Design learning activities that provide leadership and mentorship opportunities.

can be enhanced by acknowledging diverse learning styles. A *learning-style preference* is a preference for a particular style of learning, based on a previous learning experience or the way an individual has learned to approach a learning situation (Anderson, 2016). The four learning style preferences are as follows:

1. *Visual preference* is a preference for information in graphic formats (e.g., maps, charts, flowcharts), as opposed to text format.
2. *Auditory preference* is a preference for information that is language based (heard or spoken).
3. *Reading or writing preference* is the preference for information in text format.
4. *Kinesthetic preference* is a preference for concrete, experienced-based information (Cusatis Phillips, 2016).

Personality Traits

Online learning may be experienced differently for introverts and extroverts. Shy and introverted students may have greater opportunities for participation in the online classroom and may even prefer online learning (Bender, 2012), but they may be more likely to disapprove of coursework that requires working in a group with other students (Pavalache-Ilie & Cocorada, 2014). Extroverted students may be more likely to participate in communication using various forms of media and may enjoy the social aspects of online learning and more frequent interaction (Blau & Barak, 2012; Bolliger & Erichsen, 2013). Faculty can begin learning about students' personality traits in course introductory activities and by sending individualized emails to encourage students to share their learning styles and preferences for communication. Early opportunities to build rapport with online students can enhance their satisfaction with online learning and their relationships with faculty.

Application of Learning Styles to Improve Instruction

In a comprehensive meta-analysis of learning-style preferences and the application of learning styles to improve instruction, Pashler, McDaniel, Rohrer, and Bjork

(2008) found no evidence that matching learning-style preferences to teaching methods improved learning. They did find that students, when asked, verbalized a preference for how learning material is presented to them. Many researchers have recognized that students learn in different ways; however, there is also a lack of evidence to support that students only learn in those preferred ways (Leite, Svinicki, & Shi, 2010; Pashler et al., 2008).

To address the diverse learning preferences of online students, we recommend that faculty adopt a consistent course design to provide predictability across the curriculum, as well as provide a variety of teaching methods, course activities, and assessments. This will empower students to identify their learning-style preferences early in the curriculum and use that knowledge to achieve positive outcomes (Dapremont, 2014). However, we would also encourage students to learn using a variety of different styles to increase their adaptability in different learning environments. Studies have also shown that the most effective learners are able to adapt to the style that the learning situation requires (Bhagat, Vyas, & Singh, 2015). **Table 3-4** includes additional recommendations for addressing diverse learning preferences in the online classroom.

Student Motivation

As adult learners, online nursing students need to see the relevance and applicability of education to their lives. Postlicensure students advance their education in nursing for a variety of personal and professional reasons, including to gain employment, advance their career, or achieve certain goals they have set for themselves. Motivation is a key element for self-regulated learning and a prerequisite for meaningful learning (Cusatis Phillips, 2018). Self-regulation is how students activate and sustain their cognitive, affective, and behavioral abilities to achieve their academic

Table 3-4 Recommendations for Diverse Learning Preferences in the Online Classroom

- Adopt a consistent online course design across the curriculum to provide predictability.
- Utilize a variety of teaching methods, course activities, and assessments.
- Engage students in active learning; encourage them to explore new learning experiences.
- Use a variety of learning materials and media, such as assigned reading, audio, video, and podcasts.
- Develop problem-solving activities and encourage peer interaction in these activities.
- Consider integrating learning (low-stakes) quizzes, interactive websites, or online case-study activities that help students learn technology.
- Engage students in both individual and group course activities.
- Allow students choices and options to further explore topics of interest.
- Provide appropriate support for all students as they engage in online learning.
- Use email and private course messaging to check in with individual students and foster conversation outside of the classroom.
- Consider posting questions via Flipgrid or using social media to provide additional opportunities for interaction and social engagement.

Table 3-5 Recommendations for Enhancing Motivation in Online Students

- Develop course activities that help students identify their goals for learning.
- Provide mentorship opportunities with peers and faculty that enhance career development.
- Engage students in active learning that involves real-life examples.
- Demonstrate a meaningful rationale for tasks.
- Develop activities that help students solve real problems.
- Foster student agency by offering choices for discussion topics, project ideas, and experiential learning assignments.
- Deliver meaningful feedback that is constructive, encouraging, and supportive.
- Provide multiple opportunities for students to reflect on their progress toward their goals.
- Share motivational quotes to foster student motivation.
- Maintain a neutral presence.
- Address any potential conflict among students.
- Collaborate with academic advisors to support student success.

---

goals (Schunk & Zimmerman, 2012). Self-regulated learning can be achieved when students are motivated to learn and actively engage in the learning process. This is important because online learning requires a great deal of autonomy, independent thinking, and self-motivation. To be most successful, online students also have to manage their time well and utilize strong organizational skills. Considering that online learning is largely self-directed, faculty make considerable efforts to understand what will motivate students.

Self-determination is an intrinsic, self-sustaining form of motivation that can drive students to seek autonomy, perceived competence, and relatedness as they reach their academic goals (Ryan & Deci, 2000). Autonomy involves feeling confident that they can make their own decisions and choices in the learning experience, and perceived competence gives students the confidence to know they have the requisite skills to succeed. To enhance the perceived competence of online students, faculty are encouraged to (a) offer a balance between strict requirements and freedom in online discussions, (b) provide clear expectations and class routines, (c) deliver effective feedback, and (d) provide opportunities for students to get meaningful feedback from their peers (Jacoby, 2018; Kim, Glassman, & Williams, 2015). *Relatedness* refers to students' sense of belonging in class and involves the expression of care and respect within the learning community, which is discussed in more detail later in this chapter. **Table 3-5** includes recommendations for enhancing motivation in online students. Each of these strategies has been shown to promote individual competence and engagement in online learning as they build on principles of andragogy as discussed in Chapter 2.

Humanistic Education

Humanistic education, including humanism and caring, is an educational approach in which the teaching–learning process emphasizes the value, worth, dignity, and integrity of all individuals (Candela, 2016). As a learning theory, humanism is built on the premise that education motivates students to develop to their full potential so that they can progress toward self-actualization (Candela, 2016; Valiga, 2016). Faculty members who use the approach of humanism in nursing education emphasize *affective* aspects of development, promoting students' sense of responsibility, cooperation, and mutual respect (Candela, 2016).

Caring is a central tenet within the nursing profession. A widely accepted definition of caring is "when the one caring connects with and embraces the spirit of the other through authentic, full attention in the here and now, and conveys a concern for the inner life and personal meaning of another" (Sitzman & Watson, 2014, p. 17). One of the first ways that nurses learn and practice caring interventions is through educational interactions. Educators convey caring values through student dialogue and modeling, thereby demonstrating caring as a core value in nursing and in nursing education, whether that is in a face-to-face classroom or online classroom (Bevis & Watson, 2000; Sitzman, 2010).

We believe that demonstrating care and compassion in our interactions with students in the online classroom has a meaningful impact on their learning experiences. In fact, we consider caring as a primary intervention in the classroom, "where students believe they are safe to express their questions, ideas, or emerging thoughts" (Lewis et al., 2006, p. 32). When creating an online learning environment that promotes self-development, faculty may take the following actions (Candela, 2016):

- Model caring, empathy, and genuineness while being consistently respectful of self and others.
- Identify yourself as a co-learner in the educational process.
- Help students recognize and develop their own unique potential by facilitating their growth.
- Offer praise and support for positive contributions and evidence of growth.
- Encourage students to draw on and share their personal and professional experiences.
- Require students to identify their own needs, set goals for learning, and perform evaluations.
- Engage students in active learning and reflection on their experiences.

Similar to other teaching strategies, we appreciate opportunities to evaluate the effectiveness of caring interventions in the online classroom, particularly through feedback obtained directly from students. Previous evidence suggests that caring values can be applied to faculty–student relationships to develop effective transpersonal relationships, primarily through affirming behaviors and delivering caring feedback (Mastel-Smith, Post, & Lake, 2015). In a study that explored nursing students' perceptions of caring presence in the online classroom, students reported that they "felt" a caring presence in the online classroom in relation to how online faculty interacted with them (Post, 2017). Two primary findings emerged related to (1) what students valued in the online classroom and (2) how students perceived faculty caring. Students valued making connections with faculty that made them feel like a priority; some shared that the communication and connections with faculty in the online classroom are as strong as, if not stronger than, those in face-to-face classes. They valued timely communication from faculty members and multiple methods for connecting with them, including email, phone, and virtual conferencing. Students also shared that they valued faculty presence and caring when they were actively engaged, "involved and reading … responding or summarizing the discussions, giving feedback, making themselves available" (Post, 2017, p. 56). Overall, students appreciated that faculty gave the feeling "of another person being there" (Post, 2017, p. 56).

Student-Faculty Relationships

Effective online teaching relies on strong, well-developed interpersonal skills. Faculty members who take an interest in students, are sensitive to their feelings and challenges, convey respect for them, proactively address their anxiety, and demonstrate their availability to students have an ability to create good relationships with students (DeYoung, 2015). Studies indicate that students actually learn more in classrooms and clinical settings where teachers are student centered and empathetic (Cook, 2005). Students have also reported that strong interactions with faculty have resulted in the highest levels of learning (Boston, Diaz, & Gibson, 2019; Swan et al., 2000). In the online classroom, students appreciate when faculty demonstrate respect for students' knowledge and previous life and work experiences and when students are recognized for sharing their points of view. Some of the strategies that we implement to develop meaningful relationships with online nursing students are listed in **Table 3-6**.

Table 3-6 **Strategies Faculty Use to Develop Meaningful Relationships With Online Students**

- Demonstrate empathy for the life challenges that students experience.
- Be flexible with assignment due dates when extenuating circumstances arise.
- Demonstrate respect for previous work and educational experiences.
- Use students' past experience to build knowledge.
- Challenge student thinking in nonjudgmental and supportive ways.
- Recognize the value of the contributions that students bring to course activities.
- Acknowledge when the expertise that students contribute helps you learn.
- Honor the ability of students to do the work while balancing work and family.
- Demonstrate warmth in email and course communications; use students' first names.
- Send course announcements that recognize family time and life–work balance.
- Offer encouragement, and celebrate course milestones and student successes.
- Be available for students via email, phone, and video conferencing.
- Address performance concerns privately to provide students private spaces to learn.
- Ask students to provide feedback on course activities; value their experiences.
- Post general comments or group announcements about sensitive topics.
- Provide opportunities for individual mentorship.
- Connect with students by sharing personal stories and professional experiences.

Promoting a Sense of Belonging

A sense of belonging (SoB) is a valued concept in campus-based learning that is firmly connected to improved student attainment, increased learner satisfaction, and reduced attrition rates (Peacock & Cowan, 2019). For students, SoB involves feelings of being accepted, needed, and valued. It also includes the need to fit in and be connected to a group, class, or institution (Vaccaro, Daly-Cano, & Newman, 2015). In the online classroom, like other traditional classrooms, the lack of an SoB will have a significant impact on the ability of students to be successful. Developing connections and relationships with peers and faculty while developing their confidence, self-efficacy, and self-esteem can support students' success and help them achieve their goals (Peacock & Cowan, 2019).

Respect

Practicing and modeling respect are essential in any learning environment, particularly those that are discussion based (Brookfield & Preskill, 2005). Respecting others involves spending time getting to know them and treating them as distinctive individuals who have experiences and backgrounds that are uniquely their own. As online faculty, we can demonstrate respect by asking them to tell their stories, helping them identify their passions, and supporting them as they build their confidence in the online classroom and in their learning. When we mentor online faculty members who are new to teaching in postlicensure education, we spend a great deal of time discussing the diversity of the nurse's experience and background, both personally and professionally. As a measure of respect, it is important that all students feel valued for the skills and qualifications they possess.

For example, postlicensure nursing students are RNs with a variety of expertise and varied years of nursing experience. Some may have decades of nursing experience, yet it has been a long time since they were in a college classroom, or it may be the first time they are in an online classroom. They may find the experience of posting an online discussion or participating in an online group activity as daunting, anxiety producing, or even threatening, which can affect their ability to be successful (Whittaker, 2015). To be effective, online education must uniquely serve all students, including those with significant experience (Auricchio & Káganer, 2015). For example, Kendall and Kendall (2017) made a strong point in their discussion of an executive leadership class when they identified that "making the mistake 'whether out of ignorance, laziness, or oversight' of treating an executive as if they don't have the requisite experience will risk their learning and their satisfaction" (Kendall & Kendall, 2017, p. 62).

Social Presence: Teacher Immediacy

Formal online learning relies on good instructional design, a learning management system supported by technology, and a facilitator who sets the tone for participation and fosters social presence and teacher immediacy (Gunderson, Theiss, Wood, & Conti-O'Hare, 2014). In traditional face-to-face classrooms, students can engage with faculty in a variety of ways, including discussing issues before and after class, asking questions during class, and meeting privately during office hours (Gunderson et al., 2014). In online classes, students need opportunities to engage with faculty and build a relationship that will support their learning experience. It is up to the faculty to develop a sense of community in the online classroom and create opportunities for engagement that instill confidence in students. Social presence and teacher immediacy are not new strategies in education. The theory of social presence, the "degree of quality" or state of "being there" when using remote or distance communication, was developed by Short, Williams, and Christie in 1976. Teacher immediacy involves actions or behaviors that reduce the physical or psychological distance in interpersonal communication (Mehrabian, 1967). The following strategies are just a few ways that we try to reduce the physical distance to connect with online students, including the use of synchronous meeting times, using a phone call, and providing additional support during challenging times.

Synchronous Meeting Times

Holding synchronous meeting times or specific virtual office hours can be a helpful strategy for providing students with immediate feedback and support. We have learned that it can provide a sense of security for students to know that there is an option to meet virtually at a specific time. However, when we have scheduled optional synchronous meeting times and virtual office hours, they typically have low attendance. In a survey of online students, only 36% reported that they would value meeting synchronously two to three times during a course (Clinefelter & Asianian, 2015). Given the diverse work schedules and family commitments of our online students, synchronous meeting times have not been overly successful. In fact, there have been times when scheduling an optional session has created anxiety for students who could not attend, even though the session was not required. Because the outcomes of holding synchronous meeting times for online courses are varied, this is a strategy that we recommend assessing with each class.

Individual Phone Calls

One strategy that has worked well to initiate social presence and immediacy in the online program has been to schedule a phone call with students during the first week of class in their first course. To make students feel welcome and to help them overcome any early anxiety or feelings of isolation, a phone call can help faculty and students establish rapport and begin developing their relationship. Students have the chance to engage individually with faculty as they learn more about the course and have the opportunity to ask any questions they may have. The phone call has worked exceptionally well to set the tone for the class and get students off on the right foot. Faculty learn more about who students are and what challenges or goals they may have for the course. The call also helps students understand that the faculty member is a real person who is interested in their success and development (Gunderson et al., 2014). The initial call can include topics such as the following: review of due dates and course expectations, discussion of any challenges with technology or logging into class, sharing of student resources and how to find information, discussion of what the student can expect in terms of communication from the faculty member and the best means of contact, and any questions the student has.

Student Support During a Crisis

At the time of this writing, we are experiencing a global pandemic as a result of the 2019 novel coronavirus (COVID-19) pandemic. The students in our online program are licensed RNs who work and have been on the front lines caring for the community. In addition to the stress they may be experiencing at work, some have reported their home lives and routines being in flux as a result of having children out of school who require instruction and support. Some students have experienced illness or have family members who have also required extra support and care. Students have also reported having significant employment and economic challenges arise in their families as a result of the pandemic. As online faculty who teach postlicensure nursing students, it is not unusual for us to continually balance the academic rigor and expectations for quality engagement in the academic program with the flexibility and support that are needed for nurses to be successful. However, this has been an unprecedented time that has caused us to reflect deeply on what students truly need from us to be successful, as well as what we can realistically expect from ourselves. The pandemic has necessitated flexibility. We have shared some strategies that we have used to support students during the pandemic in **Table 3-7**.

In summary, we believe that developing a strong understanding of the unique characteristics of online students can lead to meaningful relationships between faculty and students and positive learning outcomes for students. By staying close to our foundation of caring and compassion in nursing, we can extend these values into the practice of online nursing education.

Table 3-7 Strategies for Supporting Students During a Crisis

- Post regular announcements to recognize the challenges that they may be experiencing and offer course reminders.
- Email students individually to let them know you are there for them; offer support.
- Encourage students to communicate with you about specific challenges they are having with assignments and due dates; offer flexibility during extenuating circumstances.
- Explain to them what your experience has been with the changing situation in your own family or in the community in order to humanize the experience, but at the same time, avoid burdening them with too much detail about personal struggles.
- Recognize other factors that may be influencing the time they have to complete coursework, such as increased hours at work or having children and other family members at home during the day; share strategies that may help.
- Offer resources, such as reminders to connect with their academic advisor, distance librarian, writing support, and student services.
- Schedule *optional* virtual chats to connect with students individually or as a group to build community and share experiences.
- Create *optional* discussion board threads to discuss the pandemic and share resources.
- Suggest a phone call if the student is struggling and may need more connection or support.

(continues)

Table 3-7 Strategies for Supporting Students During a Crisis   *(continued)*

- Schedule an *optional* virtual "town hall" for all students in the program to discuss challenges and opportunities and offer support.
- Coach students to persist by reminding them that the term will be completed soon and that they will have a break between terms; help them look ahead.
- Notify team members when students are struggling so that others can reach out with support (e.g., academic advisor, faculty advisor).
- Celebrate students' success in meeting deadlines, completing projects, and persisting.
- Demonstrate care, compassion, and flexibility.
- Reduce workload by requiring one discussion reply in discussions instead of two.
- Give a week off, if possible, to allow students to catch up.

Best-Practice Recommendations for Online Teaching

- Implement teaching and learning strategies that honor students as adult learners.
- Develop a strong understanding of the unique characteristics of your student population in order to achieve a student-centered approach to quality online teaching.
- Create opportunities to learn students' stories and help them identify their learning needs.
- Prioritize strong interpersonal relationships with online students that demonstrate caring and empathy, respect for differences, sensitivity to culture and individuality, and an interest in their well-being.
- Promote a sense of belonging by demonstrating respect for students' experience and background and by valuing their contributions.
- Implement strategies that will reduce the physical distance between you and your online students, such as scheduling synchronous meeting times, offering a phone call, and providing additional support during challenging times.

References

American Association of Colleges of Nurses. (2017a). *Fact sheet: Degree completion programs for registered nurses: RN to master's degree and RN to baccalaureate programs.* https://www .aacnnursing.org/Portals/42/News/Factsheets/Degree-Completion-Factsheet.pdf

American Association of Colleges of Nursing. (2017b). *Nursing shortage.* https://www.aacnnursing .org/Portals/42/News/Factsheets/Nursing-Shortage-Factsheet-2017.pdf

American Association of Colleges of Nursing. (2019). *Fact sheet: Enhancing diversity in the nursing workforce.* https://www.aacnnursing.org/Portals/42/News/Factsheets/Enhancing-Diversity-Factsheet .pdf

Anderson, I. (2016). Identifying different learning styles to enhance the learning experience. *Nursing Standard, 31*(7), 53–63. http://doi.org/10.7748/ns.2016.e10407

Auerbach, D., Buerhaus, P., Staiger, D., & Skinner, L. (2017). *2017 data brief update: Current trends of men in nursing.* http://healthworkforcestudies.com/publications-data/data_brief_update_current _trends_of_men_in_nursing.html

Auricchio, G., & Káganer, E. (2015). *How digitalization is changing the way executives learn.* http://www.ieseinsight.com/docImpresion.aspx?id=1734

Bednarz, H., Schim, S., & Doorenbos, A. (2010). Cultural diversity in nursing education: Perils, pitfalls, and pearls. *Journal of Nursing Education, 49*(5), 253–260. http://doi.org/10.3928/0148 4834-20100115-02

Bender, T. (2012). *Discussion-based online teaching to enhance student learning: Theory, practice, and assessment.* Stylus Publishing.

Bevis, E. O., & Watson, J. (2000). *Toward a caring curriculum: A new pedagogy for nursing.* Jones and Bartlett Learning.

Bhagat, A., Vyas, R., & Singh, T. (2015). Students awareness of learning styles and their perceptions to a mixed method approach for learning. *International Journal of Applied & Basic Medical Research, 5*(Suppl. 1), S58–S65. http://doi.org/10.4103/2229-516X.162281

Blau, I., & Barak, A. (2012). How do personality, synchronous media, and discussion topic affect participation? *Journal of Educational Technology & Society, 15*(2), 12–24.

Boston, W., Diaz, S.R., & Gibson, A.M. (2019). An exploration of the relationship between indicators of the community of inquiry framework and retention in online programs. *Journal of Asynchronous Learning Networks, 13*(3), 67–83. https://files.eric.ed.gov/fulltext/EJ862358.pdf

Bolliger, D. U., & Erichsen, E. A. (2013). Student satisfaction with blended and online courses based on personality type. *Canadian Journal of Learning and Technology, 39*(1), 1–23.

Brookfield, S. D., & Preskill, S. (2005). Discussion as a way of teaching: Tools and techniques for democratic classrooms (2nd ed.). Jossey-Bass.

Candela, L. (2016). Theoretical foundations of teaching and learning. In D. Billings & J. Halstead (Eds.), *Teaching in nursing: A guide for faculty* (pp. 211–229). Saunders.

Clinefelter, D. L., & Aslanian, C. B. (2015). *Online college students 2016: Comprehensive data on demands and preferences.* The Learning House. https://www.learninghouse.com/wp-content/uploads/2017/09/OnlineCollegeStudents2015.pdf

Cook, L. J. (2005). Inviting behaviors of clinical faculty & nursing students' anxiety. *Journal of Nursing Education, 44,* 156–161.

Cusatis Phillips, B. (2018). Understanding the learner. In M. H. Oermann, J. C. DeGagne, & B. Cusatis Phillips (Eds.), *Teaching in nursing and role of the educator: The complete guide to best practice in teaching, evaluation, and curriculum development* (2nd ed., pp. 29–44). Springer.

Dapremont, J. (2014). Black nursing students: Strategies for academic success. *Nursing Education Perspectives, 35*(3), 157–161.

DeYoung, S. (2015). *Teaching strategies for nurse educators* (3rd ed.). Pearson.

Dusst, E., & Winthrop, R. (2019). *Top 6 trends in higher education.* Brookings Institution. https://www.brookings.edu/blog/education-plus-development/2019/01/10/top-6-trends-in-higher-education/

Espinosa, L. L., Turk, J. M., Taylor, M., & Chessman, H. M. (2019). *Race and ethnicity in higher education: A status report.* American Council on Education. https://1xfsu31b52d33idlp13twtos-wpengine.netdna-ssl.com/wp-content/uploads/2019/02/REHE-Exec-Summary-FINAL.pdf

Fang D., Li, Y., Turinetti, M., & Trautman, D. E. (2018). *2017–2018 enrollment and graduations in baccalaureate and graduate programs in nursing.* American Association of Colleges of Nursing.

Gunderson, B. J., Theiss, M. A., Wood, L. K., & Conti-O'Hare, M. (2014). Using a telephone call to increase social presence in online classes. *Nursing Education Perspectives, 35*(5), 338–339. http://doi.org/10.5480/11-569

Hershan, R., & Lauderdale, C.L. (2018). *Trends in higher education: 2018 outlook: The rising need for sustainable financial, operational, and academic models.* https://www.alvarezandmarsal.com/sites/default/files/article/pdf/trends_in_higher_education_2018_outlook.pdf

Inside Track. (2019). *Top 10 higher education trends to watch for in 2019.* https://www.educationdive.com/news/9-higher-ed-trends-to-watch-in-2019/545330/

Irvine, D. (2010). How to reward a multigenerational and culturally diverse workforce. *Workspan, 4*(10), 63–68. http://www.worldatwork.org /waw/adimLink?id=36840

Jacoby, L. (2018). What motivates students in the online communication classroom? An exploration of self-determination theory. *Journal of Educators Online, 15*(2).

Jenzabar. (2019). *8 higher education trends you need to be ready for in 2019.* https://www.jenzabar.com/blog/eight-hot-higher-education-trends-for-2019

Keating, S. B. (2018). A proposed unified curriculum. In S. B. Keating & S. S. DeBoor (Eds.), *Curriculum development and evaluation in nursing education* (pp. 171–184). Springer.

Kendall, J. E., & Kendall, K. E. (2017). Enhancing online executive education using storytelling: An approach to strengthening online social presence. *Decision Sciences Journal of Innovative Education, 15*(1), 62–81. http://doi.org/10.1111/dsji.12121

Kim, Y., Glassman, M., & Williams, M. S. (2015). Connecting agents: Engagement and motivation in online collaboration. *Computers in Human Behavior, 49,* 333–342.

Kolb, A. Y., & Kolb, D. A. (2005). *The Kolb learning style inventory: Version 3.1. 2005 technical specifications.* Experience Based Learning Systems, Inc.

Leite, W. L., Svinicki, M., & Shi, Y. (2010). Attempted validation of the scores of the VARK: Learning Styles Inventory with multitrait–multimethod confirmatory factor analysis models. *Educational and Psychological Measurement, 70*(2), 323–339. http://doi.org/10.1177/0013164409344507

Lewis, S. H., Rogers, M., & Naef, R. (2006). Caring-human science philosophy in nursing education: Beyond the curriculum revolution. *International Journal for Human Caring, 10*(4), 31–38.

Lipscomb, V. (2010). Intergenerational issues in nursing: Learning from each generation. *Clinical Journal of Oncology Nursing, 14*(3), 267–269. http://doi.org/10.1188/10.CJON.267-269

Mastel-Smith, B., Post, J., & Lake, P. (2015). Online teaching: Are you there, and do you care? *Journal of Nursing Education, 54,* 145–151. http://doi.org/10.3928/01484834-20150218-18

Mehrabian, A. (1967). Attitudes inferred from non-immediacy of verbal communications. *Journal of Verbal Learning and Verbal Behavior, 6*(2), 294–295. http://doi.org/10.1016/0022-5371(67)80113-0

National Academy of Medicine. (2011). *The future of nursing: Leading change, advancing health.* https://www.nap.edu/download/12956

National League for Nursing. (2016). *Achieving diversity and meaningful inclusion in nursing education.* http://www.nln.org/docs/default-source/about/vision-statement-achieving-diversity.pdf?sfvrsn=2

National Center for Education Statistics. (2019). *Enrollment and employees in postsecondary institutions, Fall 2017; and financial statistics and academic libraries, Fiscal year 2017.* https://nces.ed.gov/pubs2019/2019021REV.pdf

National Council of State Boards of Nursing. (2017). *National nursing workforce study.* https://www.ncsbn.org/workforce.htm

Oster, M. (2019). *The state of higher education in 2019.* Grant Thornton. https://www.grantthornton.com/-/media/content-page-files/nfp/pdfs/2019/2019-GT-State-of-Higher-Education-report.ashx

Pardue, K., & Morgan, P. (2008). Millennials considered: A new generation, new approaches, and implications for nursing education. *Nursing Education Perspectives, 29*(2), 74–79. http://doi.org/10.1515/ijnes-2013-0024

Pashler, H., McDaniel, M., Rohrer, D., & Bjork, R. (2008). Learning styles: Concepts and evidence. *Psychological Science in the Public Interest, 9*(3), 105–119. https://doi.org/10.1111/j.1539-6053.2009.01038.x

Pavalache-Ilie, M., & Cocorada, S. (2014). Interactions of students' personality in the online learning environment. *Procedia—Social and Behavioral Sciences, 128,* 117–122. http://doi.org/10.1016/j.sbspro.2014.03.128

Peacock, S., & Cowan, J. (2016). From presences to linked influences within communities of inquiry. *International Review of Research in Open and Distributed Learning, 17*(5), 267–283.

Penn State University. (2017). *Center for Collegiate Mental Health.* https://sites.psu.edu/ccmh/files/2018/01/2017_CCMH_Report-1r3iri4.pdf

Popkess, A. M., & Frey, J. L. (2016). Strategies to support diverse learning needs of students. In D. Billings & J. Halstead (Eds.), *Teaching in nursing: A guide for faculty* (pp. 15–34). Elsevier.

Post, J. (2017). Online teaching: How students perceive faculty caring. *International Journal for Human Caring, 21*(2), 54–58.

Robinson, J. A., Scollan-Koliopoulos, M., Kamienski, M., & Burke, K. (2012). Generational differences and learning style preferences in nurses from a large metropolitan medical center. *Journal for Nurses in Staff Development, 28*(4), 166–172.

Rumay Alexander, G. (2016). Multicultural education in nursing. In D. Billings & J. Halstead (Eds.), *Teaching in nursing: A guide for faculty* (pp. 263–281). Elsevier.

Ryan, R. M., & Deci, E. L. (2000). Intrinsic and extrinsic motivations: Class definitions and new directions. *Contemporary Educational Psychology*, *25*(1), 54–67. http://doi.org/10.1006/ceps.1999.1020

Sailsman, S., Rutherford, M., Tovin, M., & Cianelli, R. (2018). Cultural integration online: The lived experience of English-as-a-second-language RN-BSN nursing students learning in an online environment. *Nursing Education Perspectives*, *39*(4), 221–224. http://doi.org/10.1097/01.NEP.0000000000000301

Schunk, D. H., & Zimmerman, B. (2012). *Motivation and self-regulated learning: Theory, research, and applications*. Routledge.

Short, J., Williams, E., & Christie, B. (1976). *The social psychology of telecommunications*. London, England: John Wiley & Sons.

Sitzman, K. (2010). Student-preferred caring behaviors for online nursing education. *Nursing Education Perspectives*, *31*(3), 171–178.

Sitzman, K., & Watson, J. (2014). *Caring science, mindful practice: Implementing Watson's human caring theory*. Springer.

Stanley, D. (2010). Multigenerational workforce issues and their implications for leadership in nursing. *Journal of Nursing Management*, *18*, 846–852. http://doi.org/10.1111/j.1365-2834.2010.01158.x

Swan, K., Shea, P., Fredericksen, E., Pickett, A., Pelz, W., & Maher, G. (2000). Building knowledge building communities: Consistency, contact and communication in the virtual classroom. *Journal of Educational Computing Research*, *23*(4), 359. https://www.learntechlib.org/p/91328/

U.S. Department of Labor, Bureau of Labor Statistics. (2018). *Employment projections 2018–2028*. https://www.bls.gov/news.release/pdf/ecopro.pdf

Vaccaro, A., Daly-Cano, M., & Newman, B. M. (2015). A sense of belonging among college students with disabilities: An emergent theoretical model. *Journal of College Student Development*, *56*(7), 670–686. http://doi.org/10.1353/csd.2015.0072

Valiga, T. M. (2016). Philosophical foundations of the curriculum. In D. Billings & J. Halstead (Eds.), *Teaching in nursing: A guide for faculty* (pp. 118–129). Elsevier.

Villarruel, A., Washington, D., Lecher, W., & Carver, N. (2015). A more diverse nursing workforce. *The American Journal of Nursing*, *115*(5), 57–62. http://doi.org/10.1097/01.NAJ.0000465034.43341.b1

Whittaker, A. (2015). Effects of team-based learning on self-regulated online learning. *International Journal of Nurse Education Scholarship*, *12*(1), 1–10. http://doi.org/10.1515/ijnes-2014-0046

Wros, P., Wheeler, P., & Jones, M. (2014). Curriculum planning for baccalaureate nursing programs. In S. Keating (Ed.), *Curriculum development and evaluation in nursing* (3rd ed., pp. 245–284). Springer.

Successful Academic Progression and Online Nursing Students

Melissa Robinson and Henny Breen

"The real voyage of discovery consists not in seeking new landscapes, but in having new eyes."

Marcel Proust

Overview

The purpose of this chapter is to discuss factors that affect successful academic progression for online nursing students. To illustrate a holistic approach to the successful progression of online students, we present a revised version of an interprofessional model that was developed by our team and previously disseminated in the *Journal of Community & Public Health Nursing*. This model supports online nursing students in our institution and can be applied to other online programs, including graduate programs. The model includes a set of strategies used to support the student from the initial point of contact with the institution through the successful completion of the degree. An emphasis is placed on understanding the unique needs and goals of students in an online postlicensure program who are motivated to advance their education while successfully balancing coursework with family commitments and a busy work schedule.

Background

Since 2011, when the Institute of Medicine, currently known as the National Academy of Medicine, published its landmark report *The Future of Nursing*, in conjunction with the Robert Wood Johnson Foundation, successful academic progression for nurses has been a national initiative. The report called for increasing the number of nurses with a bachelor of science in nursing (BSN) degree in the workforce to 80% and doubling the number of nurses with doctoral degrees. Several factors have influenced the demand to educate more nurses with higher levels of nursing education, including a well-documented nursing shortage, an effort on behalf of healthcare organizations to achieve Magnet status, and a focus on high-quality patient care outcomes (American Association of Colleges of Nursing [AACN]), 2017; Buerhaus, Staiger, & Auerbach, 2008). Increasingly, nurse employers are motivated to support nurses as they achieve higher levels of nursing education. Some employers have changed the eligibility requirements for hire to a BSN or higher. Although online education has influenced the progress toward advancing the education of nurses in practice, more efforts are needed to support a highly educated nursing workforce. Current national workforce data indicate that only 55% of registered nurses (RNs) are prepared with a BSN or graduate degree (AACN, 2017).

Motivation for Higher Levels of Nursing Education

Nurses are motivated to earn higher degrees by a variety of personal and professional reasons. Historically, nurses have pursued continuing education and life-long learning opportunities to stay current with healthcare changes, attain higher levels of education in nursing, or advance professionally (Megginson, 2008). Life or work experiences often convince or motivate adults to seek out learning opportunities. The nurse's readiness to learn often develops from real-life problems and the realization that new knowledge is needed (Candela, 2016). Most recently, nurses have responded to employers' requirements for higher levels of education and their call to move into leadership roles; advance in their specialty; or take the next step toward advanced practice, academia, or research (Wros, Wheeler, & Jones, 2014). Nurses are also driven by personal goals and professional commitment, and they advance their education at a variety of times during their careers. Regardless of age or years of experience, nurses continue to recognize the importance of advancing their education to secure meaningful employment and prepare for the profession.

Barriers to Degree Advancement for Nurses

RNs often report barriers as they make the decision to transition to baccalaureate education. Some express fears or anxiety as they anticipate a lack of recognition for previous educational accomplishments or transferability of previous credits (Megginson, 2008), as well as concerns about the time commitment and expenses associated with educational advancement (Sarver, Cichra, & Kline, 2015). Many nurses anticipate challenges with time management and balancing higher education with family commitments and work responsibilities. Additional obstacles include concerns related to advances in technology, planned retirement, and a perceived lack of benefit (Nininger, Abbott, & Shaw, 2019; Warshawsky, Brandford, Barnum, & Westneat, 2015). These are common concerns seen repeatedly in the literature surrounding adult education, in general, and they contribute to challenges in retaining students through degree completion (Hardin, 2008).

Student Persistence

Student persistence and *student retention* are terms that are often used interchange-ably in higher education. According to the National Center for Education Statistics (2019), *student retention* refers to institutional measurements, and *student persistence* refers to student measurements. Said another way, the institution has the responsi-bility to retain students, whereas students are responsible for persisting through de-gree completion. As educators begin to recognize the similarity of learning regardless of delivery mode, they also believe that problems with retention and progression are a more significant challenge in online programs as compared with traditional face-to-face programs (Allen & Seaman, 2011; Bawa, 2016; Moore & Fetzner, 2019). A review of the existing literature indicates that up to 40% to 80% of college students drop out of online classes (Bawa, 2016; Smith, 2010; Stanford-Bowers, 2008).

In a recent study from Arizona State University and the Boston Consulting Group (2018) that included six institutions offering face-to-face and online courses, three reported higher retention and graduation rates for students who took at least one online course compared with students who took only face-to-face courses. The study indicated that first-time freshmen at Houston Community College were re-tained at rates 9–10 times higher, and graduated up to 17 percentage points higher, than students who took only face-to-face courses. With such vast differences in student characteristics and the types of modalities available to students in higher education, additional research will reveal strategies to support student retention and progression.

Although the literature indicates a variety of reasons for attrition in online classes, students who provide a reason for their withdrawal have cited personal, work-related, or program-related reasons (Willging & Johnson, 2009). Online stu-dents are at risk for attrition at any point during program completion, including during the admission process, during any given semester, or at any point in their progression. Strategies that support student persistence with academic progression are essential. McClenney and Waiwaiole (2005) suggested that improving student retention rates is a collective responsibility that includes the faculty, staff, and ad-ministrators in the institution, as well as students, working together to promote students' success with academic progression.

Holistic Academic Progression for Nurses: An Interprofessional Model

Although we acknowledge the importance of supporting the academic success of all students across the institution, we have made significant efforts to reduce many of the barriers that are unique to being successful in rigorous online degree programs. We have recognized that the success of online students begins at the time that they are choosing their academic program and continues as they build early relationships with members of our interprofessional team. Student success continues with strong academic support from professional advisors and online faculty throughout the ed-ucational experience and culminates with the achievement of the BSN degree. To build on the success of our students, our team worked collaboratively to formalize the holistic approach we were using to support the academic progression of online nursing students. We believe this approach could be adopted and/or modified by other postlicensure online programs to improve retention and persistence rates.

The interprofessional model was originally published in an article titled "Holistic Academic Progression for Nurses: An Interprofessional Model" in the *Journal of Community & Public Health Nursing*. Initially, the model described the members of the interprofessional team supporting RN-to-BSN students during their educational experience, including outreach coordinators, admissions counselors, academic advisors, and the faculty director. We have modified the model to include a broader perspective on the various forms of support provided by online faculty members during classroom experiences and through mentorship provided to students as they progress through the program. The model, shown in **Figure 4-1**, illustrates our commitment to providing a student-centered experience (center) and the multiple forms of interaction and support that are so essential for quality online learning experiences.

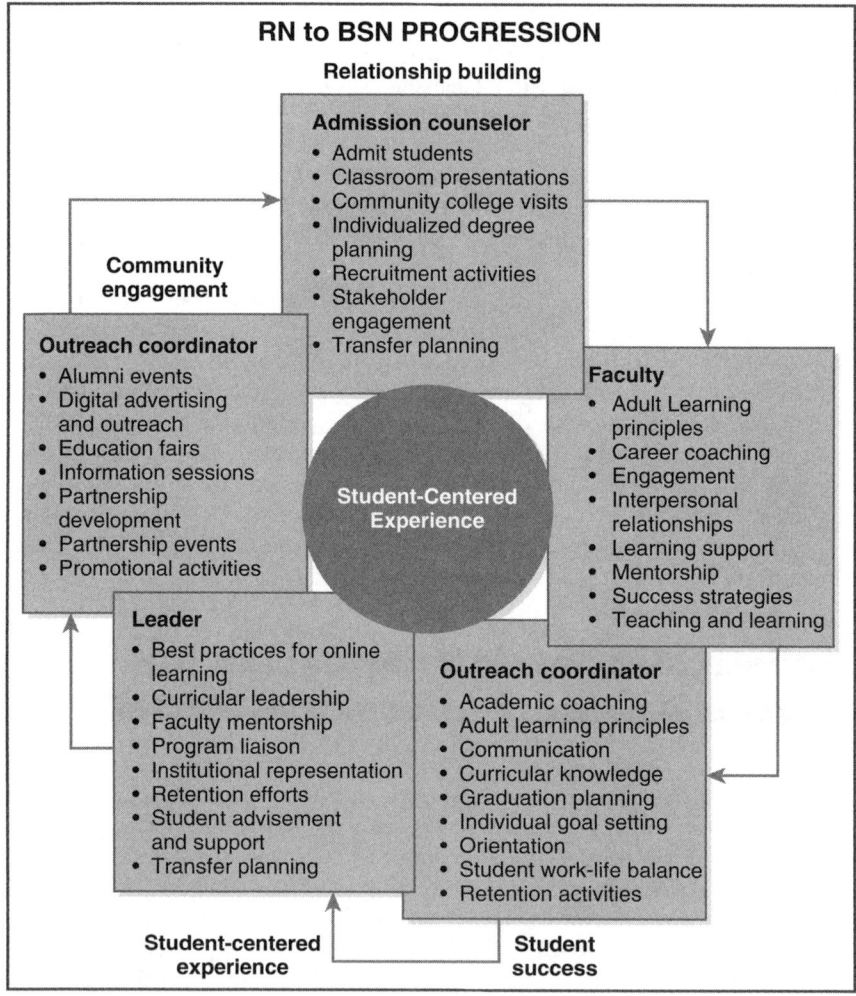

Figure 4-1 Academic progression for online nursing students: an interprofessional model

Data from the "Holistic Academic Progression for Nurses: An Interprofessional Model" previously published in *Journal of Community & Public Health Nursing*.

Program Description

The online RN-to-BSN program attracts a diverse student population, including new graduate nurses as well as nurses with varied years of practice and specialty experience in nursing. The students are geographically and generationally diverse. The average age of the RN-to-BSN student in the program is 37, and the majority are employed full time in nursing. They attend the online program while balancing career and family responsibilities. As adult learners, nurses in the RN-to-BSN program benefit from using their previous nursing education and experience as a foundation for integrating new learning, which is in keeping with our constructivist educational philosophy. Further, they benefit from being involved in planning their education. The program is designed specifically to support the success of a working nurse. The flexible online course delivery has made the program accessible to nurses across the country who remain living and working in their own communities while advancing their nursing education. Key features of the online RN-to-BSN program are listed in **Table 4-1**.

Interprofessional Team

Although each team member has distinct responsibilities, collaborative overarching strategies are effective when integrated across the student experience. For example, individualized course planning is implemented by multiple team members collaboratively with the student. Beginning with the first point of contact in the community through admission to the school of nursing and continuing throughout the program with skilled support from the academic advisor and faculty mentorship in the classroom, students experience multiple sources of academic support from the team. The roles and responsibilities of each member of the interprofessional team are discussed in the following sections.

Table 4-1 **Key Features of the Online RN-to-BSN Program**

- Community-based nursing curriculum
- Flexible, 100% online course delivery
- Online program orientation with technology support
- Opportunities for campus engagement with faculty and RN-to-BSN team
- Service-learning clinical experiences (which take place in a local or international community)
- Individualized RN-to-BSN academic advising
- Embedded online librarians and access to e-tutoring
- Emphasis on course interaction and collaboration
  - Student to student (peer interaction)
  - Student to course content
  - Student to faculty
- Unique opportunities for online nursing elective courses (emphasis on liberal arts core)
  - Evolution of Nursing (3 credits)
  - Health Disparities (3 credits)
  - Palliative Care Nursing (3 credits)
  - Trauma-Informed Care (3 credits)

Outreach Coordinator

The role of the outreach coordinator includes a focus on community engagement and relationship building by providing a consistent and personalized presence in the healthcare community. Outreach activities include, but are not limited to, creating and maintaining relationships with healthcare organizations and nurse employers, engaging with nursing school alumni and other stakeholders, and identifying initiatives that engage a variety of professional groups. The outreach coordinator is often the first point of contact for potential students and members of the community to learn about opportunities at the college.

The outreach coordinator serves an important role within the nursing school related to outreach and recruitment while working closely with the RN-to-BSN team to understand the needs of the student population and community. Specific outreach activities include serving in various vendor opportunities and conferences hosted by hospitals and professional nursing organizations, delivering in-services in the community that educate nurses on the value of earning a BSN, and hosting face-to-face and virtual information sessions about education advancement.

The addition of virtual information sessions has improved access to program information for nurses in the workforce, including those in rural and out-of-state communities. The synchronous webinars address a variety of topics related to the online program, including admission requirements, transfer planning, local and international service-learning opportunities, and elective nursing courses. Current students, academic advisors, and faculty members have participated in the webinars to share information and reflect on their experiences in the program. The webinars are strategically designed for students who are considering their program options and help students envision themselves in the program and build on institutional loyalty. Research has demonstrated that a lack of specific, accurate information at the appropriate time is one of the top reasons that adult students choose not to enroll at a higher education institution (Noel-Levitz, 2011). Thus, we have committed our attention to combining outreach, enrollment, and academia best practices. We strive to demonstrate our passion for health care, our desire to connect with adult students, and our aim of continuously cultivating new outreach opportunities.

Through collaboration and shared responsibility, it is possible to increase the visibility of the institution and engage inquiries that provide nurses with the ability to reach their goals for advanced education. For example, the outreach coordinator and admissions counselor work closely together to design and plan student recruitment, which benefits the entire college. Cross-collaboration stimulates innovation by utilizing multiple perspectives to develop meaningful actions (Baldwin & Chang, 2007). Each member can focus on building relationships in the community, which, in turn, helps the college attract prospective students. See **Table 4-2** for specific strategies implemented by the outreach coordinator that support the successful progression of online nursing students.

Admissions Counselor

The admissions counselor focuses on educating students about program requirements and their transition into a new academic environment. The counselor provides the necessary knowledge and preparation for navigating the transfer process

Table 4-2 Strategies Implemented by the Outreach Coordinator

- Assessment of the needs of the community and institution
- Engaging the healthcare community and clinical organizations
- Representing the institution at community events and professional conferences
- Implementing partnership events and information (campus, virtual) sessions
- Fostering alumni and student engagement on campus and in the community
- Collaboration on marketing activities

Table 4-3 Strategies Implemented by the Admissions Counselor

- Recruitment activities and admissions
- Relationship development (community partners, students)
- Collaboration with students on academic goals and development of course plans
- Assessment of transfer credit
- Educating students about the admission process
- Transitioning new students to the academic advisor to begin the program

between institutions or back into the academic environment. Many practicing nurses who have been away from the academic environment encounter changes in technology, questions about transfer credits, and unfamiliarity with higher education requirements, which can cause anxiety and stress when returning to school (Duffy et al., 2014). To help students overcome challenges with academic progression, the admission counselor's goal is to build a close working relationship. A level of support that is enhanced by purposeful interactions creates a foundation for program entry and student–professional expectations (Wyatt, 2011).

The admissions counselor's primary responsibility is to recruit and admit students to the institution. The counselor plays a crucial role in influencing students' decision to enroll, helping them commit to their academic goals, and building confidence in their ability to earn the BSN. Ongoing, effective communication with students is essential to educate them about degree requirements and the admission process. In this way, the admissions counselor facilitates students' transition into the institution while assisting them in moving toward matriculation. Student interactions take place in a variety of formats, either in the counselor's office or in the community, with the primary goal of providing timely follow-up on questions related to transfer planning, transfer-credit evaluations, and incomplete applications. The counselor is in constant collaboration with new students, potential students, and team members, including the outreach coordinator, academic advisor, and faculty. See **Table 4-3** for specific strategies implemented by the admissions counselor that support the successful progression of online nursing students.

Academic Advisor

The focus of the academic advisor is proactively advising students for progression in the major, implementing specific retention practices, and collaborating with the RN-to-BSN team for student success. To support progression, the advisor coordinates academic plans, educates students about their degree requirements while addressing their unique academic history, and creates a safe space for active listening and effective communication. To enhance retention, the advisor coordinates quarterly events for advisees, promotes a supportive environment by acknowledging student life events, and audits degree plans to ensure each semester's degree candidates are cleared for graduation. The advisor also coordinates student support by engaging faculty and sharing student feedback with the larger RN-to-BSN team. Authentic feedback allows faculty to adjust classroom experiences and the admission counselor to utilize student testimonials in recruitment. Ultimately, the RN-to-BSN academic advisor sets the tone for student success with an individualized and professional advising approach to supporting student progression in the program.

The role of the academic advisor has changed significantly per our academic advisor who has over two decades of higher education advising experience. In the past, faculty saw advising as a clerical task, an obligation to the college to register students, and that was all the advising that was expected of them (Harrison, 2009). As access to online education has expanded for adults advancing their education, academic advisors have adapted to a "virtual" advising model that provides students with greater access to their advisors using the communication methods that work best for them. Advances in technology allow advisors to conduct meetings at flexible times using email and virtual applications such as Skype, WebEx, and Zoom. The academic advisor also schedules individual phone appointments regularly with students.

In a study that addressed pre-nursing and nursing students' perceptions of the characteristics and qualities of effective academic advisors, students identified being knowledgeable as the most important characteristic of a nursing academic advisor, followed by fostering a caring professional relationship and being approachable (Harrison, 2009). Given that online students are not able to stop by the advisor's office at any time because of geographical differences and work schedules, cultivating a genuine sense of trust and caring is a high priority for the advisor. The advisor works diligently to create a solid connection with the student, as well as to support a strong connection to the college, which affects the advising relationship as well as retention in the program. The academic advisor works collaboratively with faculty in the program on issues related to student support and retention and when serving as an advocate for students. With knowledge of adult learning principles and best practices for academic advising, RN-to-BSN advisors get to know individual students and adapt quickly to their needs, set up processes that are focused on student success, and maintain an individualized advising model. See **Table 4-4** for specific strategies implemented by the academic advisor to support the successful progression of online nursing students.

Program Director and Online Faculty

A faculty member serves as the director of the RN-to-BSN program. The director provides leadership for the delivery of the curriculum, manages the program partnerships with community colleges and clinical organizations, and serves as a liaison for nursing and additional departments within the institution. The director serves

Table 4-4 Strategies Implemented by the Academic Advisor

- Academic advising of online students
- Individual meetings by phone, virtual access, or face to face on campus
- Collaborating with students on course planning, goal setting, registering for classes, and preparing for graduation
- Providing day-to-day student support (responding to requests, reaching out to support students, providing flexible opportunities for student appointments)
- Providing social support and advice for work–life balance
- Providing assistance with problem solving when challenges arise
- Collaborating with faculty to support student success and retention
- Advocating for college policies and procedures

on the committee that addresses admissions and the progression of students in nursing and has a key role in advocating for policies that support the success of all students, including students in the online program.

The curriculum is led by a small team of online faculty who have expertise in postlicensure education and certification in online teaching. The director maintains oversight of course scheduling, participates in mentoring and evaluation of adjunct faculty, and ensures expectations for rigor and quality assurance in online education are met. The online curriculum is taught using a course lead model to ensure consistency and utilize content expertise. The full-time faculty members are experienced online educators with a strong understanding of nursing workforce issues as well as the challenges that nurses face while balancing their education program with work and family responsibilities.

The director works closely with the interprofessional team on issues affecting outreach and recruitment in the community and on student issues that affect advising, student success, and retention. The benefits of having a nursing faculty member participate in the community include having individual discussions with nurses to share details about the curriculum, the importance of continuing education in nursing, and workforce issues, all of which can be discussed in depth. In the classroom, the online faculty members work closely with students to support their success, both academically and professionally. They assist students with prioritization of their coursework while balancing family and work responsibilities. Making themselves available to have telephone conferences, video conferencing, or face-to-face campus meetings with students and demonstrating continual online engagement are essential for achieving student satisfaction and success with online learning.

One of the strongest elements within the interprofessional model is providing a diverse representation of team members in the community. Therefore, the faculty director participates in face-to-face and virtual information sessions, presentations at community colleges, and tabling events at conferences and clinical organizations, as well as meeting with potential students and stakeholders in a variety of formats. Ongoing evaluation of student and stakeholder satisfaction, developing credibility in the outreach to the community, and creating opportunities to improve communication about the program are all essential to maintaining a reputable program and strengthening student outcomes.

Community Partnerships

In recent years, direct enrollment from associate-degree nursing programs has increased because of articulation agreements designed to support educational mobility and facilitate a seamless transfer of academic credit between associate-degree and baccalaureate nursing programs (AACN, 2014). Community colleges have provided vital access to higher education and to associate-degree nursing programs for adult students. Due to affordable prices, less strict admission requirements, and sites that are geographically available, community colleges have served a valuable role in higher education and in the community (Robinson, Mole, Hiller, Swenson, & Harrington, 2018). To facilitate academic progression between institutions, it is recommended that faculty representatives work collaboratively to develop formal partnership agreements that reduce institutional barriers to progression (Hodges & Selena-Salis, 2016). We have formalized the process for articulation and dual enrollment in community college coadmission agreements. The goals of the formal coadmission agreement include the following:

1. Facilitate community college student progression to baccalaureate education and the RN-to-BSN program through consistent program communication, curricular coordination, and focused academic advising.
2. Develop individualized academic plans for community college nursing students that recognize their diverse academic experiences.
3. Increase the number of community college nursing graduates who progress to the RN-to-BSN program and graduate with a baccalaureate degree.

Currently, we have developed 12 formal partnerships with community colleges across Oregon, which are supported by close collaboration between nursing programs. During an annual partnership summit, program leaders and nurse faculty from each of the institutions are invited to share updates from their respective schools. Throughout the year, the team provides community college classroom visits for admissions counseling, transfer planning, and advising sessions that support students in setting goals and making proactive decisions about progression into the baccalaureate program. It has been effective for admissions counselors to make those visits with faculty members who can also share details about the nursing curriculum and current nursing workforce issues.

In 2006, the first of 12 coadmission agreements was signed between Linfield College and Chemeketa Community College (CCC). The agreement created a pathway for successful progression from associate-degree nursing education to baccalaureate education. As of this writing, 18 recent graduates of the CCC nursing program are currently enrolled in at least one course at Linfield College in pursuit of earning a BSN. Furthermore, under the guidelines of the coadmission agreement, an additional 13 CCC students who are enrolled in the associate-degree program are currently coadmitted to Linfield College. The agreement has successfully supported academic progression between the two nursing programs, and it has also made a difference in the local healthcare community by providing access to education for new graduate nurses who seek employment within a large hospital system. As many hospital systems seek Magnet recognition, they are requiring nurses to achieve their BSN prior to employment. The partnership between Linfield and CCC increases

Table 4-5 Strategies Implemented by the Program Director and Online Faculty

Program director	■ Program and team leadership ■ Mandatory online program orientation ■ Community partnership development ■ Outreach, recruitment, and advising of prospective students in the community ■ Advising current and prospective students ■ Collaborative problem-solving ■ Institutional representation and advocacy
Online faculty	■ Career coaching ■ Certification in online teaching ■ Curriculum development ■ Continual online engagement ■ Interpersonal relationships ■ Learning support and access to resources ■ Mentorship ■ Specialization in adult education ■ Success strategies (time management, prioritization, life/work balance) ■ Teaching and learning

opportunities for local nurses to stay in their community and gain employment in Magnet-status hospitals.

See **Table 4-5** for specific strategies implemented by the program director and online faculty to support the successful progression of online nursing students.

Program Evaluation: The Interprofessional Model

Program evaluation is a systematic assessment of all components of an academic program (Ellis, 2016). Online nursing programs use a variety of evaluation data and outcomes to measure quality and effectiveness. Evaluation data of interest to faculty, employers, students, and other stakeholders can result in program improvement (Hamner & Bentley, 2003; Moore, 2005). The Sloan Consortium (Sloan-C) Pillars have set a standard for institution-wide online learning program assessment and evaluation for many years. The Sloan-C challenges institutions to continually evaluate and improve the quality, scale, and breadth of online education, according to their own distinctive missions and the effectiveness of learning in and student and faculty satisfaction with their online programs (Moore & Fetzner, 2019). Sloan-C also encourages programs to share knowledge and best practices to improve the quality of online learning so that it will "become the norm" in higher education (Moore, 2005).

The following sections include examples of evaluation data used to assess the effectiveness of the interprofessional model, including (a) measurements of student persistence; (b) student feedback describing their experiences with academic advising; and (c) input gathered from community college advisors, faculty, and directors related to their satisfaction with services provided by the academic program. Course and faculty evaluation are discussed in Chapter 6.

Measurements of Student Persistence

Online nursing students in our program can begin coursework in the major at three different entry points during the year. They are also permitted to take a semester off during the program if needed as a result of personal circumstances (i.e., work, family, personal) and complete the program at the pace that it works best for them. We have found that providing flexibility in degree planning is the most effective way to support successful academic progression for online students who are in the nursing workforce. For the purposes of measuring student persistence, we assess retention and graduation rates over the time it takes them to complete the BSN degree (**Table 4-6**).

Student Survey: Feedback From Students on Academic Advising

We have used surveys to solicit feedback from online students about their experiences with academic advising. Student feedback obtained through course evaluations and student surveys is a primary source of knowledge used to understand how various elements influence program effectiveness and student success (Ellis, 2016). Professional advising and student-centered support are primary elements of the interprofessional model that is used throughout the online student's academic experience. Academic advising is an integral part of a successful college experience and has been directly linked to higher persistence to graduation (Christian & Sprinkle, 2013; Sanders & Killion, 2017).

Table 4-6 Measurements of Student Persistence

Average persistence rate* for students beginning the first course in the RN-to-BSN major in the fall

2014	2015	2016
Completed BSN in **1** academic year	Completed BSN in **2** academic years	Completed BSN in **3** academic years
89.4%	92.5%	91.6%

Average persistence rate* for students beginning in the first course in the RN-to-BSN major in the spring or summer

86.4%	88.5%	92.2%

*Persistence rate = % of students still enrolled (retained) plus % of students who graduated with a BSN.
Data from Linfield College Fact Book, 2018

In a recent survey conducted to evaluate student experiences with advising in the online RN-to-BSN program, anonymous feedback was obtained from 111 online students. Overall, students indicated satisfaction with (a) the availability of their advisors, (b) individualized degree planning, and (c) a supportive presence provided by their advisor during the program. Additionally, three of the student comments acknowledged the value of strong academic planning early on in the admission process:

> I think the advising team really understands that we working nurses are pulled in many directions and don't have the same time we did in our RN program to follow up with the different aspects of completing on on-line program . . . my advisors [sic] helped me expedite my application and organize financial aid . . . these little things were so helpful in getting me started on the right foot.
>
> It leaves no questions [academic planning] . . . I had a game plan before I started my program.
>
> While I was sure I wanted to pursue an online BSN, Linfield became my first choice because of the ease of the application process . . . no huge database to navigate, accessibility of advisors and academic planners.

The accessibility of the academic advisors emerged as a consistent theme described by students in their feedback. They appreciated that advisors are timely in their communication and provide multiple opportunities for communication, including email, phone calls, and face-to-face appointments:

> My advisor is accessible and responds quickly to my questions. . . . She has kept me informed about what I need to do with regards to registration and my academic plan.
>
> My advisor always answers promptly and is helpful even when I'm asking redundant or stupid questions . . . which happens when I get overwhelmed and tired and can't figure it out on my own.

Students described advising experiences that provided individualized degree planning that made them feel like their education was "personalized" and that they were "actually known and heard" when they interacted with them. One student reflected on the importance of individual preferences in the course-planning process:

> Seeking professional advice, I found more than just advice at the time of need I found an understanding and kind friend! Thank you for helping me to be successful!
>
> I appreciated that there was a plan and an order. I did not have to research which class to take when, and when each were [sic] offered. It was just outlined for me. There was an elective that I just was not excited about. I contacted my advisor, obtained options, and found a class that fit me much better.

Another student shared the unique circumstances of life and work that can create challenges to being successful in a rigorous education program:

> I work [the] full-time night shift and have two young children. Going back to school was extremely intimidating with all I have on my plate. Since day

1 with my advisor [sic] she has helped make this process as easy as possible. She is always available to answer my questions and she sends me emails reminding me about registration . . . I couldn't stay on top of this without her!

Students who responded to the survey also described a supportive advising presence that influenced their success in the program:

Advising is on the *professional* level!

The support! I had some serious life-altering events occur during my schooling at Linfield, and my advisor was phenomenal with helping me through the process! She went out of her way to check on me, to make sure I had everything in line to get an incomplete in the courses, so I could finish my classes at a later time! I couldn't have done it without her help!

I definitely think that the advisors are probably one of the best aspects about Linfield. Especially doing the program online, having someone there for support is comforting.

[One of the best aspects is] the encouragement that the advisor provides to me as a student throughout my RN to BSN education.

Community Partner Survey

An important component of partnership development in the community and continuous quality improvement is to obtain feedback from various external stakeholders about the services provided by the institution and specifically by the online program. Recently, our team conducted a confidential survey to obtain input from advisors, faculty, and directors at our community college partners. A sample of the survey questions is presented in **Table 4-7**. The survey was conducted using a Likert scale with the following options: (a) agree, (b) neutral, (c) disagree, and (d) not applicable. Feedback on the survey indicated that our partners reported a high level of satisfaction with the partnership between institutions, agreed that the responsibilities and purpose of the partnership were well defined, and reported a high level of satisfaction with the services provided to their institution, including students, advisors, and directors.

Outcomes of Program Evaluation

The interprofessional, holistic approach to supporting academic progression has resulted in high rates of student persistence, student satisfaction, and community partner satisfaction. Although our priority is to support students, the collaborative model has also resulted in higher levels of work satisfaction among staff and faculty, which is also valuable. The primary elements of community engagement, relationship building, and student-centeredness provide a foundation for the success of the online program. Our goal is to continue to reevaluate specific strategies to ensure academic success and satisfaction among students, staff, faculty, and our community partners.

A major benefit of program evaluation includes the opportunity to identify priorities for ongoing program development, which for our program include the

Table 4-7 Sample Survey Used to Evaluate Community Partnerships

1. What best describes your role in the partner institution?
   a. Advisor
   b. Faculty
   c. Program director
   d. Other (open-ended)
2. The purposes of the partnership agreement between Linfield College and my institution are well defined.
3. The responsibilities of Linfield College and my institution are well defined.
4. I feel comfortable contacting Linfield College with questions or concerns.
5. When requesting service (i.e., information, support) from Linfield College, I have been satisfied that the service requested is timely and accurate.
6. I am satisfied with the frequency of communication and timing of communication from the Linfield RN-to-BSN program.
7. The following outreach activities provided by Linfield College are effective in serving the needs of students at my institution:
   a. Classroom presentations
   b. Tabling events/information sessions
   c. Promotional materials (i.e., program information sheets)
   d. Linfield college online program web pages
   e. Admissions counseling and advising
8. The Linfield College transfer grid for our institution is an effective tool for student advising.
9. Overall, I believe that our institution is satisfied with our partnership agreement with Linfield College.
10. Overall, I believe that my institution is likely to recommend that other institutions develop partnerships with Linfield College.
11. Please provide any additional feedback that you would like to share. (open-ended)

following: (a) Prioritize student retention and support; (b) develop relevant and engaging curricular opportunities for nursing students of all levels; (c) advocate for institutional policies that support the online, adult student population; (d) identify opportunities to expand partnership development in local, state, and regional communities; (e) examine the potential for new degree programs that will positively affect the healthcare community, including graduate programs; and overall, (f) utilize innovation and collaborative practices that will contribute to more nurses achieving higher levels of education within the state and nationally.

Best-Practice Recommendations for Online Programs

- Address barriers that online nursing students experience in order to proactively plan for student success and degree attainment.
- Use early interactions with online students to begin socializing them to the online community and the institution.

- Work collaboratively with online students to create individualized academic plans that support successful progression.
- Develop formal processes for interprofessional team collaboration that will enhance student, staff, and faculty experiences in online education.
- Create advising structures for students that include professional academic advisors as well as faculty advisors.
- Develop mechanisms for program evaluation that include experiences with the professionals supporting the student's entire experience with the program and institution.
- Use evaluation data to perform continuous program improvement and identify opportunities for program development.

Acknowledgment

The authors would like to recognize the following team members for their contributions in supporting online nursing students and developing the interprofessional model: Jessica Mole, Joanne Swenson, Reese Hiller, and Anna Harrington-Chaudhary.

References

Allen, E. I., & Seaman, J. (2011). *Going the distance: Online education in the United States*. http://www.onlinelearningsurvey.com/reports/goingthedistance.pdf

American Association of Colleges of Nursing. (2014). *Articulation agreements among nursing education programs*. http://www.aacnnursing.org/News-Information/Fact-Sheets/Articulation-Agreements

American Association of Colleges of Nursing. (2017). *Degree completion programs for registered nurses: RN to master's degree and RN to baccalaureate programs*. https://www.aacnnursing.org/News-Information/Fact-Sheets/Degree-Completion-Programs

Arizona State University & the Boston Consulting Group. (2018). *Making digital learning work: Success strategies from six leading universities and community colleges*. https://edplus.asu.edu/sites/default/files/BCG-Making-Digital-Learning-Work-Apr-2018%20.pdf

Baldwin, R. G., & Chang, D. A. (2007). Collaborating to learn, learning to collaborate. *Association of American Colleges & Universities, 9*(4). https://www.aacu.org/publications-research/periodicals/collaborating-learn-learning-collaborate

Bawa, P. (2016). Retention in online courses: Exploring issues and solutions—A literature review. *SAGE Open*, 1–11. http://doi.org/10.1177/2158244015621777

Buerhaus, P. I., Staiger, D. O., & Auerbach, D. I. (2008). *The future of the nursing workforce in the United States: Data, trends, and implications*. Jones & Bartlett.

Candela, L. (2016). Theoretical foundations of teaching and learning. In D. Billings & J. Halstead (Eds.), *Teaching in nursing: A guide for faculty* (pp. 211–229). Saunders.

Christian, T. Y., & Sprinkle, J. E. (2013). College student perceptions and ideals of advising: An exploratory analysis. *College Student Journal, 47*, 271–291.https://eric.ed.gov/?id=EJ1022274

Duffy, M. T., Friesen, M. A., Speroni, K. G., Swengros, D., Shanks, L. A., Waiter, P. A., & Sheridan, M. J. (2014). BSN completion: Barriers, challenges, incentives, and strategies. *The Journal of Nursing Administration, 44*(4), 232–236. http://doi.org/10.1097/NNA.0000000000000054

Ellis, P. (2016). Systematic program evaluation. In D. Billings & J. Halstead (Eds.), *Teaching in nursing: A guide for faculty* (pp. 463–507). Saunders.

Hamner, J. B., & Bentley, R.W. (2003). A systematic evaluation plan that works. *Nurse Educator, 28*(4), 179–184. https://journals.lww.com/nurseeducatoronline/Abstract/2003/07000/A_Systematic_Evaluation_Plan_That_Works.9.aspx

Hardin, C. J. (2008). Adult students in higher education: A portrait of transitions. *New Directions for Adult and Continuing Education, 144*, 49–57. https://eric.ed.gov/?id=EJ824818

Harrison, E. (2009). What constitutes good academic advising? Nursing students' perceptions of academic advising. *Journal of Nursing Education, 48*, 361–366. https//doi.org/10.3928/0148 4834-20090615-02

Hodges, B., & Selena-Salis, A. (2016). Building connections: A prototype template for 2-year to 4-year program articulation agreements in public health education. *Pedagogy in Health Promotion: The Scholarship of Teaching and Learning, 2*(1), 48–53.

Linfield College. (2018). *Fact book.* https://www.linfield.edu/research/fact-book-online.html

McClenney, K. M., & Waiwaiole, E. N. (2005). Focus on student retention: Promising practices in community colleges. *Community College Journal, 75*(6), 36–41. https://eric.ed.gov/?id=EJ873952

Megginson, L. A. (2008). RN-BSN education: 21st century barriers and incentives. *Journal of Nursing Management, 16*, 47–55. http://doi.org/10.1111/ j.1365-2934.2007.00784.x

Moore, J. (2005). The Sloan Consortium quality framework and the five pillars. http://www.mit.jyu .fi/ope/kurssit/TIES462/Materiaalit/Sloan.pdf

Moore, J., & Fetzner, M. (2019). The road to retention: A closer look at institutions that achieve high course completion rates. *Online Learning, 13*(3). http://dx.doi.org/10.24059/olj.v13i3.1650

National Academy of Medicine. (2011). *The future of nursing: Leading change, advancing health.* https://www.nap.edu/download/12956

National Center for Education Statistics. (2019). *Home page.* https://nces.ed.gov/

Nininger, J. M., Abbott, M. R., & Shaw, P. (2019). Eradicating barriers to advancement from RN to BSN: An exploratory study. *The Journal of Continuing Education in Nursing, 50*(1), 15–19.

Noel-Levitz. (2011). *2011 marketing and student recruitment practices at four-year and two-year institutions.* https://www.noellevitz.com/documents/shared/Papers_and_Research/2011/2011 MARKETINGANDRECRUITMENTPRACTICES.pdf

Robinson, M., Mole, J., Hiller, R., Swenson, J., & Harrington, A. (2018). Holistic academic progression for nurses: An interprofessional model. *Journal of Community & Public Health Nursing, 4*, 211. http://doi.org/10.4172/2471-9846.1000211

Sanders, M., & Killion, J. (2017). Advising in higher education. *Radiologic Science, 22*(1), 15–21.

Sarver, W., Cichra, N., & Kline, M. (2015). Perceived benefits, motivators, and barriers to advancing nursing education: Removing barriers to improve success. *Nurse Education Perspectives, 36*, 153–156. http://doi.org/10.5480/14-1407

Smith, B. (2010). *E-learning technologies: A comparative study of adult learners enrolled on blended and online campuses engaging in a virtual classroom* (Doctoral dissertation). Retrieved from ProQuest Dissertations.

Stanford-Bowers, D. E. (2008). Persistence in online classes: A study of perception among community college stakeholders. *MERLOT Journal of Online Learning and Teaching, 4*, 37–50. https://www.scirp.org/reference/ReferencesPapers.aspx?ReferenceID=1296237

Warshawsky, N. E., Brandford, A., Barnum, N., & Westneat, S. (2015). Achieving 80% BSN by 2020: Lessons learned from Kentucky's registered nurses. *Journal of Nursing Administration, 45*, 449–456. http://doi.org/10.5480/14-1407

Willging, P. A., & Johnson, S. D. (2009). Factors that influence students' decision to drop out of online courses. *Journal of Asynchronous Learning Networks, 13*(3), 115–127. https://eric.ed.gov /?id=EJ862360

Wros, P., Wheeler, P., & Jones, M. (2014). Curriculum planning for baccalaureate nursing programs. In S. Keating (Ed.), *Curriculum development and evaluation in nursing* (3rd ed., pp. 245–284). Springer.

Wyatt, L. G. (2011). Nontraditional student engagement: Increasing adult student success and retention. *Journal of Continuing Higher Education, 59*(1), 10–20. https://eric.ed.gov/?id=EJ915953

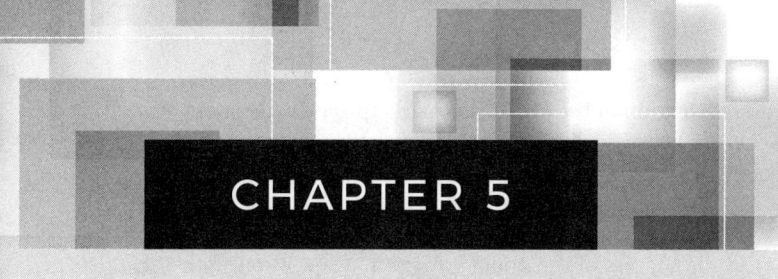

CHAPTER 5

Leadership of Online Nursing Programs

Melissa Robinson and Henny Breen

"The key to successful leadership today is influence, not authority."

Ken Blanchard

Overview

The purpose of this chapter is to discuss leadership of online nursing programs. Dedicated program leadership that includes formal and informal roles within the institution is described. Leadership development that emphasizes collaboration and systems thinking is presented as an opportunity to address challenges with acceptance of online education and contribute to institutional governance structures.

Background

Dedicated leadership for online nursing programs within higher education is critical to ensure quality online program learning outcomes and provide day-to-day operational support. Online faculty members may serve in leadership roles that include part-time administrative appointments or assigned workloads; coordinators, directors, or program leads; or full-time administrative positions dedicated to providing leadership for online programs. It has been our experience that having faculty appointed for various leadership roles within the online program has been effective, including the roles of program coordinator, service-learning coordinator, and course lead, which we discuss in this chapter.

In addition to program leadership, successful online education programs require institutional commitment. Dr. Gloria Pickar, the president of Compass Knowledge Group, has consulted with several institutions as they prepared to launch new online programs. She recommended that administrators focus on three major areas: marketplace, curriculum and instruction, and infrastructure (Hill, 2009).

Dr. Pickar described evaluation of the audience (marketplace) as the most important step in the assessment process, which includes developing an audience profile and gauging the potential for growth (Hill, 2009). In addition to considering an external audience that includes online students and our academic and practice partners, we have recognized the importance of working closely with internal audiences that have a part to play in the success of the online program. A few of our internal audiences include the administration, our faculty colleagues outside of the online nursing program, and the marketing department. As administrators consider curriculum and instruction, they are encouraged to align the online program to effectively target the needs of working, professional adults (Hill, 2009). Adult online students require flexible admission requirements, relevant online learning experiences, and qualified online faculty to be successful with online learning. Lastly, successful online programs require a supportive infrastructure. A few of those structures include high-quality recruitment and admission processes, accessible technology support, advising and retention support, small class sizes of 15–25 students, and program orientation (Hill, 2009; Nilson & Goodson, 2018).

Acceptance of Online Education

The acceptance of online education is a primary consideration for all program leaders and particularly for those in traditional liberal arts institutions like ours. Online education is most successful when institutions consider online education as "education" rather than "online education" (Foley, 2020). Online programs should be considered as different from traditional programs when it comes to the audience and the goals to deliver education that is relevant, efficient, and accessible in an online format. At the same time, online programs should be considered the same as traditional programs when it comes to educational standards and the support and integration of students within the institution. Unfortunately, many institutions still view online learners as distinct and separate from students attending traditional and residential programs (Lederman, 2009). The reality is that online education has been around for over 20 years, and the majority of students now expect that online learning will be a part of their higher education experience. Some students, such as nurses seeking postlicensure nursing degrees, would be excluded from advancing their education without online programs, based on geographical barriers and work commitments in their communities. Therefore, it is important for program leaders to be aware of the barriers to acceptance of online education within their institutions.

A 2019 survey of faculty attitudes on technology conducted by Gallup and Inside Higher Ed reported that faculty members remain skeptical of online education, but their opinions are becoming less negative (Jaschick & Lederman, 2020). The survey also found the following (Jaschick & Lederman, 2020):

- Of faculty members, 46% reported teaching an online course for credit, up from 39% in 2016 and 30% in 2013.
- Online teaching is still new to faculty: 41% have taught online courses for less than 5 years, and only 25% have taught online courses for more than 10 years.
- More than three-quarters of faculty reported that teaching online has improved their teaching, including helping them think more critically about engaging students in course content and using multimedia more effectively.

- Of faculty members, 39% fully support increased use of educational technologies, up from 32% in 2018 and 29% in 2017.
- Of faculty members, 60% believe academic fraud is more common in online courses than in face-to-face courses, whereas the rest believe fraud occurs equally in both settings.

While the number of distance programs and online courses continues to grow, chief academic officers don't believe the acceptance of the online learning modality has improved. In fact, in the most recent survey of online education conducted by the Babson Survey Research Group, "Online Report Card–Tracking Online Education in the United States," only 29.1% of chief academic officers believed their faculty accept the value and legitimacy of online education, which was lower than the percentage previously reported in 2004 (Allen & Seaman, 2016). Their perception was that faculty believed that the learning outcomes for online education were inferior to the learning outcomes in face-to-face education.

In a synthesis of 68 empirical studies published between 1995 and 2015 about online teaching, faculty reported concerns about perceived barriers to student success in online classes, their ability to use the technology required in online teaching, and the quality and integrity of the online classroom (Wingo, Ivankova, & Moss, 2017). Additionally, faculty expressed concerns about how online teaching would be evaluated, particularly in the tenure and promotion process, and how it would affect their image and reputation within the institution (Wingo et al., 2017). In the following sections, we discuss the strategies we have used to enhance the legitimacy of the online nursing program within the institution while providing day-to-day operational support for the program.

Dedicated Program Leadership

We have found that the online program is most successful when it is supported by informal leaders who consistently advocate for the program across the institution, in addition to the formal leaders with assigned roles and responsibilities. In our program, formal leadership roles include a program coordinator, a service-learning coordinator, and a course lead assigned to every online course. Each of the roles has been filled by faculty members who have workloads assigned to teaching in the online program.

Collaborative Leadership Model

The qualifications and leadership skills of program leaders are critical to program effectiveness (Ellis, 2016). Because of the nature of the nursing profession, nurse leaders are particularly skilled at taking on a number of roles within the institution. At any given time, they may be functioning as educators, clinicians, researchers, and administrators. Strong interpersonal skills, mutually respectful communication, and collaboration within an interprofessional environment are foundations of nursing practice (American Association of Colleges of Nursing, 2008). Nurses are experienced at influencing change, serving as diplomats and integrators, bringing out the best attributes in individuals and groups, and developing teams (Grossman & Valiga, 2017). We have recognized that a couple of leadership attributes have been particularly effective in the leadership of the online nursing program: systems thinking and collaboration.

Systems thinking is a cohesive approach to leadership that views all key processes as parts of an overall system, rather than in isolation (Furst-Bowe, 2012). Because governance models in higher education often involve faculty, staff, and students having a voice in decision making, we have been strategic in our efforts to participate actively in the governance structure so that the online program is represented. One of the challenges within higher education is not only navigating the ongoing external forces, such as the increasing competition of online nursing programs and diminishing financial resources, but also the internal forces discussed previously regarding the acceptance of online education. A systems perspective has allowed us to recognize that any change to one aspect of the institution will have an impact on many other areas of the institution (Furst-Bowe, 2012). In that way, we can provide advocacy for the online program while gaining perspectives on the needs and challenges for other parts of the institution. When faculty leaders can collaborate with internal partners at all levels of the institution, they share accountability for the strategic growth and success of the institution while simultaneously considering the needs of the institution and the program they represent (Cowen, 2018).

Representing the online program within the governance structures of the institution is critical to the overall delivery and success of the program. It is also a way for faculty members to improve the visibility and credibility of the online program in an effort to improve the acceptance of online education within the institution. It has been our goal to contribute to the governance structures in ways that do not slow down decision making, which can be an outcome of some governance structures, but instead contribute to leadership that is inclusive and nimble and therefore results in timely quality improvements for students and the institution (Cowen, 2018). The faculty leaders in our online program serve on a variety of standing committees and work groups within the school of nursing and institution. A few examples of participation in governance structures include serving as members of committees involved in strategic enrollment planning, budget planning, curriculum, promotion and tenure, faculty senate or executive committee, evaluation or quality assurance, and accreditation.

The outcomes of the online program have improved through the consistent commitment of faculty leaders to engaging in the collaborative model within the online program and across the institution. Faculty leaders should be well versed in the leadership literature to develop as systems thinkers and collaborative team members. We have been intentional in our efforts to develop our leadership abilities, both as individuals and as a team. Some of the resources that we have utilized to develop our qualifications in leadership are included in **Table 5-1**. In the sections that follow, we share a description of the formal leadership roles held by faculty to ensure effective delivery of the online nursing program.

Coordinator of Online Programs

In an effort to ensure that the online program is integrated within the institution and to provide operational support for the online program, administrators may choose to appoint a faculty leader (director, associate dean) from the online program or create an administrative position for leadership of the online program. Although our online program is highly collaborative, we have also found that having formal

Table 5-1 Leadership Development Resources

Book/Resource	Author(s)
The Growth and Development of Nurse Leaders	Angela Barron McBride
Reframing Academic Leadership	Lee G. Bowman and Joan V. Gallos
Servant Leadership Roadmap: Master the 12 Core Competencies of Management Success With Leadership Qualities and Interpersonal Skills	Cara Bramlett
Daring Greatly: How the Courage to Be Vulnerable Transforms the Way We Live, Love, Parent, and Lead	Brené Brown
Quiet: The Power of Introverts in a World That Can't Stop Talking	Susan Cain
Pure Heart Leadership: An Authentic Approach to Leadership	Shana Garrett
The Tipping Point: How Little Things Can Make a Big Difference	Malcolm Gladwell
The New Leadership Challenge: Creating the Future of Nursing	Sheila Grossman and Theresa M. Valiga
Servant Leadership: A Journey Into the Nature of Legitimate Power and Greatness	Robert K. Greenleaf
Consensus-Oriented Decision Making: The CODM Model for Facilitating Groups to Widespread Agreement	Tim Hartnett
The Truth About Leadership: No Fads, Heart-of-the-Matter Facts You Need to Know	James M. Kouzes and Barry Z. Posner
Our Iceberg Is Melting: Changing and Succeeding Under Any Conditions	John Kotter and Holger Rathgeber
Leaders Eat Last: Why Some Teams Pull Together and Others Don't	Simon Sinek
Multipliers: How the Best Leaders Make Everyone Smarter	Liz Wiseman

The CliftonStrengths Assessment Tool (Gallup, 2020)
https://www.gallup.com/cliftonstrengths/en/strengthsfinder.aspx

The Leadership Framework Self-Assessment Tool (NHS Leadership Academy, 2012).
https://www.leadershipacademy.nhs.uk/wp-content/uploads/2012/11/NHSLeadership
-Framework-LeadershipFrameworkSelfAssessmentTool.pdf

structures identified for leadership has been effective in ensuring quality experiences for students, staff, and faculty.

The coordinator of the online program works collaboratively with the faculty to provide oversight of the curriculum and with the interprofessional team for day-to-day delivery of the program. The roles and functions of the interprofessional team members are discussed in Chapter 4. The coordinator functions as an advocate for the online program within the institution and represents the program in the community by supporting recruitment efforts, building relationships with academic and practice partners in the community, and representing the institution at various outreach events and conferences. The coordinator also works with online faculty to develop policies and procedures that enhance the quality and delivery of the online program, which is discussed in Chapter 6. A description of the role of the coordinator of the online nursing program is included in **Table 5-2**.

Table 5-2 **Role Description: Coordinator of Online Nursing Programs**

The role of the online program coordinator (director, associate dean) works closely with the online program team and the dean of nursing to provide curricular oversight, faculty support, and day-to-day operational support for the online program.

Responsibilities:

- Interviews potential adjunct faculty and makes recommendations to the dean of nursing related to qualifications and appropriateness for teaching in online programs
- Facilitates orientation and mentorship assignments for new faculty teaching in the program
- Collaborates with faculty on curriculum development, program evaluation, and student issues
- Evaluates online teaching and makes recommendations about future teaching assignments
- Assesses and makes recommendations for faculty development and teaching qualifications for the online program
- Schedules online courses based on program enrollment, anticipated needs, and strategic plan
- Reviews and approves syllabi for online nursing courses
- Reviews and approves all textbook selections for the online program
- Collaborates with the admissions department on issues affecting recruitment and admission
- Collaborates with the registrar on issues affecting transfer courses and admission/graduation requirements
- Collaborates with the online academic advisors to support students, solve problems, and implement retention strategies
- Serves as faculty advisor to online students
- Develops and ensures delivery of the online program orientation
- Facilitates team meetings to support program functions and group processes
- Collaborates with the service-learning coordinator to support experiential learning objectives
- Represents the online program in the school of nursing and institutional governance structures

Service-Learning Coordinator

One of the key elements of the Commission on Collegiate Nursing Education (CCNE) Standards for Accreditation of Baccalaureate and Graduate Nursing Programs (2018) requires that all students are afforded the opportunity to develop professional competencies in practice settings, including students in distance-education programs. Key element III-H of the accreditation standards requires planned clinical practice experiences that (a) enable students to integrate new knowledge and demonstrate attainment of program outcomes, (b) engage in interprofessional collaborative practice experiences, and (c) benefit from opportunities to be evaluated by faculty (CCNE, 2018). Experiential learning in our online program includes direct and indirect practice experiences that have been developed for online nursing students, as discussed in Chapter 11. Some of the experiences are virtual, and others take place in the community throughout the program, including a service-learning practice experience in the final capstone course.

To provide oversight of the service-learning program and ensure that online students have opportunities to meet the professional competencies of the degree program, we have developed the service-learning coordinator role. The faculty member serving in the role of service-learning coordinator works collaboratively with the program coordinator and other online faculty members to develop meaningful practice experiences for online students. The service-learning coordinator also works collaboratively with internal stakeholders, including the service-learning and international program offices within the institution, and with external stakeholders, including the local and international community organizations that serve as academic practice partners. The service-learning coordinator serves as the course lead for the experiential learning course, mentors full-time and adjunct faculty to support their work with students and community partners, and ensures that all experiential learning activities include specific objectives that align with course and program outcomes, as well as assessment and evaluation conducted by faculty. **Table 5-3** includes a description of the role of the service-learning coordinator in the online program.

Course Lead

The course lead in the online program is responsible for the design, development, and delivery of the online course and for ensuring that the faculty members who teach in the course are prepared and mentored throughout the course. The course lead is a full-time faculty member with leadership experience as well as experience and certification in online teaching. In addition to preparing each section of the course and mentoring faculty, the course lead serves an important role related to problem solving of student challenges as they arise and working collaboratively with the online team to support student retention. The course lead is responsible for providing faculty appraisals of online teaching and evaluating each course. As a result of collaboration across the curriculum, the course-lead model has provided a great deal of consistency and satisfaction among students and faculty. The responsibilities and qualifications of the course lead are included in **Table 5-4**.

Table 5-3 Role Description: Service-Learning Coordinator

The service-learning coordinator coordinates the service-learning program for all students, including those serving in international communities. It is recommended that the service-learning coordinator serves as the course lead for the experiential learning course.

Responsibilities:

Community Service Learning:

- Coordinates community service-learning program
- Provides up-to-date information about service learning to be included in the online program orientation
- Facilitates planning discussions in the semester prior to service-learning experience
- Supports students between semesters as needed to coordinate service-learning experiences
- Mentors online program faculty in the service-learning experience and expectations for student learning in the local community or in the international community
- Updates service-learning documentation as needed in consultation with the program coordinator and/or International Programs Office staff
- Provides annual service-learning reports as needed

International Service Learning:

- Coordinates the international service-learning program
- Maintains the service-learning web page that provides information for international service-learning opportunities
- Addresses student questions about international service opportunities
- Coordinates relationships with external international programs to develop a variety of service options for students to choose from, to ensure expectations of the international program are met, and to ensure the international experiences meet student learning needs
- Facilitates compliance with International Program Office procedures (e.g., insurance, documentation)
- Consults with International Program Office regarding international travel and safety
- Processes and approves applications from students who wish to participate in the international service-learning experiences, with input from the online program team
- Advises students regarding the application process and next steps as they prepare to travel
- Facilitates course scheduling to ensure for effective student participation or online course release while they are out of the country

Qualifications:

1. Master's degree in nursing required; doctoral degree in nursing or related field preferred.
2. Experience and certification in online teaching, as approved by the dean of nursing or designee.
3. Full-time faculty role with workload assigned to the online nursing program.
4. Course lead for the experiential course preferred.
5. Experience in coordinating service learning preferred.

Table 5-4 Course Lead in the Online Program: Responsibilities and Qualifications

Responsibilities:

1. Provides leadership in coordinating the content of the assigned online course with faculty teaching additional sections of the course
2. Provides orientation and mentorship to faculty on course content, learning activities, best practices for online teaching, and student success factors
3. Develops the course using best practices for online education and the achievement of course outcomes
4. Submits course syllabus and textbook orders according to established deadlines
5. Oversees implementation of course outcomes by all faculty members teaching in the course through frequent and clear communication
6. Collaborates with the program coordinator to identify qualified adjunct faculty members to teach the course
7. Collaborates with the program coordinator to perform annual peer appraisal of online teaching of adjunct faculty members teaching the course

Qualifications:

1. Master's degree in nursing required; doctoral degree in nursing or related field preferred
2. Experience and certification in online teaching, as approved by the dean of nursing or designee
3. Full-time faculty role with workload assigned to the online nursing program
4. Expertise in assigned course content

Summary

Institutional commitment and dedicated leadership are essential to ensure the effectiveness of online nursing programs. Online nursing faculty members are well prepared to serve in leadership roles that support the day-to-day operations of online programs. They are also uniquely qualified to influence challenges with the acceptance of online education and contribute in multiple areas of leadership within the governance model for the institution.

Best-Practice Recommendations for Online Programs

- Develop formal leadership roles for online programs that include well-defined responsibilities.
- Create opportunities for online faculty members to develop leadership qualifications and effectiveness.
- Participate in the governance structures of the institution to represent the online program through advocacy, collaboration, and decision making.

References

Allen, I. E., & Seaman, J. (2016). *Online report card: Tracking online education in the United States.* Babson Research Group.

American Association of Colleges of Nursing. (2008). *The essentials of baccalaureate education for professional nursing practice.* https://www.aacnnursing.org/portals/42/publications/baccessentials 08.pdf

Commission on Collegiate Nursing Education. (2018). *Standards for accreditation of baccalaureate and graduate nursing programs.* https://www.aacnnursing.org/Portals/42/CCNE/PDF/Standards -Final-2018.pdf

Cowen, S. S. (2018). Shared governance does not mean shared decision making. *The Chronicle of Higher Education.* https://www.chronicle.com/article/Shared-Governance-Does-Not/244257

Ellis, P. (2016). Systematic program evaluation. In D. Billings & J. Halstead (Eds.), *Teaching in nursing: A guide for faculty* (pp. 463–507). Saunders.

Foley, C. (2020). *From the desk: Director says online education is a university's "heart and lungs."* https:// news.iu.edu/stories/2020/02/iu/inside/19-from-the-desk-director-says-online-education-is -universitys-heart-and-lungs.html

Furst-Bowe, J. (2012). Systems thinking: Critical to quality improvement in higher education. *Quality Approaches to Higher Education, 2*(2), 2–4. http://asq.org/edu/2011/12/best-practices /systems-thinking-critical-to-quality-improvement-in-higher-education.pdf

Gallup. (2020). *The CliftonStrengths Assessment Tool.* https://www.gallup.com/cliftonstrengths/en /strengthsfinder.aspx

Grossman, S., & Valiga, T. M. (2017). *The new leadership challenge: Creating the future of nursing.* F. A. Davis.

Hill, C. (2009). *Seeing where the distance education opportunities lie.* https://www.facultyfocus.com /free-reports/distance-learning-administration-and-policy-strategies-for-achieving-excellence/

Jaschick, S., & Lederman, D. (2020). *2019 survey of faculty attitudes on technology: A study by Inside Higher Ed and Gallup.* https://www.insidehighered.com/booklet/2019-survey-faculty-attitudes -technology

Lederman, D. (2019). *Professors' slow, steady acceptance of online learning: A survey.* https://www .insidehighered.com/news/survey/professors-slow-steady-acceptance-online-learning-survey

NHS Leadership Academy. (2012). *The Leadership Framework Self-Assessment Tool.* https://www .leadershipacademy.nhs.uk/wp-content/uploads/2012/11/NHSLeadership-Framework-Leadership FrameworkSelfAssessmentTool.pdf

Nilson, L. B., & Goodson, L. A. (2018). *Online teaching at its best: Merging instructional design with teaching and learning research.* Jossey-Bass.

Wingo, N. P., Ivankova, N. V., & Moss, J. A. (2017). Faculty perceptions about teaching online: Exploring the literature using the technology acceptance model as an organizing framework. *Online Learning, 21*(1), 15–35. http://doi.org/10.10.24059/olj.v21i1.761

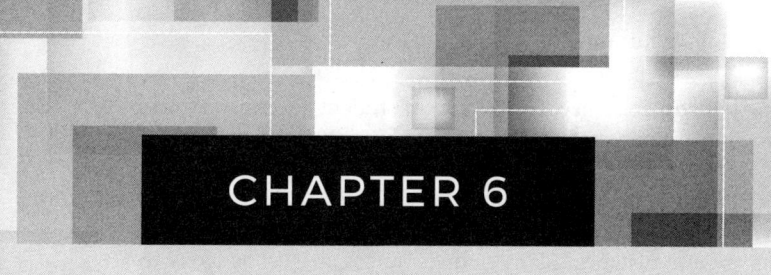

CHAPTER 6

Quality Assurance in Online Nursing Programs

Melissa Robinson and Henny Breen

"Learning is not attained by chance, it must be sought for with ardor and diligence."

Abigail Adams

Overview

While distance education has expanded rapidly to provide nurses with access to advanced degrees through diverse degree programs, faculty members have been challenged to create policies and procedures that support the quality assurance that is needed to advance online education. Additionally, academic administrators and faculty colleagues of nursing want assurance that online degree programs are meeting high expectations for student learning and outcomes. The purpose of this chapter is to share our approach to integrating quality assurance into online nursing programs through policy development and the use of standards for online teaching.

Background

Quality assurance and monitoring are essential in nursing education, and online education is no exception. Ongoing attention to quality assurance can lead to decision making that is supported by evidence and ensures that regulatory and accreditation standards for online nursing education are met. As online education started to rise in popularity, early studies focused on student satisfaction, the convenience of online education, the potential for isolation among faculty and students, challenges with technology, and student-support issues to determine the evidence of quality (Billings, 2007). As technology and understanding of student and faculty experiences in online education improved, research and evaluation studies shifted to better understanding the strategies needed to support student success and best practices in online education (Billings, Dickerson, Greenburg, Yow-Wu, & Talley, 2013).

Further, it is important to note that although we use the terms *distance education* and *online education* interchangeably, there is a difference in terms of geography. Not all online students are at a distance. Many online courses are just as likely to attract students living on campus as those who live at a distance (McAfooes, 2020). This is consistent with our experience and can be a source of contention within the institution if enrollment declines in face-to-face classes.

Currently, what constitutes quality in online education offers some variation but also provides some distinct guidance for administration, faculty, and instructional design professionals. Some of the most consistent quality indicators reported in the literature are (1) student satisfaction, (2) online student retention, (3) high-quality course design, and (4) good teaching. Consistent with our experience teaching in an online nursing program that is part of a traditional liberal arts college, doubts remain regarding the quality of online courses, despite the continued growth of online education and evidence to the contrary (Allen & Seaman, 2016).

To address the importance of high-quality learning for online students and to provide assurance to our administrators, faculty colleagues, and other stakeholders, we have developed a set of policies, procedures, and other quality measures to ensure the online program is meeting high expectations for student learning and outcomes. In the following sections, we share some of the ways that we approach quality assurance from an institutional, program, and faculty perspective.

Institutional Support for Quality Online Education

Institutional support is essential for the delivery of quality online education. We know that students can learn as much or more from online courses as from traditional ones (Nilson & Goodson, 2018; Swan, 2019; U.S. Department of Education, 2010). Therefore, institutional leaders can feel confident investing in online education programs and supporting online education with human, fiscal, and physical resources. When they do make the investment, it is important to connect online education to the mission, priorities, and strategic plan of the institution (Chaloux & Miller, 2019; McAfooes, 2020).

If online programs are being added or if the growth of online programs is part of the strategic plan, administrative restructuring may be needed to integrate online programs within the traditional structure. The delivery of high-quality online programs includes structures designed to recruit and retain students; supporting and developing online faculty; providing technological tools; and dedicated support from instructional designers, student support services, academic advisors, distance librarians, and other support staff and learning resources. The administration must also consider the need for faculty to have development in best practices for online education (Manz Friesth, 2020).

High-quality online programs and diverse online course offerings can strengthen the reputation of the institution, which can also lead to positive enrollment and revenue outcomes (Nilson & Goodson, 2018). On the other hand, poor online learning experiences can leave students feeling disengaged and closed off to future learning and directly affect student attrition (Alexiou-Ray & Bentley, 2015;

Ragan & Schroeder, 2019). An institutional commitment to an ongoing evaluation of program outcomes can result in program improvements.

Quality in Online Programs

Our approach to ensuring quality in online education starts with the principles of good teaching. We believe that the primary difference in online teaching versus traditional face-to-face classroom teaching is the modality of where the process of teaching and learning occurs, and the expectations for high-quality teaching and learning should be consistent. The *Seven Principles for Good Practice in Undergraduate Education*, first published by Chickering and Gamson in 1987, have endured in higher education across the United States and Canada. Designed to maximize student learning, the principles have direct application to the online classroom (**Table 6-1**).

The principles shown in Table 6-1 evolved over time as a result of technology being recognized as a resource for learning and integrated into higher education (Chickering & Ehrmann, 1996). Further, problem-based learning, engagement in real-world problems, and active learning were recognized as strong elements of quality teaching (Merrill, 2001), and the importance of respect for diverse talent and ways of learning was acknowledged (Graham, Caglitay, Lim, Craner, & Duffy, 2001). As the role of faculty development and professional instructional design in online education was becoming increasingly important, Puzziferro and Shelton (2009) revisited and affirmed the basic principles of good practice in teaching. It was their assessment that the landscape of higher education was constantly evolving, along with our values. Thus, learning was no longer a product to be delivered but, rather, one that is experienced by the learner (Puzziferro & Shelton, 2009).

To ensure quality based on the evidence of the need to develop consistent online course design, the Quality Matters Rubric was used as a resource. The Quality Matters (QM) Rubric has been used by many institutions to build quality online courses into their online education programs. The QM Rubric is part of a national subscription-based program that involves professional training and support for individual subscribers and institutional subscribers (Quality Matters, 2020). The QM organization offers professional development to train faculty and peer reviewers to focus on course design, implement course improvement, and achieve certification for online courses. The QM Rubric is evidence based,

---

Table 6-1 Seven Principles of Good Practice in Undergraduate Education

1. Good practice encourages student–faculty contact.
2. Good practice encourages cooperation among students.
3. Good practice encourages active learning.
4. Good practice gives prompt feedback.
5. Good practice emphasizes time on task.
6. Good practice communicates high expectations.
7. Good practice respects diverse talents and ways of learning.

Chickering, A. W., & Gamson, Z. F. (1987). Seven principles for good practice in undergraduate education. *AAHE Bulletin*, 3–7.

frequently linked to quality in higher education literature, and intended to encourage consistency in online course design, and it encourages conversations among colleagues about quality within institutions and across disciplines (Baldwin, Ching, & Hsu, 2018).

Six national and statewide evaluation instruments for online course design in higher education, including the QM Rubric, were reviewed by Baldwin et al. (2018), who prioritized a list of 12 criteria including items such as ensuring learning objectives are available and course activities are used to build community. They were found in all evaluation instruments that build quality into consistent online course design. These criteria for quality are consistent with our approach. The only difference is that we look for learning outcomes for each course and learning objectives for each module within the online course. We would also add that student-to-content and student-to-instructor interactions are supported not only by providing contact information but also in terms of timely responses to student communications.

Assessment and Evaluation of Online Learning

Faculty and administrators need to consider how to regularly use assessment tools to evaluate learning effectiveness and student satisfaction with their experience to ensure continuous quality improvement (McAfooes, 2020). Administrators should ensure that the online programs are integrated into the overall institutional evaluation plan. The specific purposes of program evaluation may include the following: (1) how various elements of the program interact and influence program effectiveness; (2) the extent to which the mission, goals, and outcomes of the program are met; (3) a rationale for decision making that leads to quality improvements; and (4) an ability to identify what resources can be used to improve the program's quality and effectiveness (Ellis, 2016).

A continual program evaluation plan can also ensure that the institution is meeting the standards of accrediting bodies, including state boards of nursing, professional nursing accreditation, and regional accrediting bodies. Institutions use a variety of tools for assessment and program evaluation, including course and program evaluations, student satisfaction surveys, community partnership surveys or focus groups designed to evaluate services and programs, metrics documenting student success, external program review, and more. A few examples of program evaluation used by our institution include course evaluations, student persistence rates, and an academic program review.

Course Evaluation

One element of program evaluation is integrating course evaluations into every online course in order to obtain input from students about their experience. **Table 6-2** provides a sample of a standard course evaluation given at the end of every online course. Students are given a Likert scale for their responses: strongly agree, agree, neutral, disagree, and strongly disagree. They also have a chance to provide narrative comments at multiple phases of the evaluation.

Table 6-2 Sample Course Evaluation

1. Provides a coherent syllabus that makes course learning outcomes clear
2. Holds class regularly and punctually
3. Organizes class sessions effectively
4. Makes clear the relationship between course activities and the goals of the course
5. Encourages students to make connections across classes, subjects, or disciplines
6. Holds students to high expectations
7. Effectively integrates course resources into class (course resources might include textbooks, articles, videos, online activities, simulations, etc.)
8. Demonstrates enthusiasm for the subject matter
9. Explains course material clearly
10. Encourages student questions and viewpoints
11. Facilitates active learning (might include small-group activities, discussions, demonstrations, simulations, presentations)
12. Gives assignments with clear instructions and expectations
13. Grades students according to established criteria
14. Regularly provides graded assignments to assess student progress
15. Returns graded work within a reasonable time
16. Provides instructive feedback on assigned work
17. Is available to students outside class (might include office hours, appointments, emails, etc.)
18. Encourages students to seek help when needed
19. Overall, the instructor taught the class well
20. Overall, the course was a valuable learning experience

As online faculty, we have made a strong commitment to ongoing course improvement based on the input we receive from students each semester. We use announcements to provide encouragement to students to complete evaluations, assuring them that their input is confidential, valued by their faculty, and used to make ongoing course improvements. Because students are the primary stakeholders in the learning experience, we acknowledge that the more students can be empowered to be involved in the evaluation process, the more meaningful and useful the results will be (Wandersman et al., 2012).

Student Persistence Rates

Student persistence with online learning, which was discussed in more detail in Chapter 4, is an important element of our evaluation plan for student success in the online nursing program. Factors associated with student persistence in an online program include satisfaction with online learning, a sense of belonging to the learning community, motivation, peer and family support, time management skills, and increased communication with the instructor (Hart, 2012). If support factors are not present in sufficient quantity, the student may be at risk of course failure or withdrawing from an online course or the entire program. A review of the existing literature indicates that up to 40% to 80% of college students drop out of online classes (Bawa, 2016). The interprofessional model, also presented in Chapter 4, represents another approach to quality assurance that has been effective in our online program.

Academic Program Review

Conducting an academic program review is a valuable way to introduce quality control to online programs by gaining important perspectives from an expert in the field who is external to the institution (Dunn & Halonen, 2017). Prior to the restructuring of the online program within our institution, the administration hired a consultant to perform a comprehensive review of the online program. The review included an assessment of the institutional infrastructure, including enrollment services, academic advising, distance library and information technology (IT) support, student support services, and instructional design support. The consultant also assessed curricular issues and evaluated program outcomes. Overall, it was a helpful way to identify next steps and perform strategic goal setting related to the online programs.

Quality Assurance Specific to the Online Nursing Program

Online programs require dedicated leadership to ensure adequate representation within the institution as well as day-to-day operational support for online program delivery. The leadership of online nursing programs is discussed in Chapter 5. In the following sections, we provide some examples of policies we have developed collaboratively and advocated for within the School of Nursing and at the institutional level to ensure a quality program. The policies are based on best practices and evaluation criteria. Advocacy is often an important role for the program leadership in online programs. Depending on the institution, challenges may arise related to the differences in the student populations served by the institutions, for example, traditional, residential students versus online, "adult," degree-seeking students. Despite the awareness that institutional support is critical to the success of online students, online program administrators have reported challenges with a lack of understanding from the institution regarding online students' needs and circumstances (Parkes, Gregory, Fletcher, Adlington, & Gromik, 2015). The differences in needs and circumstances, if misunderstood, can result in the inability to maintain the quality and integrity of the online program. Therefore, policies that maintain the integrity of the program and promote student success are critical.

Preparation for Online Teaching

Given our belief that online teaching is a specialized form of education and to ensure only qualified faculty taught in the program, a policy was developed that all full-time faculty need to be certified in online teaching (**Table 6-3**). This was critical, given the leadership role they took on in course development and support for adjunct faculty as course leads, as discussed in the leadership chapter.

Best Practices for Online Teaching

Best practices for online teaching are discussed in detail in Chapter 9. **Table 6-4** highlights the best practices for online teaching in our program. They are grounded in pedagogical theories and supported by online experts, some of whom contributed to our education.

Table 6-3 Preparation for Online Teaching

Preparation: Full-time faculty and adjunct faculty must provide evidence of preparation for online teaching as detailed below:

- Full-time nursing faculty teaching in the online nursing program must complete a certificate program in online education or a comparable university course approved by the dean of nursing or designee.
- Preferred qualifications for online teaching include previous online teaching experience.
- Prior to teaching their first online nursing course, faculty are required to participate in mentorship activities with an assigned faculty mentor and/or course lead assigned to the online program.

Evaluation: The dean of nursing or designee, assigned mentor, or course lead in the online program will evaluate the online teaching of the faculty member using the process for peer appraisal of online teaching.

- A peer appraisal of online teaching will be conducted at the completion of teaching the first online course.
- For full-time faculty, the peer appraisal of online teaching will be used to improve online teaching effectiveness, to develop professional development plans, and as one form of performance data for faculty evaluation.
- For adjunct faculty, the peer appraisal of online teaching will be conducted annually and used to improve online teaching effectiveness, to develop mentoring activities, and to influence rehire decisions.

Table 6-4 Best Practices for Online Teaching

Prior to the First Day of Class:

- Review the course syllabus, outcomes, content, calendar, and assessments.
- Review the class roster.

Creating a Positive Online Learning Community:
The essential elements of successful distance learning include honesty, respect, responsiveness, relevance, openness, and empowerment (Palloff & Pratt, 2007).

- Post a personal/professional faculty biography in the Information link.
- Create an introductory forum to break the ice and have everyone introduce themselves.
- Post a short, individualized response to welcome each student to class.
- Create a discussion forum designated for student questions/faculty responses.
- Create a chat forum where students can discuss things other than the course, socialize, and develop a supportive community.
- Post a welcome announcement that conveys support and excitement about their participation in the course. A welcome should include the following:
  - Some general feedback and support for student experiences in online learning and for their progress in the curriculum
  - Specific instructions for how to get started in class
  - Instructions for where to locate resources and support
  - Contact information for faculty and your routine for responding to ques
  - tions, course messages, and emails (explain the differences and your preferences)

(continues)

Table 6-4 Best Practices for Online Teaching   *(continued)*

- Expectations for communication or netiquette
- An invitation for early participation, interaction, and questions at the start of class

Facilitation of Learning and Course Interaction:

Continual faculty engagement in the online classroom creates conditions for a maximally beneficial learning experience for students (Data from Dereshiwsky, 2013).

- Log in to the class at least 5 times per week (respond to email, messages, and questions in the discussion within 24–48 hours)
- Read all posts and moderate discussions. Suggestions for moderating discussions include the following (Data from Draves, 2007):
  - Look for openings—ask follow-up questions; ask for more information.
  - Be neutral and nonjudgmental—avoid negative feedback in the discussion.
  - Help build confidence in the discussion by creating a secure environment.
  - Hold high expectations for students and encourage everyone's participation.
  - Help with frustration and intervene with support.
- Actively engage in content discussion *regularly* to facilitate collaboration, advance dialogue, encourage deep reflection, and challenge students to think critically.
  - Make connections between course material and practice examples.
  - Focus on important concepts and course ideas; ask relevant questions.
  - Model thoughtful, well-written/well-constructed responses; utilize literature.
  - Present new information from emerging ideas and examples.
  - Rather than dominating a discussion, facilitation should reflect a presence in the discussion.

Consider multiple opportunities for interaction in the student-centered, collaborative classroom: student–instructor interaction (email, discussion, question forum, feedback, journaling, etc.), student–student interaction (group work, chats, discussion, introduction, etc.), and student–content interaction (discussion, written assignments, research, active learning activities, etc.).

Assessment, Grading, and Giving Feedback:

- Display an ongoing commitment to course outcomes and consistency across the curriculum.
- Utilize grading rubrics for discussions and assignments.
- Provide meaningful, substantive feedback when grading discussions and assignments.
- Communicate expectations for returning graded work to students (e.g., 1 week).

Constructive instructor feedback that is delivered in a positive, encouraging manner is essential for students' cognitive growth (Data from Kimball & Jazzar, 2011).

Discussion:

- Focus on content, quality, and timely collaboration/engagement in the group process.
- Provide more feedback individually when there is reduced faculty presence in the discussion.

- Ensure discussions are supported by literature, practice examples, and experience.
- Raise expectations as students progress through the course and program.

Assignments:

- Include the rubric with feedback (track changes or format that supports learning).
- Feedback should be meaningful, substantive, and reflective of an understanding of content.
- Use American Psychological Association (APA) format and consider writing skills (edit minimally; feedback should support growth).

A sandwich approach to assignment feedback (positive, negative, positive) is recommended by Kimball and Jazzar (2011), especially for beginning instructors, because it encourages learners while providing an honest, open, and direct critique. Feedback includes a positive comment about something the student did well and demonstrates genuine respect for the student (top slice in the sandwich); a critical perspective/analysis that is served constructively and aligned with the rubric related to content and writing style (middle slice); and a final expression of positive, sincere support (bottom slice). The final slice invites the student to rethink the assignment and apply the learning to the next assignment/course. The goal of this approach is to motivate the student to continue on the path of learning.

Peer Appraisal

The colleague appraisals used within our academic setting were developed for the face-to-face teaching faculty. In our tenure process, we found that our colleagues did not know how to appraise our work. As a result, we developed the peer appraisal shown in **Table 6-5** based on the best practices outlined in Table 6-5. It is also used by our course leads in the mentoring relationship and to provide appraisals for adjunct faculty who are teaching in the online nursing program.

Online Course Expectations

A clear policy that provides structure for students helps to ensure consistency in expectations. **Table 6-6** shows the policy that we hold our students to in order to ensure a positive learning environment in which students can have opposing views and learn from each other, which is in keeping with our constructivist philosophy.

Student Feedback

Ensuring quality in an online program is a collaborative effort among all stakeholders, including students. We value the input students can provide for use during our courses. It also sends a message that we are working with them to ensure a learning experience that they value. Formal course evaluations provide good anonymous

Table 6-5 Peer Appraisal of Online Teaching

1. Creating a Positive Online Learning Community			
Essential Elements	**Yes**	**No**	**Comments**
Posted a faculty biography and welcome message			
Created an introductory forum to break the ice			
Created a discussion forum for student questions			
Created a social chat area for student peer support			
Posted an introductory announcement that included the following: ■ General support for getting started in the online course; a positive welcome ■ Specific instructions for how to get started ■ Contact information for faculty ■ Expectations for communication ■ Invitation for early participation, questions, and interaction			

Feedback:

2. Facilitation of Learning and Course Interaction			
Essential Elements	**Yes**	**No**	**Comments**
Logged in to class *at least* 5 times per week to respond to questions, engage in discussions, and provide feedback to students			
Evidence that faculty has *actively* engaged in course discussions by doing the following: ■ Asking follow-up questions, asking for students to provide more information, and asking probing questions ■ Challenging students to think in different ways and question assumptions ■ Making connections between course material and/or practice examples			
■ Integrating current research and literature ■ Focusing on important concepts and ideas ■ Building confidence and encouraging interaction ■ Promoting reflection and encouraging critical thinking ■ Supporting students to help with frustrations ■ Modeling thoughtful, well-constructed responses that use literature when appropriate ■ *Facilitating discussion*, as opposed to dominating discussion			

Feedback:

3. Assessment, Grading, and Giving Feedback			
Essential Elements	**Yes**	**No**	**Comments**
Maintains commitment to course outcomes and consistency across curriculum			
Utilizes grading rubrics for discussions and assignments			
Provides meaningful, substantive feedback			
Typically returns graded work within 1 week			
Discussion feedback: ■ Focuses on content, quality, and timely collaboration ■ Ensures posts are supported by literature, practice examples, and experience ■ Expects higher achievement as course progresses Assignment feedback: ■ Returns the assignment to the student with the rubric in the gradebook (as opposed to email) ■ Includes substantive written feedback ■ Emphasizes skill development in writing and APA style			
Feedback:			

Signature (Peer Reviewer):

Table 6-6 Online Course Expectations

Online Course Expectations

- Students are expected to read the course announcements, syllabus, schedule, assignment expectations, and all other course materials at the beginning of the course and, periodically, throughout the term.
- It is expected that every member of the online learning community will have different views, opinions, and experiences in relation to the topics that are discussed. We believe that the learning experience will be enhanced if students and faculty respond to each other respectfully, politely, and with professionalism.
- The online classroom is a safe, confidential learning environment where clinical situations and scenarios are discussed for the purposes of collaborative learning.
- In addition to the time spent on coursework, students are expected to log in a minimum of 3–4 times per week to check for announcements, new discussion responses, and returned assignments. Regular and consistent engagement in class is an important part of success in the program. Please check the course syllabus for specific expectations.

(continues)

Table 6-6 Online Course Expectations *(continued)*

- Students may notice similarities in the way that online education is delivered across the curriculum, particularly related to the design of online courses. It is important to know that faculty members have a variety of teaching styles and preferences.
- Each course is designed with its own set of course outcomes or goals for learning; therefore, teaching and learning strategies vary from course to course. Refer to the syllabus for descriptions of course activities and expectations.
- The knowledge and skills gained in one course will provide a foundation for subsequent courses. The learning that occurs across the curriculum builds from simple to more complex.
- Every course includes a variety of resources that support learning: online access to the library, writing tips and APA resources, Blackboard support, e-tutoring, and more.
- In online courses, student identification is confirmed through the college ID and secure password. Faculty members use a variety of tools to assess academic integrity (i.e., plagiarism).

Communication Expectations

- It is expected that students will communicate early and consistently with faculty when there are questions, concerns, or extenuating circumstances.
- Check college email regularly (at least 3 times a week) for college and program announcements and individual communications from faculty and staff.
- Please do not forward your college email to your personal email—this will result in missed course announcements.
- Faculty members are expected to respond to emails and questions within 24–48 hours.
- It is important to check with each instructor or refer to the syllabus to understand their preferences for communication and their time line for responses.

General Guidelines for Email Communication

- Use a descriptive subject line.
- Include a greeting for the person you are writing, and sign your name with return contact information.
- Be succinct, clear, and respectful in your communication.
- Include the correct people; pause before clicking "reply all."

information but are not available to be used in a timely manner. To provide additional opportunities for students to give more informal feedback and to support ongoing course development, it is helpful to obtain feedback from students during a new assignment, when piloting a new course activity, or as final reflection so that any needed changes can be made. **Table 6-7** includes some sample prompts used to engage students in providing feedback about their learning, including the "muddiest point," which is a strategy often used in face-to-face classrooms (Mosteller, 2016).

Table 6-7 Sample Prompts to Engage Student Feedback to Enhance Quality

1. Given that this is a pilot activity for leadership development, please provide feedback regarding how you experienced having the independence to develop your own schedule for the majority of the course. If you prefer to give your feedback privately, please use the journal option.
2. As this class is coming to an end, please share your thoughts and feelings about what this virtual community meant to you and identify two lessons from this course that you will carry with you into your practice.
3. Please take the time to think back on your previous nursing program. Is there any course content that seemed redundant to you? My goal is to determine if I need to make any revisions to the course content.
4. Muddiest Point: Please share a time in the course that was most "muddy" or confusing. My goal is to determine if there are areas of the course that can be clarified.
5. This is the first time I have used this assignment. Your feedback on how this assignment contributed or did not contribute to your learning would be appreciated.

Summary

Attention to quality is critical to the success of any educational program. Ongoing quality improvement can enhance student learning outcomes, increase student persistence, and provide the structures needed to support accreditation and regulatory requirements. In this chapter, we have shared some of the policies and procedures that we have used to build quality in the online program. We have also referenced other chapters in the book that include additional quality measures.

Best-Practice Recommendations for Online Programs

- Commit to implementing quality assurance and monitoring at the institutional, program, and faculty level.
- Develop formal policies and procedures that outline the expectations for online courses and faculty qualifications for online teaching.
- Create a set of best practices for online teaching that includes mentorship and a peer-appraisal process to enhance the quality of teaching and learning in the online program.
- Define program evaluation measures that include obtaining regular feedback from students through course evaluations and classroom evaluation activities.

References

Alexiou-Ray, J., & Bentley, C.C. (2015). Faculty professional development for quality online teaching. *Online Journal of Distance Learning Administration, 18*(4), 1–6.

Allen, I. E., & Seaman, J. (2016). *Online report card: Tracking online education in the United States.* Babson Research Group.

Baldwin, S., Ching, Y., & Hsu, Y. (2018). Online course design in higher education: A review of national and statewide evaluation instruments. *Tech Trends, 62*, 46–57. http://doi.org/10.1007/s11528-017-0215-z

Bawa, P. (2016). Retention in online courses: Exploring issues and solutions—A literature review. *SAGE Open*, 1–11. http://doi.org/10.1177/2158244015621777

Billings, D. (2007). Distance education in nursing—25 years and still going strong. *Computers, Informatics, & Nursing, 25*(3), 121–123.

Billings, D. M., Dickerson, S. S., Greenburg, M. J., Yow-Wu, B., & Talley, B. (2013). Quality monitoring and accreditation in nursing distance education programs. In K. Frith & D. Clark (Eds.). *Distance education in nursing* (3rd ed.). Springer.

Chaloux, B., & Miller, G. (2019). E-learning and the transformation of higher education. In G. Miller, M. Benke, B. Chaloux, L. C. Ragan, R. Schroeder, W. Smutz, & K. Swan (Eds.), *Leading the e-learning transformation of higher education* (pp. 3–22). Stylus.

Chickering, A. W., & Ehrmann, S. C. (1996). Implementing the seven principles: Technology as a lever. *American Association for Higher Education Bulletin, 49*(2), 3–6.

Chickering, A. W., & Gamson, Z. F. (1987). Seven principles for good practice in undergraduate education. *AAHE Bulletin*, 3–7.

Dereshiwsky, M. (2013). *Continual engagement: Fostering online discussions*. WI: LERN Books.

Draves, W. (2007). *Advanced teaching online* (3rd ed.). LERN Books.

Dunn, D. S., & Halonen, J. S. (2017). Choosing an external reviewer. *The Chronicle of Higher Education*. https://www.chronicle.com/article/Choosing-an-External-Reviewer/240271

Ellis, P. (2016). Systematic program evaluation. In D. Billings & J. Halstead (Eds.), *Teaching in nursing: A guide for faculty* (pp. 463–507). Saunders.

Graham, C., Cagiltay, K., Lim, B. R., Craner, J., & Duffy, T. M. (2001). Seven principles of effective teaching: A practical lens for evaluating online courses. *Extending the Pedagogy of Threaded Topic Discussions, 2001*(1). https://www.learntechlib.org/p/94251/

Hart, S. (2012). Factors associated with student persistence in an online program of study: A review of the literature. *Journal of Interactive Online Learning, 11*(1), 19–42. http://www.ncolr.org/jiol/issues/pdf/11.1.2.pdf

Kimball, D., & Jazzar, M. (2011). *To increase learner achievement, serve feedback sandwiches*. http://info.magnapubs.com/blog/articles/teaching-and-learning/to-increase-learner-achievement-serve-feedback-sandwiches/

Manz Friesth, B. (2020). Teaching and learning at a distance. In D. M. Billings & J. A. Halstead (Eds.), *Teaching in nursing: A guide for faculty* (6th ed., pp. 392–408). Elsevier.

McAfooes, M. J. (2002). Teaching and learning in online learning communities. In D. M. Billings & J. A. Halstead (Eds.), *Teaching in nursing: A guide for faculty* (6th ed., pp. 409–436). Elsevier.

Merrill, M. D. (2001). First principles of instruction. *Journal of Structural Learning & Intelligent Systems, 14*(4), 459.

Mosteller, F. (2016). *Muddiest point*. https://studymoose.com/re-muddiest-point-essay

Nilson, L. B., & Goodson, L. A. (2018). *Online teaching at its best: Merging instructional design with teaching and learning research*. Jossey-Bass.

Palloff, R., & Pratt, K. (2007). *Building online learning communities: Effective strategies for the virtual classroom*. Jossey-Bass.

Parkes, M., Gregory, S., Fletcher, P., Adlington, R., & Gromik, N. (2015). Bringing people together while learning apart: Creating online learning environments to support the needs of rural and remote students. *Australian and International Journal of Rural Education, 25*(1), 65–78.

Puzziferro, M., & Shelton, K. (2009). Supporting online faculty—Revisiting the seven principles (a few years later). *Online Journal of Distance Learning Administration, 12*(3). https://www.westga.edu/~distance/ojdla/fall123/puzziferro123.html

Quality Matters. (2020). *Why quality matters*. https://www.qualitymatters.org/why-quality-matters/about-qm

Ragan, L. C., & Schroeder, R. (2019). Supporting faculty success in online learning: Requirements for individual and institutional leadership. In G. Miller, M. Benke, B. Chaloux, L. C. Ragan, R. Schroeder, W. Smutz, & K. Swan (Eds.), *Leading the e-learning transformation of higher education* (pp. 108–131). Stylus.

Swan, K. (2019). Enhancing e-learning effectiveness. In G. Miller, M. Benke, B. Chaloux, L. C. Ragan, R. Schroeder, W. Smutz, & K. Swan (Eds.), *Leading the e-learning transformation of higher education* (pp. 77–107). Stylus.

U.S. Department of Education. (2010). *Evaluation of evidence-based practices in online learning: A meta-analysis and review of online learning studies.* https://www2.ed.gov/rschstat/eval/tech/evidence-based-practices/finalreport.pdf

Wandersman, A., Snell-Johns, J., Lentz, B. E., Fetterman, D. M., Keener, D. C., Livet, M., . . . Flaspoor, P. (2012). The principles of empowerment evaluation. In D. M. Fetterman, A. Wandersman, & R. A. Millett (Eds.), *Empowerment evaluation principles in practice* (pp. 27–41). Guilford Press.

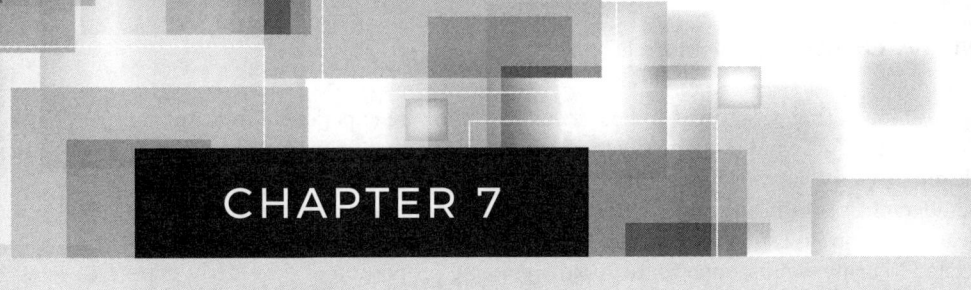

CHAPTER 7

Curriculum Development

Henny Breen and Melissa Robinson

"The curriculum is so much necessary raw material, but warmth is the vital element for the growing plant and for the soul."

Carl Jung

Overview

The focus of this chapter is program development as well as underlying theories and concepts related to nursing curriculum development given today's healthcare environment and nursing practice educational needs. Curriculum development at the program and course levels is explored, with three recommended course design models discussed.

Health care and Societal Issues Affecting Nursing Education

Many schools of nursing have made an intentional shift to clinical community settings given the recommendation of the Institute of Medicine, currently known as the National Academy of Medicine, 2011 *Future of Nursing* report. The report identified that nurses need skills in leadership, health policy, system-improvement research and evidence-based practice, teamwork, and collaboration, which goes beyond technological competence. In addition to this broad-based knowledge, competency in specific content areas, such as public health, and a greater orientation to community-based primary care and an emphasis on health promotion are required by nurses today (National Academy of Medicine, 2011).

Although there continues to be a focus on acute care experiences in hospitals in associate degree and undergraduate programs, many nursing programs at all levels are placing a heavier emphasis on community, given the changing population demographics and healthcare environment, with an emphasis on prevention and health promotion, care management, and shorter hospital stays. These changes are related to many factors, such as the rapidly growing proportion of the elderly population in the United States. According to the U.S. Census Bureau (2018), by 2030, all baby boomers will be older than 65 years of age, resulting in older people outnumbering children for the first time in history. One in every five residents will be of retirement age, with 78 million people aged 65 years and older compared with 76.7 million under the age of 18 projected for 2035. Further, the older population is becoming more racially and ethnically diverse. The proportion of those aged 65 and over in 2010 was 14.5% White, 9.4% Asian alone, 8.8% Black alone, 7.1% American Indian and Alaska native alone, 5.8% Hispanic or Latino alone, 5.5% Native Hawaiian and Pacific Islander alone, 4.4% two or more races, and 3.5% some other race. Over 38% of those over age 65 had one or more disabilities in 2010, with the most common difficulties being related to activities of daily living (West, Cole, Goodkind, & He, 2014).

Other factors that affect curricular decisions include healthcare reform, globalization, violence and threats of violence, natural disasters, and technology (Veltri & Barber, 2016). We need to constantly keep in mind the healthcare environment in determining the educational needs of current and future nurses.

Program Development

To illustrate the process for developing a new program, we will use, as an exemplar, the registered nurse (RN)–bachelor of science in nursing (BSN) program within our college. Before starting a program, it is critical to have a good understanding of the approval process within the educational institution and to consult with the regional accrediting body and state board of nursing to ensure there are no potential barriers. It is also important to gain the support of the college administrators in order to ensure that the program being planned aligns with the overall goals of the institution (DeBoor, 2018). Other essential aspects of developing an online program include support from the nursing faculty, a good understanding of the American Association of Colleges of Nursing (AACN) Essentials of Baccalaureate Education, and knowledge of practice issues as identified by state boards of nursing and the workforce in different settings.

Alignment

Multiple layers need to be attended to when designing a curriculum: the mission and vision of the college; the mission, vision, and program outcomes of the nursing program; the learning outcomes of each individual course; and the objectives of each module within each course. The ability to navigate these multiple layers is critical to the success of an online program, in addition to expertise in online curriculum development. For example, one of the mission statements for our college is as follows:

> Linfield facilitates experiential learning. Students apply theory and knowledge to lived experience in order to test and refine their understanding of a subject, clarify career goals, and discover the value of serving others.

The mission statement aligns with the School of Nursing (SON) philosophy, which states,

> Consistent with the foundational education principles of Linfield College, the School of Nursing promotes integrated learning, global and multicultural awareness, and experiential learning that fosters reflective practice essential for professional nurses in the 21st century.

As a faculty, it was important to discuss how the philosophy of our college and SON aligned with our own philosophy of nursing education to ensure that the RN-to-BSN program was in alignment. For example, if we value experiential learning, it needs to be integrated throughout the program rather than included only as a practicum add-on experience at the end of the program. The program outcomes for the RN-to-BSN program are the same as the program outcomes for the generic (prelicensure) undergraduate program. It was important to ensure they met accreditation standards and the BSN essentials and were consistent with the philosophy of the college. Decisions were made regarding the number of credits to fulfill the requirements for a BSN degree, including credits for prior learning. Our program awards 32 semester credits of nursing coursework, which includes many of the clinical courses. Students are also required to transfer in or complete prerequisite credits that meet the college's requirements for earning a bachelor's degree.

Although the program outcomes are the same as those of the prelicensure program, the course of study is much different, given the experience and previous education acquired in becoming an RN. A major difference is that there is no requirement to prepare for the national licensing exam (NCLEX) following graduation. Much of the focus is on coursework that enhances professional growth, professional communication, theoretical perspectives, community- and population-based nursing care, health promotion, and leadership (Baxter, 2018). Within our program, there is an emphasis on vulnerable populations and social justice.

Our RN-to-BSN nursing program includes the following courses that students can complete in four semesters, or they may choose to slow down their progression and complete coursework on a part-time basis. Entry into the program may occur during three different semesters (fall, spring, or summer). Some elective courses for meeting Linfield curriculum credit requirements are also offered during the January term. The core nursing courses are as follows:

Semester 1

Transition to Professional Nursing Practice (6 credits)

Semester 2

Evidence-Based Nursing (3 credits)

Professional Communication in Health Care (3 credits)

Semester 3

Nursing Leadership (3 credits)

Population-Based Nursing (3 credits)

Semester 4

Integrated Experiential Learning (6 credits)

Table 7-1 provides an example of aligning the program outcomes with the AACN Essentials of Baccalaureate Education developed in 2008 and the RN-to-BSN courses. It is important to note that work is being done at this time to update the essentials, which will include recommendations for a finite set of competencies within each identified domain, including essential areas of practice for all baccalaureate nursing students, including those in RN-to-BSN programs (AACN, 2019).

Table 7-1 Alignment of Baccalaureate Essentials to Program Outcomes and Courses

AACN Baccalaureate Essentials	Linfield School of Nursing Program Outcomes	Courses
Essential I Liberal Education for Baccalaureate Generalist Nursing Practice	Integrates knowledge from liberal arts, sciences, and nursing science as a basis for professional practice	All courses
Essential II Basic Organizational and Systems Leadership for Quality Care and Patient Safety	Uses principles of stewardship and leadership effectively and efficiently to influence the practice environment and improve health outcomes	Nursing Leadership Integrated Experiential Learning
Essential III Scholarship for Evidence-Based Practice	Applies clinical reasoning, reflective practice, and evidence-based practice in the provision of safe, quality, holistic, client-centered care	Evidence-Based Practice
Essential IV Information Management and Application of Patient Care Technology	Uses information and technology to communicate, manage knowledge, mitigate error, and support decision making to achieve healthcare outcomes for clients	Nursing Leadership Integrated Experiential Learning
Essential V Healthcare Policy, Finance, and Regulatory Environments	Demonstrates awareness of and responsiveness to the larger context of the healthcare system and effectively calls on system resources to provide care that is of optimal quality and value	Nursing Leadership
Essential VI Interprofessional Communication and Collaboration for Improving Health Outcomes	Communicates effectively and collaboratively in a professional practice	Professional Communication in Health Care

AACN Baccalaureate Essentials	Linfield School of Nursing Program Outcomes	Courses
Essential VII Clinical Prevention and Population Health	Demonstrates accountability for the delivery of standards-based nursing care that is consistent with moral, altruistic, legal, ethical, regulatory, humanistic, and social justice principles	Population-Based Nursing Care
Essential VIII Professionalism and Professional Values	Provides effective nursing care that considers diverse values, cultures, perspectives, and health practices	Professional Communication Integrated Experiential Learning
Essential IX Baccalaureate Generalist Nursing Practice	Demonstrates commitment to the nursing profession through the comportment of professional values and standards	Transition to Professional Practice

Curriculum Design

There is a great deal written about nursing curriculum for the prelicensure student. In this chapter, three models of curriculum design are discussed. The concept-based curriculum, which is becoming standard in many schools of nursing, is initially addressed. Backward design, which is an alignment design model developed by Wiggins and McTighe (2005), and an integrated course model design that has similar features, developed by Dee Fink (2013), are also discussed in this chapter. These models are a perfect fit for online nursing courses because they are based on constructivist learning theory. All three models lend themselves to designing online concept-based courses. At the end of this chapter, we provide an example of how to apply these models to a curriculum.

Concept-Based Curriculum

It is well recognized that content saturation as a result of an increasing amount of facts within each specialty focus required a change in how nursing education was delivered. In addition to content saturation, the need for higher-level thinking has led to a paradigm shift from content to concepts in curriculum development. A concept-based curriculum is understood as using core ideas (concepts) important to nursing practice to foster deeper learning through understanding how these concepts explain a variety of conditions and situations students will encounter in nursing practice (Taylor Sullivan, 2016). This is in contrast to blocking curriculum, in which the nursing curriculum is organized around clinical specialty areas, such as medical-surgical or psychiatric nursing; patient populations, such as pediatric nursing; and pathologic conditions, such as diabetes (Taylor Sullivan, 2016).

Much attention has been given to concept-based curriculum development in prelicensure nursing programs. Faculty identify concepts they consider to be core to meeting course and program outcomes. A concept-based curriculum has the potential for limitless knowledge and skill acquisition. Further, a curriculum based on concepts using exemplars to illustrate the concepts enables students to transfer and expand their knowledge and skills to different experiences, settings, and populations (Hendricks & Wangerin, 2017; Taylor Sullivan, 2016).

Close attention needs to be paid to the mapping of concepts to ensure the students' knowledge of the concept will grow in depth and breadth to avoid omission or repetition (Taylor Sullivan, 2016). Concepts in a prelicensure program are taught by course and semester, with new concepts being added, along with revisiting earlier concepts at a deeper level as the students progress through the program.

Concept-Based Curriculum in Postlicensure Programs

When our school transitioned to a concept-based curriculum, we were challenged to map concepts in the same way they were mapped in the prelicensure program. However, we found this did not work because new concepts are not introduced each semester or by course. We could not find anything in the literature that helped us in this endeavor, and we finally came to the realization that we needed to choose and integrate concepts based on the SON's community-based philosophy and the AACN (2019) Essential Requirements for Baccalaureate Education. These concepts are integrated throughout the program, and as in prelicensure programs, attention is given to ensure that the students' knowledge of the concept grows in depth as they progress through the program.

The concepts that are integrated throughout the RN-to-BSN curriculum build on the foundational concepts that students have learned in their previous diploma or associate degree programs. Therefore, the work of the RN-to-BSN program is to build on this foundation by providing new knowledge and promote professional growth by ensuring previously introduced concepts are introduced in greater depth. Students who learn conceptually need to be assessed on their ability to develop higher-level thinking skills and apply information in the context of related concepts or ideas (Giddens, 2015). Higher-level thinking moves beyond the process of linking facts together. To move to a higher level of thinking, information and concepts are organized in new ways to develop new understandings as a result of analysis of the concepts. Synthesis of the concepts is an even higher-level skill that involves the application of concepts to new settings and situations. The synthesis level is an expectation of the bachelor's level nurse. Active learning strategies are used to advance conceptual learning.

Our RN-to-BSN curriculum consists of six nursing courses taken over four semesters, as outlined earlier in this chapter. Twenty-eight concepts are integrated throughout the curriculum. The course descriptions and concepts are listed in **Table 7-2**.

The first semester consists of the transition course in which all the concepts are introduced at varying levels. For example, the concepts of community, communication, reflection, critical thinking, diversity, and health disparities, to name a few, are introduced through a learning activity that requires them to assess their local community, which includes a windshield survey and key informant interviews. They further address concepts introduced in the first semester to higher levels as they progress through the program. Numerous experiential learning strategies, such as unfolding case studies, an advocacy project, and a cultural interview, are used

Table 7-2 Course Descriptions and Concepts

Course	Course Description	Concept
Semester 1		
Transition to Professional Practice	A transition to baccalaureate nursing practice for the RN student. Builds on previous knowledge and skills applicable to the practice of professional nursing. Topics in this course include professional nursing roles of caring, advocacy, collaboration, client teaching, holistic assessment, decision making, and evidence-based practice. Students engage in health-promotion teaching activities, community assessment, and family assessment and develop their skills in utilizing information technology and professional writing.	Advocacy Assessment Caring Change Client Education Collaboration Communication Community Critical thinking Diversity Ethics Evidence-based practice Global health
Semester 2		
Professional Communication in Diverse Communities	Preparation for professional practice, including communicating with clients and collaborating with other professionals in interdisciplinary settings. Topics in this class include the use of inter- and intraprofessional communication and collaboration to produce positive working relationships, the nurse–patient relationship, culture, and patient safety. There is an emphasis on personal reflection. This class is entirely online.	Healthcare systems Health disparities Healthcare law Health policy Health promotion Information technology Leadership Populations Professionalism Quality improvement
Evidence-Based Practice	This course introduces the RN-to-BSN student to the realm of nursing research. The importance of using evidence-based research in nursing practice is discussed. A review of the current literature and a synthesis of research relevant to nursing are introduced. Students will have the opportunity to learn about various research designs and methods as well as how to critically analyze research. Students will learn how to synthesize research and communicate effectively in discussion forums and written assignments using American Psychological Association (APA).	Reflective practice Research Safety Social justice Vulnerable populations

(continues)

Table 7-2 Course Descriptions and Concepts   *(continued)*

Course	Course Description	Concept
	Ethical dilemmas in research are discussed, as well as regulating bodies that govern the practice of research in human subjects. Basic statistics are introduced in relation to nursing research.	
Semester 3		
Population-Focused Nursing	Healthcare issues and interventions from multicultural, domestic, and global perspectives. Topics include public health principles, epidemiology and disease outbreak investigation, vulnerable populations, social health determinants, and global health disparities. Students engage in collaborative and active learning activities that address population-focused advocacy and global health issues. This class takes place entirely online.	
Nursing Leadership	Principles of organizational healthcare management, healthcare policy, and the role of the nurse leader in healthcare organizations. Topics include legal and ethical issues, culture and safety at an organizational level, and management of the patient care team. There is a heavy emphasis on writing in this course, using evidence-based research and practice.	
Semester 4		
Integrated Experiential Learning	Immersion experience in nursing. Experiential learning that incorporates simulation and practice in leadership, management, and population-based nursing care. The topics in this course are selected from topics taken previously, with an emphasis on leadership, management, global health, and professional communication. This course includes clinical hours spent in a virtual community and in a face-to-face clinical placement in an acute care or community setting. The student and a coordinator will work together to secure a clinical placement in or near the community where the student lives or at an international site of the student's choice from a selection of prearranged options.	

throughout the curriculum to advance conceptual learning, cumulating in the final Integrated Experiential Learning course developed for the purpose of linking and integrating concepts for application to practice through virtual simulation and service learning. Experiential learning and a more detailed description of these strategies are discussed in Chapter 11, as well as studies we have conducted to assess conceptual learning.

Alignment Design

Although backward design as developed by Wiggins and McTighe (2005) was not developed for online education, it is an extremely useful resource when designing online courses. Indiana University has an excellent online course on how to develop courses and teach using the backward-design model. Wiggins and McTighe (2005) describe that their book *Understanding Design* is not a prescriptive program but, rather, a way of thinking in a purposeful manner about the nature of any design, with understanding as the goal. In other words, their model provides a conceptual framework. *Understanding* is defined as "an insight into ideas, people, situations, and processes manifested in various appropriate performances. To understand is to make sense of what one knows, to be able to know why it's so, and to have the ability to use it in various situations and contexts" (Wiggins & McTighe, 2005, p. 353). Understanding requires critical thinking and reflection, which are two foundational concepts to nursing.

Designing a curriculum using Wiggins and McTighe's model is thought of as backward design because the curriculum starts with looking at the big picture, with the end goals (program and course outcomes) in mind, rather than starting with interesting activities and textbooks, which educators often do. In developing online curriculum, faculty often get caught up in the technology and designing courses around the latest and most fun technology. Keeping the goal of the educational process in mind, the first step is to identify what students should know and be able to do upon graduation (program outcomes) and at the end of each course (course outcomes) and the end of each module within a course (learning objectives). Once the outcomes have been established, the kind of evidence needed to demonstrate that the students have met the outcomes needs to be decided. Once these steps have been identified, learning experiences and resources are planned that will help students be able to provide evidence that they have met the outcomes.

Integrated Design

Dee Fink (2013) has a similar model of backward design known as *integrated course model design* in which he describes significant learning as the goal. It goes beyond an understand-and-remember approach and beyond application. He developed a new taxonomy of significant learning that challenges students to make connections between course learning and current and future life experiences. The taxonomy is relational rather than hierarchical and includes foundational knowledge, application, integration, the human dimension, caring, and learning how to learn (Dee Fink, 2013). This taxonomy is particularly relevant to nursing, given the human dimension and the integration of learning. Nursing students cannot afford to think compartmentally; they need to continually integrate theory, principles, and concepts and then apply their knowledge and skills to clinical practice. Caring is another foundational concept within nursing. Both Wiggins and McTighe's and Dee Fink's course design models lend themselves to lifelong learning.

Integration of Models as Applied to an Online RN-to-BSN Curriculum

Table 7-3 demonstrates how alignment and integrated design models can be used in a concept-based nursing curriculum, drawing examples from our institution. The college mission and core themes recognize the value of theory-based experiential learning and service in addition to global and cultural understanding. This is consistent with the SON philosophy and carries it forward, including reflective practice, which is a main feature of experiential learning. This is then carried forward in the SON program outcomes, in which experiential learning is applied through course activities and service learning that promote clinical reasoning, reflective practice, and cultural awareness.

Assessment of Learning

In using a backward-design model, the decision on how to measure or assess student learning is made with the outcomes and objectives in mind. The learning activities to meet the learning objectives are then planned with the understanding of how the learning will be assessed. In our program, all learning assessment is done through the use of a grading rubric that evaluates how significant and conceptual learning advances through the semesters. In the first semester, the level of participation and application using the course content in the learning module is evaluated. Using Dee Fink's (2013) taxonomy language, evaluation would primarily include foundational, application, human dimension, and caring goals. All of these learning goals are carried throughout the program. In the second and third semesters, in addition to application, higher-level analysis is expected with increasing amounts of information from the course content, and expectations to use outside literature are integrated. In the final semester, there is an expectation for the ability to synthesize greater amounts of information, which is referred to as *integration* in Dee Fink's taxonomy.

Progression of Learning Through the Semesters

To illustrate how higher-level thinking is attained over the semesters, the concept of vulnerable populations is used as an exemplar, as follows:

>   **Semester 1:** The students are introduced to the social determinants of health (SDOH), and this new information is applied to the concept of vulnerable populations as students apply this new knowledge to assess vulnerability by learning a new skill, which is conducting a community assessment.

>   **Semester 2:** The students are introduced to the stages of change and motivational interviewing. They apply this new learning by applying both stages of change and motivational interviewing to a case study that incorporates a vulnerable patient in relation to the SDOH. This involves the integration of new knowledge (stages of change) and a new skill

Table 7-3 Example of Alignment

College Core Theme *Experiential Learning*	School of Nursing Philosophy	Program Outcome	Course	Course Learning Outcome	Module Learning Objective	Learning Activities
Linfield facilitates experiential learning. Students apply theory and knowledge to lived experience in order to test and refine their understanding of a subject, clarify career goals, and discover the value of serving others.	The School of Nursing promotes integrated learning, global and multicultural awareness, and experiential learning that fosters reflective practice essential for professional nurses in the 21st century.	Provide effective nursing care that considers diverse values, cultures, perspectives, and health practices.	Professional Communication	Demonstrate an awareness of culture in effective nurse–client relationships.	Analyze the impact of cultural health beliefs on health.	■ Conduct a cultural self-assessment using a model of cultural competence and care. ■ Interview someone of a different culture to complete a cultural assessment, followed by writing a reflective paper.

(motivational interviewing). This involves the integration of new and former knowledge through an analysis of how the information is related to vulnerable populations and facilitates higher-level thinking.

Semester 3: Students participate in weekly blog and discussion forums that require them to analyze specific social and health disparities affecting vulnerable populations, such as environmental injustice, gun violence, the opioid epidemic, vaccinations, and the connection between poverty and mental health. These activities facilitate higher-level thinking as the complexity of issues involving vulnerable populations are analyzed.

Semester 4: Students engage in a comprehensive group project in which they collaborate to develop a coalition planning document to address the vulnerable population of homeless veterans in one of the group members' communities, building on the skills they learned in the previous three semesters. Working in a small group to analyze the large amounts of information they collect, collaborating regarding that information, and making decisions about what information is important move the students from an analysis level of thinking to synthesis of the information in order to write a comprehensive coalition plan. This assignment is described in more detail in the Appendix of Chapter 11.

In summary, backward design starts with the college mission and advances to the specific learning module objectives. This ensures alignment in the curriculum design. An integrated course design is more dynamic and relational and includes a taxonomy of significant learning. The course concepts are integrated and encompass all the categories in Dee Fink's (2013) taxonomy of significant learning, with some spanning different categories as the conceptual learning deepens. A solid course design facilitates deeper and more meaningful learning.

Best-Practice Recommendations for Online Teaching

- Curriculum development and design should be based on a philosophical foundation and learning theory agreed upon by the faculty.
- A concept-based curriculum is recommended to support nursing students as they develop higher-level learning in today's complex healthcare environment.
- Within postlicensure programs, concepts can be effectively integrated through the entire nursing program, rather than allocated to specific courses.
- Alignment and integration models of course design are recommended for online curriculum planning and conceptual learning.

References

American Association of Colleges of Nursing. (2019). *AACN essentials.* https://www.aacnnursing.org/Education-Resources/AACN-Essentials

Baxter, K. (2018). Curriculum planning for undergraduate nursing programs. In S. B. Keating & S. S. DeBoor (Eds.), *Curriculum development and evaluation in nursing education* (4th ed., pp. 147–158). Springer.

DeBoor, S. S. (2018). Distance education, online learning, informatics, and technology. In S. B. Keating & S. S. DeBoor (Eds.), *Curriculum development and evaluation in nursing education* (4th ed., pp. 107–121). Springer.

Dee Fink, L. (2013). *Learning experiences: An integrated approach to designing college courses, revised and updated.* Jossey-Bass.

Giddens, J. F. (2015), The conceptual approach—Background and benefits. In J. F. Giddens, L. Caputi, & B. Rodgers (Eds.), *Mastering concept-based teaching: A guide for nurse educators.* Elsevier.

Hendricks, S. M., & Wangerin, V. (2017). Concept-based curriculum: Changing attitudes and overcoming barriers. *Nurse Educator, 42*(3), 138–142.

National Academy Medicine. (2011). *The future of nursing: Leading change, advancing health* [Policy report]. The National Academies Press. https://www.nap.edu/catalog/12956/the-future-of-nursing-leading-change-advancing-health

Taylor Sullivan, D. (2016). An introduction to curriculum development. In D. M. Billings & J. A. Halstead (Eds.), *Teaching in nursing: A guide for faculty* (5th ed., pp. 89–117). Elsevier.

U.S. Census Bureau. (2018). *Older people projected to outnumber children for first time in U.S. history.* https://www.census.gov/newsroom/press-releases/2018/cb18-41-population-projections.html

Veltri, L. M., & Barber, H. (2016). Forces and issues influencing curriculum development. In D. M. Billings & J. A. Halstead (Eds.), *Teaching in nursing: A guide for faculty* (5th ed., pp. 73–88). Elsevier.

West, L. A., Cole, S., Goodkind, D., & He, W. (2014). 65+ in the United States: 2010. *Current Population Reports.* https://www.census.gov/content/dam/Census/library/publications/2014/demo/p23-212.pdf

Wiggins, G., & McTighe, J. (2005). *Understanding by design* (2nd ed.). Pearson.

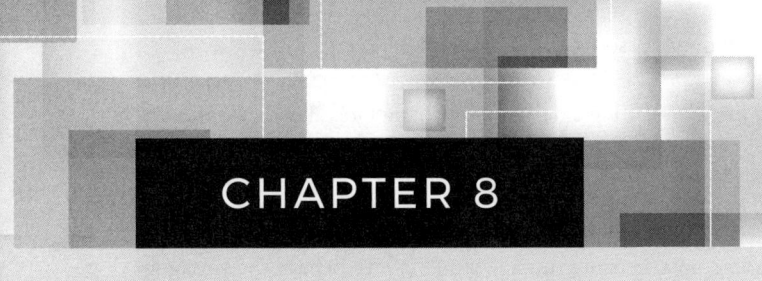

CHAPTER 8

Online Course Design

Henny Breen and Melissa Robinson

"When it comes to the design of effective learning experiences, one provocative question is worth a hundred proclamations."

Bernard Bull

Overview

This chapter addresses how to design an online course, building on the theory discussed in Chapters 2 and 7. The focus is on the integration of pedagogical theory, principles, and best practices for online course design, with examples provided throughout. Although there is some mention of how technology can be used to enhance learning, it is not the focus of this chapter. There are several sources available that the reader can access for a more "guidebook" approach to learn how to build an online course. A key feature of this chapter is the emphasis on how collaboration is an integral part of course design, consistent with our collaborative model.

Best Practices for Online Course Design

Many books and articles on online course design are "how-to" manuals on building a course online that lack reference to a theoretical foundation, or if theory is mentioned, it is not integrated into the discussion. When designing an online course, theory and an understanding of the most effective pedagogical principles should receive the same attention as they do when planning for the face-to-face classroom. Constructivist learning theories with applications in online course development include cognitive constructivism, social constructivism, collaborativist learning theory, and transformative learning theory (see Chapter 2). Models of curriculum design based on constructivist learning theory include concept-based curriculum, backward design, and integrated course design (see Chapter 7). Having a good understanding of these theories and models will provide the educator with the foundational knowledge to design a new online course or put a course taught in the face-to-face classroom online.

Pedagogical principles guide the design, implementation, and evaluation of online courses. For online postlicensure nursing students, we believe the pedagogical approaches that best serve our students include an integration of the different constructivist learning theories and models of curriculum design. Online courses need to be carefully designed and ready to go within the learning management system before the student first enters the class. This is of particular importance for working adults because they plan their schedules based not only on the workload of the course but also the course calendar. Further, they have the opportunity to review the course to ensure it is a course that meets their learning needs. This may not be as much of a factor for core curricula in nursing education because of the requirements to meet the program outcomes. However, it may make a difference in choosing elective courses.

There is some consistency in what is deemed "best practice" for online course design. The following best practices are recommended for online postlicensure nursing students, based on the literature, our experience, and the experience of our students who have provided us with ongoing feedback. Further, they are consistent with the constructivist learning theories and curriculum models we recommend for online learning and teaching. The best practices are introduced here and applied throughout the chapter.

The Learner Is at the Center of the Course Design

Before the planning of a course, it is important to know the student. In addition to knowing what the student needs to learn in terms of course content and concepts for the profession of nursing, it is important to know each student's characteristics, barriers to learning, and motivation for learning. Years of working with adult practicing nurses have taught us much about what works for them in terms of course design.

Collaborative Learning

Collaborative learning is at the heart of our online courses. Collaborativist learning theory (previously known as *online collaborative theory*), as developed by Linda Harasim, was used for a research study and found to provide an effective model to evaluate the student's ability to collaborate (Breen, 2015). The study is found in Chapter 15.

Develop a Clear and Consistent Structure

Within any program of study, it is important to have a consistent structure for all courses. It is very frustrating for students to learn a new way to navigate each course within the same program of study. It is equally important to provide a simple, consistent navigation system within each course (Johnson & Meehan, 2013).

Collaborate on Course Design

When designing a course, collaborating with at least one colleague is an excellent way to achieve high-quality course development. In many larger online institutions, it is not uncommon for online design experts known as *instructional designers* to work closely with faculty as content experts to develop an online course. We have found that collaboration is critical not only to have more than one mind working on and reviewing a course but because collaboration among all faculty who teach in the program ensures effective leveling of concepts.

Collaborative and Individual Reflection

Reflection is an integral aspect of the nursing profession, regardless of the specific nursing practice. This applies to our practice as educators as well. We engage in on-going individual and collaborative reflection to ensure each course design is meeting the intended process and outcomes for learning. Revisions are made as needed based on how well the course meets student learning needs and student feedback.

Process of Online Course Design

Backward design and integrated course models, as discussed in Chapter 7, form the framework for ensuring there is alignment between the course outcomes, assessment strategies, and learning activities. To support learner persistence, attention needs to be given to how the course is designed (Stavredes & Herder, 2014). Faculty involvement in course design is on a continuum from being minimally involved to being fully autonomous, depending on the learning institution, resulting in a number of approaches to the design process (Santelli, Stewart, & Mandernach, 2020). Course design that is faculty led is more common in smaller online programs and ranges from having minimal guidelines to some basic university guidelines and some faculty autonomy. Large online institutions tend to have a highly specialized approach that includes a standardized course design with minimal faculty autonomy (Lee, Dickerson, & Winslow, 2012). A collaborative approach, which we endorse, involves shared expertise and ideas on how the course should be organized. Faculty, instructional designers, and students may be part of the course design team (Stewart, Cohn, & Whithaus, 2016).

There are a number of different models for online course design that are important for instructional designers to be familiar with. At our institution, we designed our own courses using a combination of a simple linear instructional development process known as ADDIE, along with some important features from Dee Fink's (2013) integrated course design. The ADDIE process, as discussed by Stavredes and Herder (2014), includes the phases of analysis, design, development, implementation, and evaluation. Many other models found in the literature are variations of this linear model. **Table 8-1** provides a brief description of each phase of the ADDIE process.

Dee Fink (2013) describes the process as steps in an integrated design, as follows: (1) initial phase: build strong primary components, (2) intermediate phase: assemble the components into a coherent whole, and (3) final phase: finish important remaining tasks. The first phase is comparable to the ADDIE analysis and design

Table 8-1 The ADDIE Process

Phases of ADDIE Process	Description
Analysis	*Understand the Learner* ■ Student characteristics ■ Needs to support persistence *Understand the Purpose of the Course* ■ Within the broader curriculum
Design	*Core Elements* ■ Learning outcomes ■ Assessment strategies to demonstrate progress toward the learning outcomes ■ Assessment strategies to demonstrate achievement of the learning outcomes ■ Structure of the course ■ Sequencing of the course ■ Course materials to be used ■ Activities students will engage in
Development	*Create and Craft the Instruction for the Assessments and Course Activities* ■ Context information, such as module or unit objectives ■ Introduction ■ Syllabus ■ Calendar ■ Scaffolding
Implementation	*Launching the Course* ■ Strategies to facilitate the teaching of the course
Evaluation	*Final Evaluation* ■ Consider strategies for ongoing evaluation after implementation

phase because it involves identifying important situational factors and learning outcomes, formulating appropriate feedback and assessment procedures, and designing teaching and learning activities, ensuring they are all integrated. The intermediate phase is comparable to the remaining ADDIE phases because it includes creating a thematic structure for the course by selecting and creating teaching strategies. The final phase consists of tasks that are built into the design phase of ADDIE as well as the evaluation phase; it consists of developing the grading system and syllabus, correcting problems, and planning for an evaluation of the course and faculty teaching.

ADDIE and the integrated design processes are also consistent with the best practices discussed previously. Linear models are necessary for teaching because we believe integration is a process that starts with linear thinking and making connections. Integration, which goes beyond making connections, is critical to nursing practice and education. Integration is very much in keeping with our collaborative model, as discussed in Chapter 1, and the holistic model, as discussed in Chapter 4, because different perspectives are valued, considered, and merged as appropriate for a successful online program with very high retention and persistence rates.

The analysis section is the first step of the process and critical to the success of course design. We have devoted Chapter 3 to understanding the online nursing student and Chapter 7 to curriculum development. Chapter 7 provides an overview and example to demonstrate how a course fits within the School of Nursing's program outcomes, including course learning outcomes, module learning objectives, assessment strategies, and learning activities This chapter is focused on the design and development phases, which are integrated. Implementation is discussed in Chapter 9, which addresses online teaching strategies. Chapter 6 addresses course and program evaluations.

Collaborative Design and Development Process

We have developed a model (**Figure 8-1**) for the design and development process based on our experience, taking into account both the linear and integrated processes discussed previously. We believe ongoing reflection and collaboration are needed until the course is ready to launch. It is important to note that designing course learning outcomes is an integral part of the design process. However, in practice, learning outcomes cannot be changed once approved by the School of Nursing, and often the university curriculum committee, without going through what is often a lengthy process. The role of faculty in committee work is discussed in Chapter 5 in relation to the inclusion of online programs and in Chapter 13 in relation to faculty development and service to the institution.

Design and Development

The design of an online course can either facilitate student success with persistence or create barriers to student learning. In addition to over a decade of online teaching experience in various settings with different learning management systems, we have also been online students. We have learned that keeping it simple, consistent, and challenging, with opportunities for deep thinking, facilitates professional growth. Further, it is critical to value and respect the knowledge and skills that postlicensure students bring to the online classroom, not only in our teaching but also in how we design the course. We have learned that when we get many similar questions about an element in the course, something is amiss and needs to be corrected. This section of the chapter addresses all the core elements based on the model in Figure 8-1.

Learning Outcomes

The course learning outcomes need to be in alignment with the program outcomes, regardless of the delivery model. Course outcomes should communicate the following to learners: (1) what they are expected to know at the factual and conceptual levels, (2) the attitudes they need to develop in keeping with nursing values and ethics, and (3) the skills or competencies they will achieve as a result of taking the course (Scheckel, 2020; Stavredes & Herder, 2014). Given that many nursing programs have moved to a concept-based curriculum, decisions also need to be made

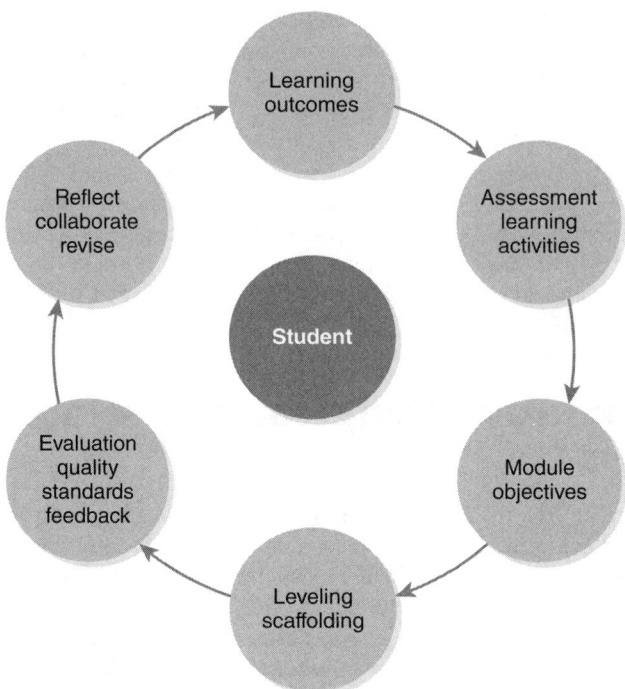

Figure 8-1 Collaborative design and development process

about which concepts to include and to what level they will be addressed (Scheckel, 2020). We have a list of concepts that are integrated throughout the online registered nurse (RN)–bachelor of science in nursing (BSN) program, as discussed in Chapter 7. The depth of understanding of the concept evolves as the student progresses through the program.

Taxonomy of Learning

A good source to use in the development of learning outcomes is the American Association of Colleges of Nursing (AACN) Essentials at the baccalaureate, master's, and doctoral levels. An understanding of both Bloom's and Dee Fink's taxonomies of learning guides the development of our learning outcomes. Benjamin Bloom led a group of researchers to initially formulate the three domains of learning in 1956. Bloom and his colleagues (Krathwohl, Bloom, & Mases, 1964) further developed the cognitive domain. The affective domain was broadened to include five behavioral categories: (1) receiving, (2) responding, (3) valuing, (4) organization of values, and (5) characterization by a value or value complex (Krathwohl et al., 1964). The psychomotor domains were further developed by Anita Harrow, among others (Hoque, 2016).

The domains of learning are well known among educators. L. Dee Fink's (2013) work is less known or used in nursing education, but we found his work to be an excellent resource for nursing education, which is also discussed in Chapter 7. See **Table 8-2** comparing Fink's integrated taxonomy of significant learning to Bloom's

Table 8-2 Taxonomies of Learning to Facilitate the Development of Learning Outcomes

	Taxonomy of Significant Learning Categories (Fink)	Taxonomy of Learning Domains (Bloom)	Verbs or Behaviors for Writing Learning Outcomes
Knowledge, Concepts	*Foundational Knowledge* Understanding and remembering information and ideas	*Cognitive Domain* Remember Understand	List, define, identify, explain summarize, describe, contrast, discuss
	Examples *Knowledge:* Describe historical persons and events and their influence on contemporary nursing. *Understanding:* Explain the contextual complexity of multicultural, domestic, and global community partnerships.		
	Application Skills; critical, creative, and practical thinking	*Cognitive Domain* Application	Apply, demonstrate, complete, illustrate, discover, manage, use, critique, imagine
	Example Apply effective therapeutic communication techniques and interviewing skills to produce positive nurse–client relationships with diverse clients across the life span.		
	Integration Connecting ideas, learning experiences, and realms of life	*Cognitive Domain* Analysis, synthesis, evaluation	Analyze, separate, order, differentiate, compare, connect, integrate, examine assess, decide, rank, recommend, support, conclude
	Examples *Analysis:* Analyze the impact of policy, finance, and regulatory environments on health care. *Synthesis:* Integrate knowledge from the liberal arts and sciences to inform nursing practice across the life span. *Evaluation:* Evaluate the reliability of evidence about the past.		
Attitude	*Human Dimension* Learning about one-self and others	*Affective Domain* Receiving, responding, valuing, organi-zation of values, characterization	Awareness of self and others, reflection

(continues)

Table 8-2 Taxonomies of Learning to Facilitate the Development
of Learning Outcomes   *(continued)*

	Taxonomy of Significant Learning Categories (Fink)	Taxonomy of Learning Domains (Bloom)	Verbs or Behaviors for Writing Learning Outcomes
	Example Reflect upon one's beliefs and values as related to professional practice.		
	Caring Developing new feelings, interests, and values	*Affective Domain* Responding, valuing, values guiding behavior	Receiving, giving, internalizing
	Example Identify as a reflective nurse in professional practice.		
Skill	*Learning How to Learn* Becoming a better student, inquiring about a subject, and self-directed learning	*Cognitive Domain* Create	Influencing, perform, modify, creating, motivated, questioning, identifying sources of information
	Example Integrate scholarship into professional writing and presentations.		
		Psychomotor Domain Using motor skills and coordinating them; dependent on the cognitive and affective domains	Begins, displays, moves, proceeds, reacts, shows, volunteers
	Example Demonstrate discipline-specific writing and information technology.		

domains of learning, along with verbs and behaviors to help in the writing of learning outcomes. An example is provided for each. In this table, we are comparing a linear process to an integrated one. Both models are excellent resources for the development of learning outcomes.

Assessment

In keeping with backward design, the next step is to develop assessment strategies that are appropriate based on the learning outcomes. The key to this element of the design process is to create a variety of strategies that will demonstrate progress toward achieving the learning outcomes (formative assessment) as well as achievement of the course outcomes (summative assessment). **Table 8-3** provides examples of formative and summative assessments.

Further, when considering the design of assessments, all three domains of learning need to be considered (Kirkpatrick & DeWitt, 2020; Stavredes & Herder,

Table 8-3 Example of Formative and Summative Assessments for Online Course Design

Learning Outcome	Formative Assessment	Summative Assessment
Prepare for the role of the professional nurse as a leader and change agent in health care	Self-Assessments ■ Leadership ■ Followership ■ Leadership skills assessment	Comprehensive leadership development plan
Objectives		
Examine the concepts of leadership, management, and followership	Collaborative discussions Blog activity	

2014). Developing the assessments at this time in the design process ensures that learning activities are in alignment with what is required to demonstrate that the learning outcomes have been met. However, the assessments may be revisited at any time during the design process.

We do want to mention that in the literature, assessment and evaluation may be considered separate concepts, and both are important aspects of course design. The main difference between the two concepts lies in how the completed work by the student is used. Faculty use the information from assessments to assess current learning that may result in a need to make revisions. Evaluation, on the other hand, involves judgment and occurs at the end of the course or program (Oermann, 2017). Kirkpatrick and DeWitt (2020) encourage educators practicing in clinical fields to "evaluate student attainment of course outcomes and defined program competencies to ensure that graduates are prepared for safe practice" (p. 451).

We believe evaluation is particularly important for prelicensure and advance practice nursing programs, given the emphasis on preparing graduates for direct patient care, clinical practice, and national licensure exams. Other postlicensure programs have more of an emphasis on the cognitive and affective domains of learning, in which grasping the role of nursing within the bigger picture of health care is important. Postlicensure programs build on prelicensure programs to advance higher-level thinking. Advance practice programs also have an emphasis on higher-level thinking, but students are required to learn and demonstrate higher-level skills in direct clinical care. For the purposes of this text, we refer to this element of the design process as *assessment.* This is not to negate that, as faculty, we need to evaluate students' work because grading is a requirement for progression. However, we want to ensure there is an emphasis on continual, progressive student learning, which requires ongoing assessment.

Dee Fink (2013) also discusses assessment as auditive versus educative assessment, a concept initially posited by Grant Wiggins in 1998. We thought it was important to highlight this distinction as something to think about compared with how assessment and evaluation are discussed in the previous paragraph. Auditive assessment mainly consists of a midterm and a final exam. It serves the purpose of providing a grade based on whether students were able to pass, indicating that they learned the content. In other words, it is a backward-looking assessment. Educative assessment, on the other hand, is ongoing, with the aim of helping students to learn better. It needs to be frequent, immediate, based on clear criteria, and delivered in a caring way.

Types of Online Assessments

There are many types of assessments that can be used within online courses—for example, authentic assessment, testing, self-assessment, reflective assessment, portfolio, WebQuests, and collaborative assessment (Dee Fink, 2013; Stavredes & Herder, 2014). **Table 8-4** includes a summary of the types of assessments that we

Table 8-4 Summary of Online Assessments

Assessment Description	Purpose	Examples
Authentic Based in the real world of nursing	Problem solving, critical thinking, clinical reasoning skills	Written formal assignment, discussion, or blog based on a case study or problem
Test Multiple choice, matching, true–false, short answer	Knowledge, conceptual understanding, application, analysis	We do not use graded tests in our program.
Self-Assessment and Reflective Assessment Reflection on personal experiences and nursing practice experiences	Attitudes, values, habits of mind	Journals, blogs, discussions, self-assessment surveys or tests to be used for a discussion
Portfolio A collection of documents representing the student's work over time	Demonstrates growth over time, showcases exemplars	Can be kept in an electronic format in the school's learning management system for assessment purposes, but students are encouraged to keep a separate binder or file at home for professional purposes
Collaborative/Peer Group work that may involve peer feedback	Teambuilding, collaboration skills	Collaborative assignment (An example is provided in Chapter 11: small-group work using a case study.)
WebQuest Inquiry-oriented strategy	Develop skills in seeking information from the web, organizing it, and presenting it to the class	Finding resources for a particular health-related problem

have found effective in online course design. When choosing a strategy, several factors need to be considered, including the philosophy of the faculty, the purpose of the assessment, the learning domain, the setting, and the effectiveness of the strategy, along with other incidental factors, such as time for preparation, implementation, and grading (Kirkpatrick & DeWitt, 2020). We also consider the concepts that are being taught. The types of assessments that best lend themselves to assessing conceptual learning among postlicensure students are authentic assessment, self-assessment, reflection, and collaborative work, which is in keeping with our constructivist approach to learning.

Integration of Assessment and Learning Activities

When planning assessment strategies, the design of learning activities must be considered because they are very much integrated into online courses. We use the discussion forums, blogs, and journals found in most learning management systems (LMSs) because they provide excellent opportunities to design integrated learning and assessment. **Table 8-5** includes common learning activities that can be created using the tools in multiple LMSs, along with the purpose of the activities.

The discussion of these tools is limited to course design in this chapter. Deeper discussion of each learning activity follows in the next chapter on online teaching strategies (see Chapter 9). We also use WebQuests, an inquiry-oriented strategy in which most or all of the information comes from the web. Students explore and gather information, analyze it, and share their findings and recommendations through collaborative discussion with their peers and faculty (Stavredes & Herder, 2014). As an example, we have used WebQuests to require students to find and assess resources for a particular health-related problem in their community.

Discussion Forums

Discussion forums are places in which students can collaborate asynchronously in response to an initial post written by faculty or possibly a student moderator. Activities created in the discussion forum "may include text, audio, video and images"

Table 8-5 The Purpose of Commonly Used Learning Activities

Learning Activity	Purpose
Discussion forum	Collaborative learning in which students develop higher-order thinking skills, including critical thinking, creative thinking, and problem solving that is supported by evidence.
Blog	Students reflect on a topic in order to engage in a critical dialogue in which diverse opinions and perspectives are shared. The blog can be designed as a less formal discussion than a traditional discussion activity.
Journal	Private interactions between the student and faculty to promote deep reflection that they may not want to share with the class.

(Vai & Sosulski, 2016, p. 20). When designing discussion forums, there are several considerations, including how many students to have in the discussion, how to construct the initial post as a question or prompt, the expectations, and how to assess the learning. When discussion groups are too large or too small, the quality of the discussion may be diminished. We have found that an average of 8–12 students provides for an opportunity to have collaboration in which the application of Vygotsky's zone of proximal development (ZPD) is most effective (Vygotsky, 1978/1997). In many online platforms, discussion groups can be set up so that students in one group can see the work of the other groups. Small, private groups of five or six students may contribute to students reading every post within their forum, but the opportunity to learn and engage with more nurses with various degrees of experience is very limited. These small, private groups should be limited to group work, not class discussions.

The construction of the discussion question or prompt is a very important consideration. The most important thing to consider is how the prompt can lead to meeting the purpose of discussions, which is collaborative learning in which students develop higher-order thinking skills. The role of the faculty in advancing this purpose should not be underestimated and is discussed more specifically in Chapter 9.

The discussion board is often considered the equivalent of a face-to-face class discussion, but there are some unique differences. Discussions often require students to support their posts with evidence from the course materials and other literature. Asynchronous discussions also allow time for students to thoughtfully respond. In many ways, this can facilitate a higher-level discussion than what is ordinarily achieved in the face-to-face classroom.

Boettcher and Conrad (2010) suggest a three-part discussion prompt that includes *what* the learners' thoughts and recommendations are and *why* the learners think what they do, including thoughts, experiences, and beliefs. The third part is having learners state what they wish they knew or what problems or challenges will follow. These suggestions are important for developing discussions that avoid simple right-or-wrong answers that may result in repetitive responses that do not advance higher-level thinking. Discussions that have a "right" answer are equivalent to short-answer knowledge questions on a test but shared with the class to be judged. Some examples of discussion questions are provided in **Table 8-6**. As a reminder, all learning activities should relate to the module learning objectives, which are designed to meet the course outcomes. Module development and learning objectives are discussed further in this chapter.

Blogs

Blogs can serve as a less formal opportunity to create interaction in the online classroom by requiring students to reflect on certain topics and share their opinions. We use blogs for controversial topics or to bring awareness to an issue. The intent is to give students the opportunity to share diverse opinions and perspectives without being judged. Students comment on their peers' blogs, but there is no requirement to carry the discussion forward as in the discussion forum. They may respectfully disagree and present their perspectives in the comments.

Blogs have been very successful in our population health course; students enjoy the less formal activity and appreciate discussing personal opinions about challenging community and public health topics (Robinson, 2017). In order to promote

Table 8-6 Discussion Question Examples

Course: Population Health

Learning Objective

Examine circumstances that make populations vulnerable and underserved.

Discussion About Economics

Analyze why the cycle of poverty is a challenge to break. Explore factors such as personal lifestyle, mental health, personal responsibility, biography, and biology. How might this information affect how you approach patient care?
Use multiple sources to support your discussion.

Course: Palliative Care

Learning Objective

Analyze ethical dilemmas identified by nurses, including truth telling, medically futile care, and palliative sedation.

Discussion About Advanced Care Planning

Discuss the essential components of advance care planning. Share any experiences that you have with this in your own family or in your clinical work. What challenges may arise when attempting to keep the patient at the center of decision making?

Use evidence to support your discussion.

Course: Professional Communication

Learning Objective

Apply reflective practice to a personal nursing practice example.

Discussion About Empathy

After viewing the videos on empathy and reading at least two of the articles:

How would you assess your ability to communicate empathy in the nurse–patient relationship? Provide an example to support your assessment. How is empathy related to emotional intelligence? What are some barriers to being able to communicate empathy that you experience, and how could they be overcome?

Be sure to cite literature to support your discussion.

Course: Nursing Leadership

Learning Outcome

Discuss different models of patient safety.

Discussion About Patient Safety Based on a Case Study

Case Study: There was a very serious close call on the pediatric outpatient unit that could have led to a child's death. Be sure to look up both chemotherapies used in this case study if you are not familiar with them. Discuss how complex adaptive systems theory, human factors, *and* the swiss cheese model provide a way to understand the near-miss. Why is this important? How should Elaine, the nurse manager in the case study, respond? How might you apply the learning from this near-miss and your understanding of what happened to your practice?

Be sure to cite literature to support your response.

meaningful discussion, students are assigned to read, listen to, or view a variety of different materials, such as YouTube videos, TED talks, podcasts, and web resources with reliable public health data to highlight prevalence. Some topics for blogs that we have used include human trafficking, rape on the reservation, rural oral health disparities, gun violence in the United States, and the opioid epidemic, to name a few (Robinson, 2017).

We have also used blogs to address a number of challenging practice issues encountered by nurses. For example, in a comprehensive leadership case study, a nurse manager is faced with terminating two nurses for ongoing incivility. The blog in response to this case study was effective for eliciting a diversity of opinions about the manger's leadership style and the impact of this action on the other staff.

Journals

Journals provide the opportunity for students to share their reflective work privately with the faculty member. It is important to base the decision on whether to use a shared or private journal on the intended learning outcome. Shared forums allow for collaborative learning, whereas private journals allow for deep personal reflections that students may not want to share with the class. For example, in our trauma-informed care course, students share some deeply personal information about trauma in their own lives through journal writing. It provides them with the opportunity to reflect on how the trauma affected them and how it may be helping or hindering their nursing practice.

Assessments and Grading Rubrics

As stated earlier, interactive learning activities are also assessed. This is much different than in a face-to-face class, where participation may be graded but rarely assessed. However, one could view any assessment as a learning activity. For example, when writing a paper, students are learning not only about the content but also about the process of academic writing. Much has to do with the quality of the feedback provided; this is discussed more fully in Chapter 9.

The use of grading rubrics in online classes is highly recommended and consistent with best practice. Important considerations for designing a grading rubric include the following: (1) the purpose of the learning activity, such as the learning process or outcome; (2) the criteria that represent meeting the requirements; (3) division of the criteria to represent distinct and meaningful levels; and (4) descriptions for each criterion and level. We share multiple examples of instructions and grading rubrics in **Tables 8-7** to **8-11**, as follows:

- Tables 8-7 and 8-9: instructions and grading rubrics that include all four considerations
- Tables 8-8 and 8-10: less formal grading criteria
- Table 8-11: rubrics that focus on feedback

A grading rubric that lists content that coincides with the instructions is intended to provide extensive feedback to the student. We commonly use such rubrics for major papers, along with tracked changes to provide feedback in context. Some tools within LMSs, such as Blackboard, Canvas, and Moodle, allow faculty and instructional designers to develop rubrics that include numeric grading as well as space for narrative feedback within the grading rubric for each criterion.

Table 8-7 Discussion Grading Rubric

Instructions: The purpose of class discussions is to collaborate with peers and the instructor on the course content to share experiences, build knowledge, reflect on ideas, and improve critical thinking. Discussions require students to apply scholarly literature, collaborate in a professional manner, and demonstrate respect for different perspectives. Evaluation is based on the following: (1) posting substantive primary posts, which are generally 200–250 words but may be longer depending on the discussion, and (2) meaningful replies to others that demonstrate thoughtful consideration of the assigned reading material, in addition to personal experiences in the practice setting. Direct quotes are to be minimally used—no more than one brief direct quote (not to exceed 15 words) per discussion—and must add substantially to the discussion. Learning to paraphrase increases critical thinking about the topic and in writing.

Criteria	Needs Improvement 0–6	Satisfactory 7–8	Excellent 9–10
Quality of Response	Primary response demonstrates a limited understanding of the discussion topics. Includes basic examples but lacks substantive information and connections to the course material.	Primary response demonstrates a satisfactory understanding of the discussion topics through well-reasoned and thoughtful reflections. Factually correct but lacks full development and strong connections to the course material.	Primary response demonstrates a strong understanding of the discussion topics. Evidence of strong critical and reflective thinking. Strong connections to the course material.
Application to Practice	Demonstrates limited connection to experiences in the practice setting or community (examples).	Demonstrates a satisfactory connection to experiences in the practice setting or community (examples).	Demonstrates excellent connections to experiences in the practice setting or community (examples).
Collaboration	Collaborates with peers without relating discussion to relevant examples and/or the course material. Comments are superficial (e.g., "I agree").	Collaborates with peers, relating their comments to relevant examples and/or the course material.	Collaborates with peers, relating the discussion to relevant examples and course material. Advances the discussion.

(continues)

Table 8-7 Discussion Grading Rubric *(continued)*

Criteria	Needs Improvement 0–6	Satisfactory 7–8	Excellent 9–10
Use of Evidence	Little to no relevant evidence used to demonstrate connections between course material and discussion.	Provides relevant evidence but does not clearly demonstrate a connection between course material and the discussion.	Provides relevant evidence of support for discussion using course material or other relevant literature.

Expectations for Participation	Expectations for participation were not met.
	    Writing includes grammatical errors or may not demonstrate proper etiquette.
		Participation was limited to 1 day or may lack replies.
		    Writing is grammatically correct.
		    Responds to peers/instructor using their names and signs all posts.
			Contributes regularly and on a timely basis.
			    Posts primary discussion by due date and at least two replies to peers on a different day.
			    Writing is grammatically correct.
			    Responds to peers/instructor using their names and signs all posts.

Table 8-8 Blog Instructions and Grading Rubric

Blog Instructions
Choose one of the blog topics for the week. You are more than welcome to be active on more than one blog; however, grading for participation in this activity will occur based on your work in one of the blogs.

Create one primary blog entry in response to the topic presented and post two comments in response to the blog entries of your peers.

The goal of the blog is to increase our awareness of critical public health issues going on in the community by engaging in an informal discussion. Please share your opinions and perspectives in a respectful and engaging manner. Blog posts should be related to the topic and should demonstrate appropriate and nonoffensive language.

There is no need to cite course material in this blog; however, please feel free to share resources, informative links, or pictures. Consider this an opportunity to be creative and share your unique and valuable perspectives.

Grading Rubric: Public Health Blog Participation

Public Health Blog	8 Points Possible
Choose one blog for participation during the assigned module.	**Grading will be based on participation that is respectful, engaging, and completed on time.**
Create one primary blog entry in response to the topic and materials presented.	**4 points**
Post two comments in response to the blog entries of peers.	**4 points**

Table 8-9 Formal Journal Instructions and Grading Rubric

Journal Instruction

Share the results of the health literacy quiz. After reviewing the information about health literacy and completing the quiz,

(1) How do you evaluate yourself on your ability to assess the needs of a patient who has a barrier related to literacy or health literacy (provide examples from your practice)?

(2) What changes might you make, given what you have learned in the module?

Criteria	Excellent 11–12	Met Requirement 9.5–11	Needs Improvement 0–9
Depth of Reflection	Response demonstrates an in-depth reflection on, and personalization of, the theories, concepts, and/or strategies presented in the course materials to date. Viewpoints and interpretations are insightful and well supported. Clear, detailed examples are provided, as applicable.	Response demonstrates a general reflection on, and personalization of, the theories, concepts, and/or strategies presented in the course materials to date. Viewpoints and interpretations are supported. Appropriate examples are provided, as applicable.	Response demonstrates a minimal reflection on, and personalization of, the theories, concepts, and/or strategies presented in the course materials to date. Viewpoints and interpretations are unsupported or supported with flawed arguments. Examples, when applicable, are not provided or are irrelevant to the assignment.

(continues)

Table 8-9 Formal Journal Instructions and Grading Rubric   *(continued)*

Components	7.5–8	6.5–7	0–6
	Response includes all components and meets or exceeds all requirements indicated in the instructions. Each question or part of the assignment is addressed thoroughly.	Response includes all components and meets all requirements indicated in the instructions. Each question or part of the assignment is addressed.	Response is missing some components and/or does not fully meet the requirements indicated in the instructions. Some questions or parts of the assignment are not addressed.
Writing	No points deducted	Up to 2 points deducted	Up to 3 points deducted
	Writing is clear, concise, and well organized, with excellent sentence and paragraph construction. Thoughts are expressed in a coherent and logical manner. There are no more than three spelling and grammar errors.	Writing is mostly clear, concise, and well organized, with good sentence and paragraph construction. Thoughts are expressed in a coherent and logical manner. There are no more than five spelling and grammar errors.	Writing is unclear and/or disorganized. Thoughts are not expressed in a logical manner. There are more than five spelling and grammar errors.

Table 8-10 Informal Journal Instructions and Grading

Instructions:

1. Take the Adverse Childhood Experiences (ACE) Quiz
2. Reflect on your ACE score. Share as much as you feel comfortable and any new awareness that you would like to share.
3. What are your reactions to how children learn and develop in early life?
4. What concerns do you have for adults who may have experienced ACEs or other types of trauma across their lifetime?
5. How does this information affect you?

Please utilize this opportunity to personally reflect on the concepts and material in this course. This is a private journal that is only visible to you and your faculty. Faculty will provide feedback for each journal activity.

Grading will be based on the following:

- Your participation should be meaningful.
- Reflections should include any new awareness, questions that are emerging, and new insights as a result of the learning in this class.
- Utilize this as a personal tool for developing your professional and reflective practice.
- Feel free to reflect on topics that expand on the topics presented, including those that interest, inspire, or challenge you.

There is no length requirement; however, the reflection should address the topics presented.

Citations are not required for this activity unless you use a specific idea from another source or have paraphrased information that requires a citation.

Table 8-11 PowerPoint Assignment Using the Instructions for the Grading Rubric

Quality-Improvement Presentation
The purpose of this assignment is as follows:

1. Apply a quality- or performance-improvement process to a problem you see either in your service-learning site or in your workplace.
2. Develop a professional presentation on quality improvement (QI).
3. Learn about and use some of the common QI tools (e.g., flowchart, fishbone diagram for root-cause analysis)

Description
Improvement requires change. There are many different kinds of changes that could lead to improvement. A QI process is just that—a means for achieving a needed improvement in how something is done. The decision to engage in a QI process is usually the result of a noted pattern of errors, a near-miss or close call, or something noticed by nurses or others that could be improved for more efficiency and improved quality of care. A QI process is not simply a major change, such as the merger of two units or a change in staffing patterns or the staff mix, because such changes do not lend themselves to the use of a QI process but, rather, the use of change theory or a change process. However, a recommendation regarding staffing may be a result of going through a QI process.

You will select a potential area for improvement in your service-learning site or workplace and develop a professional PowerPoint presentation using the model of improvement, the plan–do–study–act (PDSA) model.

The following are just some examples of changes you may want to see that lend themselves to a performance-improvement or QI process:

- Reducing the risk for an adverse event that could happen in your place of work
- Eliminating waste (e.g., materials thrown out, duplication of work)
- Improvement in workflow
- Enhancing productivity
- A procedure change
- An improvement in one of the nurse sensitive indicators

(continues)

Table 8-11 PowerPoint Assignment Using the Instructions for the Grading Rubric *(continued)*

Grading Criteria	Points	Earned	Comments
Grading Rubric *Plan* Addresses all requirements in a manner that leaves no doubt about the process that is to be improved	**15**		
Do Data identified and realistic Use graph as appropriate	**10**		
Check/Study Conclusions are concisely and clearly stated	**10**		
Act Adopt, adapt, or abandon	**10**		
Presentation Good use of pictures, color, space, bullet points, minimal APA/spelling errors	**5**		
Total	**50**		

The example in Table 8-9 is a good one to think about. Should this actually be discussed in a shared forum? This needs to be decided based on an analysis of the students in the class and the need for collaborative reflection. For example, if there is a mix of experienced and new graduate nurses, there is an opportunity for experienced nurses to reflect on their current practice and share with the inexperienced nurses. The sharing of real-world nursing experiences is highly valued by inexperienced nurses and is an application of Vygotsky's (1978/1997) ZPD. It also provides an opportunity for the experienced nurse to mentor. On the other hand, it is not uncommon for experienced nurses to feel uncomfortable sharing honestly about the ways they need to improve, so a private forum may be more appropriate. The message here is that every design tool used needs to be carefully considered, taking into account several factors, including the student population and the purpose of the activity.

In summary, assessing student learning requires careful consideration because many factors go into the design of learning activities and assessment. Several examples have been provided. However, all faculty need to reflect on the expected learning outcomes and make decisions on how students will demonstrate that they have met them and, equally important, what will be needed to guide them in working toward meeting the outcomes. Designing the course in a way that creates the most meaningful learning experiences often takes creativity, critical thinking, reflection, and collaboration—the same things we ask of our students. As these major items are being designed, the structure and sequencing of the course need to be considered, as well as the course materials.

Structure and Sequencing of the Course

Providing an orientation to the program and the technology students will be using helps students build confidence as they start their program. We created an online orientation in the LMS Blackboard Learn to introduce the students to the program; show them how to navigate the LMS; and show them how to access resources, such as academic advising support, the online library, tutoring, information technology (IT) support, and more.

Course design includes placing a focus on course navigation to ensure that students have a successful experience in the course. As faculty, it is important to attempt to put yourself in the role of the student, which is easier if you have been an online student. It is very frustrating for students if they feel they have to go on a scavenger hunt to find what they are looking for or if the classroom seems chaotic. Using the same format for all courses, with clear guidance provided through written or visual instructions, is very useful. A video walking through the course and showing students where to find things is always welcomed by students. Be sure to include the syllabus and calendar, with explicit due dates for assessed learning activities.

Faculty may teach in institutions that have consistency in how many weeks each term or semester is. This makes for consistency in the structure and sequencing of each course all year long. However, other faculty members work in settings that have a different number of weeks depending on the term. This is an important consideration in structuring and sequencing the course. For example, if one semester is 14 weeks and another semester is 7 weeks, it may make sense to develop seven modules of 1 or 2 weeks each, depending on the semester in which it is taught. This requires careful planning to consider the overall course design.

Learning Modules

We recommend that each course be divided into modules (see an example of a learning module page in **Figure 8-2**). We recommend the following for this part of the design process:

1. Develop learning objectives for the module.
2. Identify the relevant program concepts that are addressed or provide a topic outline.
3. Divide the module into weeks. The number of weeks depends on the amount of content and the work required to meet the module objectives.

To keep students engaged, we have found it necessary to have students be actively involved each week in a discussion, blog, journal, or some other activity that is graded. A consistent pattern that is predictable appears to be the most successful. An example of this consistency starts with identifying the online week. Most online programs have an identified online week, such as Monday to Sunday. Initial posts for discussions and blogs are due on Thursdays, and replies or comments are due on Sunday. All written assignments or projects are due on Sunday.

A folder for each module is an effective way for students to navigate through a course easily. Figure 8-2 provides an example from one of our courses that illustrates how the page looks when the student selects Learning Modules from the course

Learning Module 1

Introductions

Emotional Intelligence & Empathy

Week 1: Feb. 17 - 23

Week 2: Feb. 24 - March 1

Relevant Course Outcome: 1

Learning Module 2

Clinical Reasoning & Reflective Practice

Week 3: March 2 - 8

Week 4: March 9 - 15

Relevant Course Outcomes: 1, 3

Learning Module 3

Trauma Informed Care

Week 5: March 16 - 22

Week 6: March 23 - 29 (Study Break)

Relevant Course Outcomes: 1, 3

Figure 8-2 Learning module page

navigation column. When the module folder is opened, the student first sees a list of concepts, objectives, a clear "to-do" list, and assessment and learning strategies, followed by the reading assignment as illustrated in **Figure 8-3**. **Figure 8-4** illustrates the learning materials that are used for this module and the links to the assessments.

Learning Materials

Choosing learning materials for an online course may be a daunting task, given how many resources are available to choose from. It may be tempting to include too much, which will overwhelm students, thus the need to use discretion. Learning materials may include websites, webinars, videos, articles, podcasts, and relevant web courses, to name a few. It is incumbent on faculty to provide materials that support the objectives of the learning module and promote active learning. Students

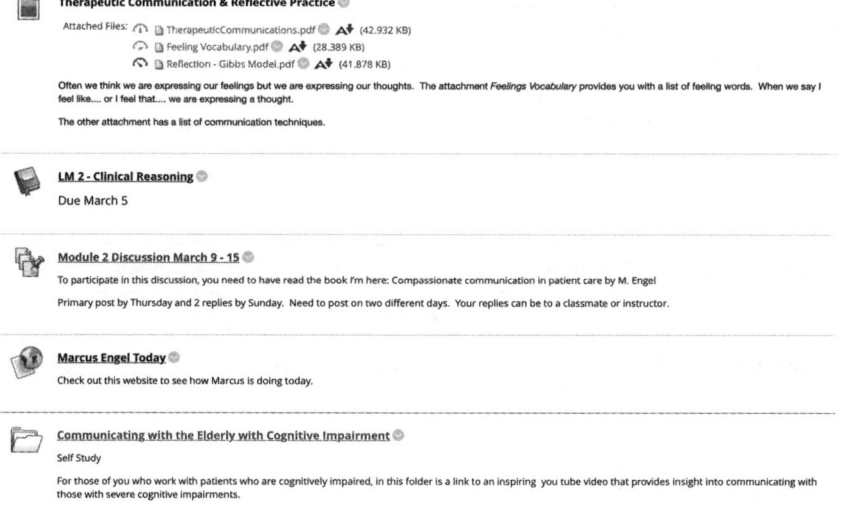

Reflective Practice & Clinical Reasoning

Concepts	Objectives
Clinical Reasoning	To be successful in this learning module, you will be expected to:
Therapeutic Communication	1. Apply clinical reasoning to a case study or practice example
Reflective Practice	2. Examine therapeutic communication 3. Apply reflective practice to a personal nursing practice example
To Do List & Assessment Activities	
To Do List	

1. Read all the information in the Learning Module
2. Finish reading the book "I'm Here"

Look ahead to the next LM as you have a paper due based on an interview. Schedule an interview.

Assessment

1. Module 2 Journal - Clinical Reasoning due by March 5
2. Participate in LM 2 Discussion based on the book "I'm Here" and Gibb's Model

Reading Assignment

Kearney-Nunnery - chapter 6 (Effective Communication chapter)

Book - I'm Here by Marcus Engel

Figure 8-3 Example of a learning module that has the identified components

Therapeutic Communication & Reflective Practice

Attached Files: ⬆ TherapeuticCommunications.pdf A⬇ (42.932 KB)
⬆ Feeling Vocabulary.pdf A⬇ (28.389 KB)
⬆ Reflection - Gibbs Model.pdf A⬇ (41.878 KB)

Often we think we are expressing our feelings but we are expressing our thoughts. The attachment *Feelings Vocabulary* provides you with a list of feeling words. When we say I feel like.... or I feel that.... we are expressing a thought.

The other attachment has a list of communication techniques.

LM 2 - Clinical Reasoning

Due March 5

Module 2 Discussion March 9 - 15

To participate in this discussion, you need to have read the book I'm here: Compassionate communication in patient care by M. Engel

Primary post by Thursday and 2 replies by Sunday. Need to post on two different days. Your replies can be to a classmate or instructor.

Marcus Engel Today

Check out this website to see how Marcus is doing today.

Communicating with the Elderly with Cognitive Impairment

Self Study

For those of you who work with patients who are cognitively impaired, in this folder is a link to an inspiring you tube video that provides insight into communicating with those with severe cognitive impairments.

Figure 8-4 Learning materials and links to the assessments

who are engaged in reading, listening, or watching are active participants in the learning process (Vai & Sosulski, 2016). We have also used interactive activities that require students to participate by answering questions or participating in a quiz to earn a certificate. Many organizations, such as the Federal Emergency Management Agency (FEMA) and ACEs Connection, provide these kinds of activities that support active learning and learning outcomes.

Some faculty like to include PowerPoint presentations, which we prefer not to use because they often miss the context for learning, which is more richly discussed in books and articles. Narrated presentations mimic classroom lectures, making them a form of passive learning and contrary to our educational philosophy. Exceptions to this are carefully considered. It is important to include instructions on how to use the learning materials as needed. For example, advising students on how long a video or podcast is lets them know how much time to set aside (Stavredes & Herder, 2014).

In Figure 8-4, you will note that the last folder is for self-study materials. This is an effective way to provide learning materials that are consistent with the module objectives but are more specialized. Students may choose to explore them depending on their nursing practice environment.

Leveling and Scaffolding

When designing the course, faculty need to simultaneously pay attention to leveling and scaffolding. For example, if the course builds on a previous course, it is incumbent on the faculty to have a good understanding of how and to what depth a concept was explored, understood, and applied in order to level their course appropriately. Again, this drives home the message of how important collaboration is to the success of an online program.

Conceptual scaffolding is particularly important because conceptual understanding deepens as students progress through the program and individual courses. Consistent with constructivist learning theory, students are guided to link prior knowledge to new learning and to use critical thinking and questioning of their underlying assumptions and beliefs, thereby transforming their thinking (Stavredes & Herder, 2014). **Table 8-12** provides an example that demonstrates how the concept of leadership is leveled and scaffolded over two semesters.

Table 8-12 An Example of Scaffolding the Concept of Leadership

Semester 3	
Learning Activity	**Assessment**
Contrast the concepts of leadership, management, and followership.	Self-assessment (formative)
Share results and compare to previous learning and experience with the three concepts.	Collaborative discussion (formative)
Review case study chronicling the experiences of a nurse manager to address patient safety, leadership theory/styles, change, etc.	Collaborative discussion and blogs (formative)
Review the leadership skills required of clinical nurses at different levels through reading assignments and YouTube videos.	Comprehensive personal leadership development plan that includes identifying competencies, skills, and goals
Plan for service-learning experience for semester 4.	Collaborative discussion with service-learning coordinator (formative—not graded)

Semester 4	
Develop a service-learning plan in the community, negotiating the service and schedule.	Present plan in collaborative discussion (formative)
Draft an initial idea/plan for a QI project based on work or service-learning experience.	Collaborative discussion with faculty (formative)
Implement as much as possible and report on the QI project.	PowerPoint assignment (summative)
Interview a nurse leader, addressing issues such as change, leadership style, holding staff accountable, ethical decision making, etc.	Write a formal paper reporting on the interview findings, assessment of the nurse leader, and application of leadership theory and principles (summative)
Engage in service learning in the community by working with a vulnerable population, using nursing knowledge and skills in working with the chosen organization. Provide leadership to the staff in regard to health-related issues as appropriate, depending on the service-lea rning site.	Two formative journals Journal prior to starting Journal midway through the experience Final journal in which they reflect on their leadership, among other concepts (summative) Collaborative discussion (formative)
Personal leadership development	Report on progress made on goals developed in semester 3 (formative)

Evaluation

Asking for feedback from students when a course is taught for the first time provides valuable information. Feedback about the ease of navigating the course is particularly helpful. It is not uncommon to teach a course about three times before it is completely to your satisfaction. You can anticipate spending 20–30 hours preparing your course if you have taught a face-to-face version before and are familiar with the LMS. More time will be needed if this is the first time you have taught an online course (Boettcher & Conrad, 2016). Each time you teach the same course, you must carefully review the course to ensure your content is current; to confirm that internal and external links are functional; and most importantly, to make changes based on student feedback not only in terms of content, as appropriate, but also design.

Best-Practice Recommendations for Online Teaching

- Keep the student at the center of the design.
- Provide online students with collaborative and individual learning experiences.

- Use formative assessments throughout the course based on learning activities that meet the module objectives, which in turn will facilitate students' ability to meet the course outcomes.
- When designing the course, collaborate with instructional designers and other faculty to enhance creativity and ensure alignment or leveling of the course.
- Engage in ongoing reflection throughout the online course design process to truly provide an integrative design.

References

Boettcher, J. V., & Conrad, R. M. (2016). *The online teaching survival guide: Simple and practical pedagogical tips.* Jossey-Bass.

Breen, H. (2015). Assessing online collaborative discourse. *Nursing Forum, 50*(4), 218–227. https://doi.org/10.1111/nuf.12091

Dee Fink, L. (2013). *Creating significant learning experiences: An integrated approach to designing college courses.* Jossey-Bass.

Hoque, M. E. (2016). Three domains of learning: Cognitive, affective and psychomotor. *The Journal of EFL Education and Research, 2*(2), 45–52.

Johnson, A. E., & Meehan, N. K. (2013). Faculty preparation for teaching online. In K. H. Frith & D. B. Clark (Eds.), *Distance education in nursing* (3rd ed., pp. 33–52). Springer.

Kirkpatrick, J. M., & DeWitt, D. (2020). Strategies for evaluating learning outcomes. In D. M. Billings & J. A. Halstead (Eds.), *Teaching in nursing: A guide for faculty* (6th ed., pp. 353–373). Elsevier.

Krathwohl, D. R., Bloom, B.S., & Mases, B. (1964). Taxonomy of educational objectives. In *Handbook II, affective domain* (pp. 66–91). David McKay.

Lee, C., Dickerson, J., & Winslow, J. (2012). An analysis of organizational approaches to online course structures. *Online Journal of Distance Learning Administration, 15*(1). https://www.westga.edu/~distance/ojdla/spring151/lee_dickerson_winslow.html

Oermann, M. (2017). *A systematic approach to assessment and evaluation of nursing programs.* National League for Nursing.

Robinson, M. (2017). Using blogs to increase awareness of public health issues. *Journal of Nursing Education, 56*(8), 514–515.

Santelli, B., Stewart, K., & Mandernach, J. (2020). Supporting high quality teaching in online programs. *Journal of Educators Online, 17*(1). https://files.eric.ed.gov/fulltext/EJ1241555.pdf

Scheckel, M. (2020). Designing courses and learning experiences. In D. M. Billings & J. A. Halstead (Eds.), *Teaching in nursing: A guide for faculty* (6th ed., pp. 353–373). Elsevier.

Stavredes, T., & Herder, T. (2014). *A guide to online course design: Strategies for student success.* Jossey-Bass.

Stewart, M. K., Cohn, J., & Whithaus, C. (2016). Collaborative course design and communities of practice: Strategies for adaptable course shells in hybrid and online writing. *Transformative Dialogues: Teaching & Learning Journal, 9*(1), 1–20.

Vai, M., & Sosulski, K. (2016). *Essentials of online course design: A standards-based guide* (2nd ed.). Routledge.

Vygotsky, L. (1997). Interaction between learning and development. In M. Gauvain & M. Cole (Eds.), *Readings on the development of children* (Vol. 2, pp. 29–36). W. H. Freeman and Company. (Reprinted from *Mind and society*, pp. 79–91, by L. Vygotsky, 1978, Cambridge University Press.)

Wiggins, G. (1998). *Educative assessment: Designing assessments to inform and improve student performance.* Jossey-Bass.

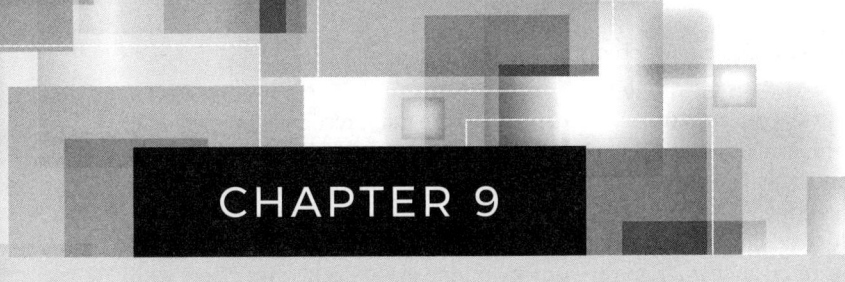

CHAPTER 9

Online Teaching Strategies

Henny Breen and Melissa Robinson

"Online discussions have more depth and meaning. In the current political climate, people are so divided and don't care why others might have a different attitude about something. Since students are able to share the experiences that have shaped and molded them, we can respect each other and maybe even challenge our own thought processes to incorporate the new ideas into our current belief systems."

(Online RN-to-BSN student)

Overview

This chapter begins with a brief discussion about the requirements for faculty to be prepared to teach online. A more thorough discussion of faculty preparation, from the perspective of faculty professional development, is found in Chapter 13. This chapter addresses the role of faculty in a learner-centered online classroom that is built on constructivist pedagogy and adult learning principles. Strategies for teaching are provided, along with examples.

Faculty Preparation for Teaching Online

Within nursing, there is a beginning acknowledgment that having content and clinical expertise is not enough to teach effectively. Education and nursing are two unique disciplines, and expertise in one does not result in expertise in the other. The American Association of Colleges of Nursing (AACN) and the National League of Nursing (NLN) both acknowledge that graduate-level evidence-based curriculum design and teaching methods are needed to form the foundation for academic practice. The NLN establishes nursing education as a specialty area of practice through its certified nurse educator (CNE) credentialing program recognizing academic nurse educators as an advanced practice role (Booth, Emerson, Hackney, & Souter, 2016). We concur with Booth et al. in advocating for pedagogical preparation for academic nurse educators.

For faculty teaching online, we believe this pedagogical preparation is essential for developing and teaching a rigorous, quality online class. Faculty members who want to transition from face-to-face teaching to quality online teaching need to have a solid foundation in education theory that is learner centered. We believe that online teaching is a specialty within the advanced practice role of academic nurse educators that requires further preparation in how to apply constructivist pedagogy to the online learning environment. Engaging in ongoing self-reflection prior to and during the teaching process is critical for faculty to develop expertise in online teaching. Palloff and Pratt (2007) challenge online instructors to engage in a transformative process of reflection, just as they would require of their students. Chapter 13 addresses the process of self-reflection. Reflective questions that we continually ask ourselves related to teaching online are found in **Table 9-1**.

Much has been written about teaching strategies that facilitate learner-centered teaching. However, less has been written about the skills needed by faculty to make the transition to learner-centered teaching—and even less as it applies to online teaching. The following section addresses that need in addition to providing several examples of teaching strategies that we have found effective in facilitating a learner-centered online classroom for nursing students.

Learner-Centered Teaching

Learner-centered teaching is based on constructivist theory, in that learners discover and transform complex information to make it their own. It is an inquiry-based approach that involves active, collaborative, and cooperative learning. Faculty guide and facilitate learning, with more of the focus on learning and less on teaching (Weimer, 2013). This requires a different set of skills that may be difficult to develop because they may not be as intuitive when making the transition to online teaching. It is also important to note that not all faculty want or need to make the transition and may not be suited for online teaching (Smith, 2005).

Table 9-1 Reflective Questions Related to Teaching

1. Am I getting too comfortable by relying on a specific set of strategies and methods?
2. Do I need to move out of my comfort zone to use different strategies and learning activities to meet the needs of different learners as the demographics of online learners change?
3. Am I facilitating discussions that are open to different perspectives?
4. What can I learn from the literature and other scholars about meeting the learning needs of diverse students in terms of age, generation, background, previous education, culture, and prelicensure versus postlicensure?
5. Are my current strategies and methods providing students the ability to meet the course outcomes?
6. Are there additional ways that I can seek feedback from students about their experiences in my classes?

Faculty who do not have a solid belief in the tenets of constructivism will likely struggle with trusting the process of active learning. Faculty who use lectures, whether in the face-to-face classroom or online through narration as their primary mode of teaching, demonstrate a belief in passive learning, in which students need to acquire new knowledge based on the expertise of the teacher passing on knowledge. However, constructivist faculty believe that information may be received passively, but understanding cannot be. Understanding comes from active learning in which the students make connections between prior knowledge, new knowledge, and the processes involved in learning (Candela, 2020; Harasim, 2017). At the same time, we do not endorse a radical approach to constructivism in which no teaching instruction takes place.

Concept-Based and Competency-Based Teaching

Nursing faculty who have made the transition to conceptual teaching may have an easier time making the transition to learner-centered teaching. Inherent within conceptual teaching is letting go of the need to "cover everything" and, rather, facilitate new learning while building on previous learning. Faculty choose concepts related to nursing practice from which students discover common principles that can be generalized to various contexts, along with discovering the relationship between concepts. Conceptual teaching facilitates the process of conceptual learning by linking new information to past learning, which in turn deepens and expands conceptual understanding. Given the continuous advances in health care, it is clear that nurses need to be skilled in conceptual thinking and clinical reasoning to adapt to these changes (Giddens, 2020). Conceptual teaching requires an understanding of constructivist pedagogy.

Faculty may also be concerned about competencies, given that many organizations, such as the ANA and Quality and Safety Education for Nurses (QSEN), have developed competencies. These competencies are represented through concepts or domains that reflect concepts (Giddens, 2020). To clear up confusion between what it means to be concept based versus competency based, Giddens (2020) provides a clear distinction while acknowledging that they share the same origin. The differences lie in the application and the outcome. *Competencies* describe the intended outcome, whereas *concepts* refer to the learning process because they are used as the framework to build knowledge. Competencies are observable and measurable skills that integrate knowledge, values, and beliefs that are assessed over time.

The Faculty Role in Constructivist Teaching

The faculty role is to provide a safe and organized environment for learning in which key principles or values of constructivist learning pedagogy are applied.

Scaffolded Teaching

Scaffolded learning is also known as the *zone of proximal development* (ZPD), a concept created by Vygotsky (1978/1997). The ZPD "is the distance between the actual developmental level as determined by independent problem-solving and the level of potential problem-solving under adult guidance or in collaboration with more capable peers" (Vygotsky, 1978/1997, p. 8). Faculty are responsible for guiding the learner through the zone by designing learning opportunities (scaffolds) that guide the student through the scaffolds in a way that provides context, motivation, and the foundation from which the new understanding can occur. These scaffolds are gradually removed as the student progresses and is able to demonstrate comprehension and skill independently (Harasim, 2017). At that point, the student may take on the role of a mentor or a "more capable peer" in the teaching process.

Active Learning and Teaching

Active learning refers to students being engaged in a way that promotes analysis, synthesis, and evaluation of course content (Harasim, 2017). This requires faculty to be highly skilled in encouraging and guiding students to participate in a way that promotes reflecting on course content and how it fits with their current knowledge, evaluating new information, and transforming that information and applying it to their practice as appropriate.

A study examining the types of interactions that are most predictive of students' sense of community included introduction, collaborative group projects, sharing personal experiences, entire class discussions, and exchanging resources (Shackelford & Maxwell, 2012). The students' sense of connectedness and learning were enhanced by faculty drawing in participants, creating an accepting climate for learning, keeping students on track, diagnosing students' misperceptions, looking for areas of consensus when there is disagreement, reinforcing student contributions, and injecting their own knowledge and confirming student understanding (Shea, 2006). Some of the instrumental requirements include setting time parameters, due dates, deadlines, clear course topics and instructions, and guidelines on how to effectively and appropriately participate in and contribute to the discussion.

It is not uncommon for faculty new to online teaching to engage in passive teaching strategies without being aware they are doing so. For example, they provide narrated PowerPoint presentations or some other form of video lecture for students. We have found that a faculty reliance on textbooks and lectures often leads to knowledge-based questions that inhibit students from moving through the inquiry process. This is not to say that these kinds of passive activities are never done, but all learning tasks need to be carefully considered, keeping in mind the educational purpose. For example, a 10-minute lecture may be required when introducing a new or complex concept, which is then used to promote discussion.

Providing articles and links to sources that can be found in the library rather than having students find the source themselves may curtail the exploration phase and students' ability to critically examine the literature for the most relevant information. Students who seek resources for themselves increase their information technology skills. At the same time, it is important for faculty to remember the importance of scaffolding information and skills to increase the students' competence in finding, assessing, and using relevant information. **Table 9-2** provides teaching suggestions to facilitate active learning.

The faculty role is critical in setting up opportunities for students to do the work of developing the skills needed to solve problems and address other issues

Table 9-2 Active Learning and Teaching Suggestions

1. Assign a podcast, recorded lecture, voiceover PowerPoint presentation, or reading material. (*passive*)
   - Assign guided questions or a learning quiz (pre or post) on the material. (*active*)
   - Develop a case-study assignment that involves solving a specific problem or developing an action plan for care. (*active*)
   - Facilitate an interactive, collaborative discussion on the topic. (*active*)
   - Engage students in a small-group activity, such as a role-play or debate. (*active*)
2. Assign study material focused on specific concepts: health disparities, vulnerable populations, equity versus equality, and advocacy. (*passive*)
   - Facilitate an interactive discussion that requires students to share their personal observations on the issues in their own community. (*active*)
   - Create an assignment for students to work in pairs to analyze the policy issues in their community that affect vulnerable populations and develop an advocacy statement. Require students to use tools such as a wiki, blog, or Google doc. (*active*)
   - Develop an individual reflective activity for students to examine their assumptions, beliefs, and values about the study material and their experience. (*active*)
3. Assign a novel or movie related to a certain topic (e.g., leadership, public health, mental health, death and dying). (*passive*)
   - Create a book club activity to discuss the concepts addressed in the novel. (*active*)
   - Require that students generate discussion questions and facilitate small-group discussions. (*active*)
   - Create an assignment that allows students to develop and share a creative "artifact" that depicts the meaning of the book or the influence it had on them (e.g., piece of art, music, poetry, photography). (*active*)
4. Assign a set of evidence-based resources to examine a specific topic. (*passive*)
   - Require that students conduct library research to locate assigned sources. (*active*)
   - Provide access to a library page, and explain how to contact the distance librarian and other resources for support. (*active*)
   - Offer synchronous support sessions and virtual chats; provide audio announcements and/or video feedback. (*active*)
5. Assign a set of learning materials (e.g., textbook, video, articles) addressing professional development in nursing. (*passive*)
   - Create an individual assignment that requires students to develop a set of goals for leadership development. (*active*)
   - Develop a résumé activity that requires students to update and share their résumés with an assigned partner, and provide feedback and mentorship. (*active*)
   - Develop a social media activity (e.g., Twitter, LinkedIn) that requires students to create a professional profile, seek networking opportunities, and engage in areas of interest related to public health, education, or policy (local, national, global). (*active*)

(continues)

Table 9-2 **Active Learning and Teaching Suggestions**   *(continued)*

6. Additional active teaching strategies:

- Draw attention to important scaffolded concepts.
- Keep students on track and reinforce student contributions.
- Provide clear instructions on how to appropriately participate in and contribute to the discussions.
- Create a learning community with a common purpose, yet provide opportunities to pursue individualized interests related to students' goals and nursing practice.
- Model the skills expected of students through their own responses in discussions and feedback.

related to nursing practice. It is an inquiry-based approach in which students take responsibility for identifying what they need to know and finding resources.

Develop a Community of Learners

Online educators need to develop a community of learners in which active participation between and among learners and faculty can occur. Creating a sense of community that is based on a common purpose is of particular importance to overcome the sense of isolation that can occur for online students. The students need to interact with faculty members, peers, and course content. These three types of interactions function in an interdependent manner because they each potentially contribute to and benefit from each other (Shackelford & Maxwell, 2012). There have been a number of studies supporting that a sense of community can be created online and is significantly associated with perceived learning, especially when there is a strong faculty teaching presence (Garrison, 2007; Harasim, 2017; Shea, 2006).

As faculty working with postlicensure students, we see ourselves as learners as well within the community of learners using the collaborative process. Collaboration is a key principle of social constructivism. Faculty need to be able to differentiate between cooperation and collaboration in teaching and guide students in moving from cooperative work to collaborative work (Breen, 2013). This means that students are encouraged by faculty, in purposeful ways, to share alternative viewpoints and challenge new ideas. This can be done by assigning individual research to address a specific topic, with the results shared with the class or small group, followed by collaborative discussion.

Community of Inquiry

A common framework used for online learning, teaching, and research is the community of inquiry (CoI) model depicted in **Figure 9-1**. It incorporates three types of interaction and was developed by Randy Garrison, Terry Anderson, and Walter Archer from 1999 to 2001 (Anderson, 2018). The CoI model has three elements: social presence, cognitive presence, and teaching presence (Anderson, 2018). In the past two decades, it has been a commonly cited model for online educational research (Bozkurt et al., 2015). The three elements are described separately; however, they interact interdependently for educational purposes (Garrison, 2007).

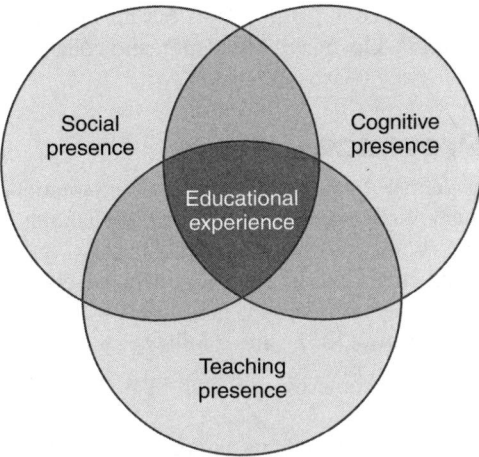

Figure 9-1 Community of inquiry model

Data from Garrison, Anderson, & Archer, 1999

Social Presence

Social presence refers to the students being connected to each other in a meaningful way that builds trust. This trust is necessary in order for students to share their different perceptions, ideas, and feelings without the fear of being judged. Social presence often starts with students posting a picture in their student profile and an introductory discussion. This introduction can set the stage for building a community of learners by purposively thinking through what students should be asked to share. For example, students in a class with prelicensure students may be asked to share where they are in their educational journey, whereas students in a first-year postlicensure or graduate-level class may be asked to share when they became registered nurses (RNs) and what area of nursing they work in. This sets the stage for students to discover what they have in common and things they may want to learn from others. Sharing about their families, pets, and what they like to do for fun also builds community by allowing students to see each other as "real" people.

Faculty also begin to develop a strong social presence with their students by having a written or video introduction in which they not only share why they are teaching the course but also their own educational journey and their teaching style. Faculty introductions should also welcome the students to the class with enthusiasm and make it evident that they care about their students and their success. This can be done by including when and how students can connect with them in realtime and how soon they can expect a response to a question. It is also very important for faculty to welcome each student by individually acknowledging something that they shared in the introductory discussion and to encourage students to welcome each other.

Social presence goes beyond the introduction and is woven throughout the course, with the purpose of meeting educational objectives (Shea, 2006). In keeping with constructivist pedagogy, students are encouraged to incorporate their professional and personal experiences, with specific examples, to apply learning, which not only establishes cognitive presence but also further establishes a social and emotional connection. Open communication and collaborative discussions are hallmarks of social presence (Garrison, 2007).

Cognitive Presence

Cognitive presence is defined by Garrison (2007) as "exploration, construction, resolution and confirmation of understanding through collaboration and reflection in a community of inquiry" (p. 65). The CoI model is based on the practical inquiry model (PIM), which describes four levels of cognitive presence that can be observed in students' online discussion postings. These levels of cognitive presence, as described by Sadaf and Olesova (2017), are as follows:

1. *Triggering* as students become aware of a problem through initiating the inquiry process
2. *Exploration*, which refers to students exploring a problem by searching for relevant information and attempts to explain
3. *Integration* as students interpret or construct possible solutions
4. *Resolution*, which refers to students applying or defending possible solutions with new thoughts or ideas.

The triggering and exploration phases exemplify low levels of cognitive presence, whereas engaging in integration and resolution allows students to build on each other's ideas and synthesize information to provide solutions. These phases are not linear; students may move back to previous phases before reaching resolution (Swan, Garrison, & Richardson, 2009). Garrison, Anderson, and Archer (2010) noted that several studies found that moving through the process of inquiry to completion was challenging, and discussions often did not move past the exploration phase. Moving through the inquiry process to completion was found to be directly related to the role of faculty in facilitating student learning through triggering questions, effective assessment, and pushing students to go beyond observing and sharing.

Before moving to teaching presence, we want to recognize that different theories and models illustrate similar ways of understanding how knowledge is constructed. For example, Harasim's (2017) online collaborativist theory identifies that three phases—idea generating, idea organizing, and intellectual convergence—lead to knowledge building and application. Adult learning theory helps us prioritize understanding students' motivations for learning. Theoretical pedagogy is critical in guiding faculty members to intentionally connect theory to their teaching practice. The bottom-line question for us is the following: How do we facilitate and motivate students to engage with the course content, relevant outside research, their peers, and faculty to construct knowledge and apply it to nursing practice?

As a result, we define *cognitive presence* as the ability of a community of learners in an online classroom to construct meaning through engaging with the course content, outside research, individual reflection, and collaborative reflection to explicitly take into account the individual work that also needs to be done in conjunction with the collaborative work.

Teaching Presence

Teaching presence includes the planning that goes into course design, as discussed in Chapter 8, and what is done when interacting with students through facilitation and direct instruction. How the course is designed facilitates discussions and provides direct instruction to establish teaching presence. Numerous studies confirm the importance of teaching presence for successful online learning in relation to student satisfaction, perceived learning, and sense of community (Garrison, 2007). Without an active teaching presence, the higher levels of cognitive presence are rarely developed (Garrison et al., 2010)

There is overlap between social and cognitive presence. Social presence is enhanced by building positive relationships with students by being open, approachable, respectful, and patient. A sense of belonging is enhanced by addressing students by name, encouraging participation, and recognizing progress and achievement. Not only do these efforts made by faculty promote social presence, they are also motivators to promote student persistence (Boston et al., 2009; Stavredes, 2011). Cognitive presence can be enhanced when faculty members promote a sense of purpose by monitoring student performance on a regular basis, being engaged in the discussions, and providing constructive and timely feedback that encourages professional growth as students grapple with complex topics.

The Learner in the Community of Inquiry Model

Anderson (2018) acknowledges that there have been recommendations for additional presences, such as vicarious, emotional, and autonomy presence, that he has not endorsed. He asserts that they already exist in the original model but notes that further definition within social presence may address these recommendations. However, Anderson is supportive of adding *learner presence* to the model based on a large study conducted by Shea and Bidjerano (2010). Learner presence represents elements of online self-regulation, such as self-efficacy, cognition, behavior, and motivation. Shea and Bidjerano (2010) examined the relationship between learner self-efficacy and how they rated the quality of their learning in online learning environments and found a positive relationship between the CoI framework and learner presence. Adding this presence allows for the CoI model to evolve beyond a teaching model to a teaching and learning model in which teachers need to match their teaching to the capacity of the learner (Anderson, 2018).

Paz and Pereira (2015) proposed that *regulated learning* be added to the teaching presence in the CoI model to demonstrate the overlap between cognitive and teaching presence because it focuses on the coregulation of learning and metacognition by both faculty and students. Adding this to teaching presence acknowledges the role of both learners and faculty in the teaching process, which is in keeping with Vygotsky's (1978/1997) ZPD and collaborativist learning theory. However, the categories within *regulated learning* found by the study conducted by Paz and Pereira seem to coincide with group-process issues with collaborative group work because they include confirming understanding of tasks, assessing work process, suggesting improvements, and reminding and encouraging others to contribute to the work, to name a few.

The main point of adding regulated learning to cognitive presence in the CoI model or adding learner presence as a fourth presence is that there is an acknowledgment of the need to consider both teaching and learning because they inform each other in the online learning environment. Both of these additions are congruent with our understanding that the three interactions of student to content, student to student, and student to faculty and the three presences of the CoI model inform each other.

Teaching Strategies to Demonstrate Presence and Engagement

Helping students move through the process of inquiry is much more demanding, requiring strong online teaching skills. In today's political and social environment of "alternate truths" and media saturation, it is essential that students learn to critically explore and evaluate the information they encounter and the knowledge they are constructing (Anderson, 2018). This is never more evident than at the time of writing this chapter during the coronavirus pandemic of 2020. Many working nurses are coping with caring for patients without proper personal protective equipment and continual policy changes as evidence about the coronavirus evolves. This is a time when faculty and students are learning together to maneuver through a global crisis.

Postlicensure nursing students are adult learners, are increasingly self-directed, and have experiences that provide for a rich learning environment (Candela, 2020). Therefore, we see ourselves as learners and colleagues in the online learning environment with a responsibility to provide meaningful learning experiences that are relevant to the life and work experiences of students. As colleagues, it has been our preference to use our first names in working with students. However, given different students' comfort level because of cultural differences, we advise them that they may refer to us by our first name or by "Professor." Collegiality does not negate the responsibility of faculty to understand the power differential between faculty and student and the impact of this on the faculty–student relationship.

It is important for faculty to be aware of the stressors students are facing, even in the best of times, given the multiple competing demands on our students' lives. The ability to have high standards while holding students accountable yet being flexible meets the needs of adult learners. We, as educators, have found this balance challenging at times. It is important for faculty to discern when students are having difficulties with time management versus facing challenging life issues, such as a dying parent, a divorce, or caring for a child with special needs. The faculty response needs to be one of respect and compassion, whether it be holding students accountable to deadlines or granting extensions. We work closely with the professional advisor to help students persist and be successful in meeting their goals, as discussed in Chapter 4.

Faculty presence throughout the entire course is important to keep students engaged and motivated. This can be challenging because there are many demands on faculty time. Nursing students vary considerably in their ability to persist in the absence of a consistent teaching presence. We have found that one way to ensure teaching presence during particularly busy times is to monitor student participation on a weekly basis to ensure they are engaged and to reach out to those who have not participated. In the discussion, we find it helpful to first respond to those students who do not have a peer response.

Faculty provide an active teaching presence by drawing attention to important scaffolded concepts by their selection and arrangement of course materials,

---

Table 9-3 Demonstrating Presence and Engagement

1. Provide a warm welcome through the use of a video or written announcement when the course starts.
2. Post regular announcements that include encouragement, support, and reminders about due dates.
3. Respond to every student individually in the introduction forum in a way that is personal to them.
4. Let students know how and when they can reach you. Let them know if you are available by text, phone call, or email.
5. Be more available before a major assignment or small-group work to be able to assist with problems.
6. Treat emails like phone calls. Respond immediately, if possible, to show respect for the student's time.
7. Establish personal connections.
8. Check weekly for students who have not engaged, and reach out by email and/or a phone call.
9. Offer video meetings on a regular basis.
10. Respond to individual students who are struggling with individualized support, such as a video conference.
11. Draw attention to important concepts.
12. Help students manage their time.
13. Be present in discussion forums.
14. Grade on time, and give meaningful feedback. If behind on grading, advise students when they can expect to see their grades.
15. Provide opportunities for students to complete assignments that meet course outcomes in a way that is respectful of their learning needs and applies to their nursing practice.

---

highlighting specific course content, and providing responses in the discussions. Faculty may also summarize discussions by highlighting patterns. Further, faculty model the skills they expect of their students through their own responses and feedback (Cormier & Siemans, 2010).

Faculty need to be able to sustain a strong presence through facilitation of the discussions and direct instruction (Garrison, 2007). Further, Edwards, Perry, and Janzen (2011) found that exemplary online faculty maintained high expectations and challenged students to think more deeply while also finding opportunities to affirm their personal worth by letting students know that they were succeeding. Exemplary online faculty recognized their students' potential and encouraged them. **Table 9-3** lists some strategies that we have found helpful in demonstrating presence and engagement that also illustrate that we care about our students and their success.

Online Collaborative Activities

Faculty need to carefully manage individual and collaborative learning activities that build on constructivist and adult education theory. For example, collaborative discussions that are relevant to nursing students' experience provide opportunities for meaningful interaction that recognizes their experience. Online activities can be offered synchronously or asynchronously.

Synchronous online activities are those learning activities that take place in realtime through the use of video or audio-conferencing technology. We have found synchronous activities to be helpful in providing instructions or clarifying a complex topic and addressing questions. Synchronous activities should be recorded so that students who could not attend can listen to the recording on their own time. Asynchronous activities involve students engaging in the same activities at different times and locations. We have found that asynchronous activities are one of the many advantages of online learning because of the flexibility to complete coursework based on the student's schedule.

Group Work

Group work in the online learning environment can be particularly frustrating for both faculty and students, which often results in avoiding it. Different styles of how students work contribute to the challenges. For example, some students like to start early, and others wait until the last minute. Some students like to take control, not trusting their peers, whereas some students prefer to let others do the majority of the work. Further challenges involve living in different time zones and having different work schedules. Therefore, it is very important to be purposeful in planning how the group work will be set up, keeping in mind the leveling of coursework in the program of study and the learning outcomes you want to achieve.

We have found that the key to successful group work is providing clear instructions and assigning individual work that needs to be done first so that every group member comes prepared to fully collaborate in the group experience. When students initially begin working in a group that requires a final product, faculty need to provide information on the purpose of group work and guidance on how to work collaboratively. It is important to closely monitor the group process to ensure that students are working well together.

Harasim's (2017) collaborativist theory and the CoI model are different, yet similar ways of understanding how students may collaboratively move through the knowledge-construction process. The collaborativist theory has not been used for research purposes to the extent that the CoI model has. Chapter 15 presents an extensive study that assesses online collaborative discourse in discussions and group work using collaborativist theory (formerly referred to as *online collaborative theory*).

Asynchronous Discussions

Special attention is given to online discussions in this chapter because of the integral part they have in online education. Online discussions provide a space for open-ended thinking, exchange of information, and collaborative reflection, allowing students to make connections between theory and practice and promoting peer learning (Arend, 2009; Liu, 2019). The purpose of online discussions is to provide an opportunity for students to explore different concepts, apply course material to real life, or dig deeper into a concept or topic (Arend, 2009). Many online instructors find that the built-in time for reflection in asynchronous discussions encourages more critical and reflective thought (Arend, 2009).

Constructing the discussion forum and the importance of the trigger questions or discussion prompts are addressed in Chapter 8. Keeping in mind Bloom's or Fink's taxonomy, as discussed in Chapter 7, will guide faculty in ensuring their questions are at the appropriate cognitive level. Examples at different cognitive levels are provided in Chapter 8. In a discussion forum, faculty pose questions or a discussion prompt, and students are required to provide a substantial response. Some learning management systems provide the option to hide student responses until the student has posted an initial response. This may be an institutional policy or at the faculty member's discretion as a way to avoid the potential of plagiarism or encourage individual reflection on the course content prior to collaborating with the class. However, it is important to consider if the goal is to have individual reflection followed by collaborative reflection or to allow students to reflect on other students' responses before they begin their own. Faculty may consider having a combination of both options in the course.

Online discussions replace the interactive discussions that are often a part of face-to-face teaching. However, as stated previously, the asynchronous nature of online discussions provides the opportunity for more reflection and the opportunity to address concepts in greater depth through collaborative learning. It is important to provide clear instructions regarding how to participate in a way that encourages collaboration. Some suggestions to consider include the following:

- Expectations for the initial post, such as cognitive level (analysis, synthesis, application) and length
- Number of references to support the discussion and whether they are required only for the initial post, replies, or both
- What is meant by a substantial response and carrying the discussion forward
- Number of replies
- Any requirements regarding whom to reply to (e.g., some institutions require students to respond to faculty posts in the discussion)
- Will peer responses be hidden until the initial response is posted?

Some faculty or students may refer to discussions as assignments, which we discourage because it detracts from the collaborative learning. **Table 9-4** provides an example of information that can be provided to students to help explain the difference between collaborative discussions, group work, and individual assignments.

Facilitating Reflective, Critical, and Analytical Thinking

The ability to facilitate learning and knowledge of how to develop a high-quality online course were found to be the most important skills for online faculty to develop by researchers Kyong-Jee and Bonk (2006). In a later study, Arend (2009) looked at how asynchronous discussions influenced critical thinking among students. The nature of text-based online communication makes it particularly useful for critical thinking by allowing for more reflective and less spontaneous discourse (Garrison & Anderson, 2003). **Table 9-5** identifies a combination of facilitation skills that Arend (2009) found in her study and skills we have identified through our experience. We believe these skills contribute to higher levels of not only critical thinking but also reflective and analytical thinking.

Critical thinking is the careful evaluation of information and how to interpret it to make good judgments. Bandman and Bandman (1994) defined *critical thinking* as "the rational examination of ideas, inferences, assumptions, principles, arguments, conclusions, issues, statements, beliefs, and actions" (p. 5). Analytical thinking is

Table 9-4 Online Collaborative Discussions, Group Work, and Individual Assignments

All assignments in online learning are developed for the purpose of meeting the course outcomes. It is helpful to understand that online learning is often collaborative and that the goals of online discussions are different from those of the individual assignments.

Discussions and online blogs are typically 1 week long. The purpose is to collaborate asynchronously with other students and the instructor on course content in order to share knowledge, reflect on ideas, and improve critical thinking. Therefore, the learning is collaborative. Understanding, application, and analysis of course content is shared so that all members of the group benefit from each other. No final product is required. Individual contribution to the collaborative process is evaluated and graded based on the online grading rubrics designed by the faculty member.

Group assignments are similar to discussions because the work is collaborative among a smaller group of students. The main difference is that a final product, such as a paper or presentation, is produced. The group may decide to meet in realtime (synchronous) to complete some of the group work. Depending on the group assignment, the collaborative process leading to the final product may or may not be evaluated for a grade.

Individual assignments, such as reflective journals, case studies, and written papers, are private between the student and faculty member. Students work independently, and the work is evaluated and graded by the faculty member.

Ultimately, all of the assignments that take place throughout the course are designed to assist the student in meeting the course outcomes that are identified in the course syllabus.

Table 9-5 Facilitation Strategies That Enhance Critical, Reflective, and Analytical Thinking

- Use explicit instructions concerning how to participate in the discussions.
- Use discussions frequently, and have them account for a healthy percentage of the final grade.
- Create a safe environment, and encourage participation.
- The quality of faculty responses, not frequency, contributes to higher-level thinking.
- Use purposeful responses, such as the Socratic method, that encourage students to move through the inquiry process.
- Maintain a neutral stance, especially when the topic is controversial.
- Extend the discussion with comments such as, "Some in this debate would say … whereas others … What are your thoughts?"
- Affirm the value of simply participating, even if you disagree.
- Post follow-up questions that are meant to encourage students to search elsewhere on the Internet for answers.
- Avoid evaluative statements, such as "I agree," which tend to end the discussion.
- Avoid questions with correct answers.
- Avoid directing students to a "right answer" in an open-ended discussion.

part of critical thinking. It is the step-by-step approach to breaking down complex problems or processes into their parts to identify causes and patterns. Reflective thinking involves consideration of the larger context and the meaning and implications of an experience or action (Kearney-Nunnery, 2020). Reflective thinking also helps develop an attitude of inquiry, question assumptions, and gain new perspectives for change and improvement.

Socratic Method

The Socratic method is valuable for advancing critical and reflective thinking in students through an application and analysis of information that requires clarity, logical consistency, and self-regulation (Oyler & Romanelli, 2014). Socratic questioning is purposeful questioning that probes beneath the surface and helps students to:

- Discover the truth of their own thinking.
- Develop deeper understanding.
- Develop sensitivity to clarity, accuracy, relevance, and depth.
- Arrive at judgments through their own reasoning.
- Analyze their thinking, including its purpose, assumptions, perceptions, inferences, concepts, and implications in arriving at judgments through their own reasoning.

Critical thinking and Socratic questioning are connected in that critical thinking involves metacognition and regulation of one's own thoughts (Oyler & Romanelli, 2014). Asynchronous online discussion is one of the most valuable formats for Socratic discourse because it allows for reflection and ongoing research before responding and allows for multiple learners to reply simultaneously (Kingsley, 2011). Within an online discussion, responses to Socratic questioning are shared, with the potential of the class moving through the phases of the inquiry process as discussed within cognitive presence aspect of the CoI model. **Table 9-6** provides some examples of Socratic questions that can be used in an online discussion.

Table 9-6 **Examples of Socratic Questions**

1. Can you be more specific?
2. Can you provide an example to illustrate your point?
3. You made an interesting point, but I am wondering how it relates to . . . ?
4. Could you elaborate on what you mean?
5. I noticed that several of you use the term "drug seeking." I wonder what impact that has on your thinking about people who suffer from addictions?
6. Can you find any evidence to support that people living in poverty tend to have poor parenting skills?
7. Interesting comment; I wonder how you view your position in comparison with the views of the other students in this class who think quite the opposite?
8. This is such an important perspective; how do you see this reflected in the patient population that you work with?
9. Thank you for sharing your experience; can you be more specific about what you have witnessed in your community?

It is important to maintain a neutral stance. Faculty should not be evaluating discussion posts either positively or negatively in the discussion forum. Statements like "I agree" from a faculty member will often close the discussion and prevent students from presenting an opposing view. Corrective statements or statements of disagreement from faculty may also close the discussion, leaving students feeling "called out" and preventing them from taking future risks in presenting their thoughts.

Facilitation Challenges

Some faculty, especially when new to online teaching, may feel the need to respond to each student within a discussion, but this can be disempowering, leading students to only look to faculty rather than develop a community of learners. It is a delicate balance between quantity and quality to ensure enough faculty presence (Arend, 2009). Some students may not be used to discussing and learning from each other when they first start taking online classes. They will need support and guidance to get used to collaborative discussions. Faculty also need to discern when it is important to intervene to deflect potential problems but at the same time not interfere with the flow of ideas. Blatant bias or misinformation may require sensitive intervention on the part of faculty to correct this for the class while at the same time remaining neutral. Individual feedback may be the most appropriate place to address such issues. The intent of most online discussions is to have students think in new ways about the course material. Higher levels of critical, reflective, and analytical thinking tend to be found when faculty have the skill to know when to participate with purposeful, neutral, and probing comments or questions.

Grading and Feedback

Quality feedback is important, regardless of the mode of learning. However, Frayer (2014) found that students perceive faculty feedback as one of the most important dimensions of the online classroom. Feedback serves the purpose of enhancing cognitive understanding of course material and provides a mechanism for motivation, interpersonal connection, and engagement (Mandernach, 2018). Providing quality feedback is a critical teaching role for online faculty, and it takes time. Faculty need to set aside time devoted to delivering quality feedback. We provide the following suggestions, along with examples of different forms of feedback, to help faculty balance their workload and, at the same time, enhance student learning and satisfaction with online learning.

Instructional Resources

In designing the course, include some learning activities that provide opportunities for learning that do not require grading. We have found some great resources available online that are interactive, and students can earn a certificate. Care needs to be taken to ensure that these resources are a good fit to facilitate meeting the course outcomes. Some examples that we have successfully used that students value include modules from the Federal Emergency Management Agency (FEMA) and Centers for Disease Control and Prevention (CDC). These agencies provide in-depth learning modules in which students can submit evidence that the work has been completed and earn a certificate.

In organizing the learning modules, give consideration to when there will be a heavier load for assessment, requiring the provision of extensive feedback. For example, you may want to integrate an assignment with automated feedback that is done the week following the due date of a major writing assignment and not have a discussion that week.

Feedback Banks

We believe that developing feedback banks or using automated-response software programs is at the discretion of faculty. They are very useful for large online classrooms. Feedback banks are responses that faculty use frequently because it saves time to copy and paste them. The concern is that they may take away the personalization that faculty like to convey. We do use less personal strategies, such as copied and pasted feedback that highlights certain learning outcomes we want to reinforce for all students, which would be combined with feedback that is more personal and specific to the student's work. For example, the comment, "Examining historical events in the context of the social and political times by using both primary and secondary sources is so important to increase our understanding of the events" was used in an Evolution of Nursing course, followed by an individualized comment about the student's specific work.

Group Feedback

Group feedback can be an effective way to provide feedback to the entire class or a small group. This could be related to seeing a common pattern of errors and used as a teachable opportunity, or it could be motivated by a desire to highlight how the class did exceptionally well. Group feedback may also come from a feedback bank developed in a previous semester and found to be relevant in a subsequent class. **Table 9-7** provides an example of group feedback in response to the work done for a module on trauma-informed care. Note that the announcement highlights some things that were done well, provides some direct teaching, and corrects some information without pointing out any errors in thinking that came through in the students' work.

Personalization

Feedback can be personalized by using students' names and making specific reference to their work or professional context. Students value feedback that is individualized, provides gentle guidance, is positively constructive, is specific, and is written in a positive tone that suggests changes that can be useful in other contexts (Getzlaf, Perry, Toffner, Lamarche, & Edwards, 2009). Adults, in particular, are sensitive to feeling respected and validated and want a clear connection between their academic

Table 9-7 Announcement—Group Feedback

Hi Class,

The Substance Abuse and Mental Health Services Administration (SAMHSA) explains that the "4 Rs" of trauma-informed care (TIC) are realization, recognition, response, and resisting retraumatization. The purpose of this journal was to raise awareness of the prevalence of trauma, to recognize that the patients you see may have experienced trauma, to understand how to respond given your role in the care of the patient, and most of all, to prevent retraumatization. It is clear from your reflections that you have become sensitive to the prevalence of trauma and the sequela. I was very touched by the work you have done this past week in working through your thinking and feelings about this sensitive topic.

I think of trauma in different ways, such as single-incident victimization and ongoing victimization. We know more and more about the impact of trauma on the developing brain and the posttraumatic stress (PTS) response, which is on a continuum from the stress response to posttraumatic stress disorder (PTSD) and can be short-lived or ongoing. We know that other mental health issues, such as addiction, can start as a coping mechanism in response to a full-blown chronic illness, along with other kinds of related issues, such as depression, anxiety, and psychosis. Trauma can lead to avoidance behaviors, as some of you mentioned, such as withdrawing from physical touch. This is such a huge topic that we cannot fully cover it, and it is not necessary for nurses. However, it is necessary to be sensitive to the issue and respond appropriately using the principles of TIC, which are not that much different from what we learned about the components of the therapeutic nurse–patient relationship, such as safety, trust, transparency, peer support and mutual self-help, collaboration and mutuality, empowerment, and voice and choice, in addition to cultural, historical, and gender issues.

Additionally, the book *Childhood Disrupted: How Your Biography Becomes Your Biology, and How You Can Heal* by Donna Jackson Nakazawa is highly recommended. It discusses how adverse childhood events (ACEs) can lead to physical health problems as well as mental health issues.

I don't think it is appropriate to probe for a history of trauma, which is why I am an advocate for universal TIC: Treat everyone with the principles of TIC, just as we do for infection control—we apply standard principles. Our thinking changes if we approach all patients as if they have a history of trauma, not knowing if they do or do not; this way, retraumatization is hopefully avoided. You don't have to know; some patients may not want to disclose, they often don't. Some of you described patients you've had, and with this new knowledge, your approach would have changed. THANK YOU for sharing your reflections. Self-reflection is a hallmark of this RN-to-BSN program.

Examining our thoughts, feelings, and behavior is so important because it can be very challenging to examine our stereotypes and biases. Consider your attitude toward a patient who comes into the emergency room for the fourth time with a drug overdose and is obnoxious and demanding or sullen and withdrawn. How do your thoughts about and response to the patient change when you know she has a history of ongoing rape by her stepdad? The reality is that we may never know that person's history, but we do know that all behavior has meaning, and treating that person with a TIC approach in the emergency room, intensive care unit, or another setting can make a difference.

Again, thank you for your thoughtful contributions to the discussion and your journal reflections.

Faculty name

Table 9-8 **Examples of Personalized Feedback**

Student name, you are making strong connections between poverty, education, and access to resources. I would like to see you take your analysis just a bit deeper. For example, what can be done when resources are so limited? How do you address this in your practice, particularly because you are seeing the struggles with mental health and not having proper resources? *Faculty name*

Student name, be sure to review the requirement in the grading rubric about applying specific data or evidence from the literature in your comments—adding something from the material can take this even further by demonstrating how you are thinking critically to connect the concepts. *Faculty name*

Student name, thank you for your thoughtful reflections in this discussion. As I think about nurses today working during this pandemic, I can't help but wonder how difficult it must be to attend to patients' fears and anxieties because they are probably experiencing their own. *Faculty name*

Student name, thank you for this insightful reflection. It is very difficult being a new grad, and this is a rough start by being put in this situation. You can now see how it was a combination of the system issues that you mentioned that also contributed to the error. I had a colleague who made a similar error while working in psych when patients would come to the cart and identify themselves, and a patient gave the wrong name and received several wrong meds. Like you, he did not know the patients. *Faculty name*

and professional work (Merriam, 2001). We know that the ability to learn and be open to feedback improves when people feel valued and respected. After receiving this kind of feedback, students will comment that they feel motivated to learn more because their confidence is increased. Examples of personalized feedback are provided in **Table 9-8**.

Grading and Timeliness

Grading in a timely manner is important not only for student satisfaction but also for student learning. Students cannot make any needed improvements to their discussion posts, for example, if they do not have the feedback to help them in this regard. Therefore, we make it a practice to grade the discussions within a few days of the close of the discussion, especially at the beginning of the course, when students are learning the expectations.

Assignments are typically graded within a week. There may be some differences in when grading needs to be completed, depending on the length of the semester and institutional policy. For example, in a 5- to 7-week semester, the turnaround time for grading and feedback needs to be much shorter for students to benefit. Faculty should let students know when to expect to see their grades and keep them updated if it is going to take longer than anticipated. There are some other considerations that faculty need to think about when it comes to assessing assignments. Grading major papers can be very challenging and time consuming. **Table 9-9** lists some recommendations for the assessment of written assignments.

Table 9-9 **Recommendations for Assessment of Written Assignments**

1. Written assignments should be planned to guide students in meeting specific course outcomes.
2. The number of required papers in an online course should be reasonable. Consider not having a discussion the week a major paper is due.
3. Written assignments should foster students' higher-level thinking about the content rather than having them summarize what they have read.
4. The directions about the purpose and format of the paper should be clear, and students should have the rubric ahead of time.
5. In evaluating papers in which students analyze issues, the criteria should focus on the rationale for the position, not the specific position.
6. Strategies for the teacher to avoid potential bias include reading papers anonymously, reading papers more than once, and grading papers in random order.
7. Consider limiting the number of papers to grade per day to avoid grading fatigue.
8. Provide personalized feedback, as discussed previously.
9. Regularly, have a colleague read graded, anonymous papers to perform interrater review and confirm grading.
10. Hide the grade from student view until several papers are graded to provide time for comparing how students are doing so that there is equity in how grades are assigned.
11. Limit your editing of papers. The focus needs to be on constructive feedback. Editing does the work for students rather than empowering them to take responsibility for their own work.
12. If issues with writing and American Psychological Association (APA) style are prevalent, refer students to the writing resources offered by the institution. Consider providing the opportunity for a rewrite.

Summary

It is important for nursing faculty to provide a learner-centered environment that facilitates a community of learners who advance in the knowledge-construction process and develop skills that can be applied to their nursing practice. Faculty members who maintain a strong teaching presence within the community of learners can effectively hold students accountable for active participation. Assessment is an intentional part of course design. Grading and providing feedback are critical components of assessment that can have the potential to motivate or deflate a student. This is why there is an emphasis on taking the time to provide quality feedback. Even a poor grade can be couched with feedback that is respectful and caring to maximize the impact on student confidence.

Best-Practice Recommendations for Online Teaching

- Theoretical pedagogy is critical in guiding faculty to intentionally connect theory to their teaching practice.
- Engaging in ongoing self-reflection prior to and during the teaching process is critical for faculty to develop expertise in online teaching.

- Online educators have the ability to develop a community of learners in which active participation between and among learners and faculty can occur.
- Faculty members who provide students with encouragement and compassion can support students as they move through the process of inquiry.
- Balancing high standards and holding students accountable with flexibility supports the success of adult learners in the online classroom.

References

Anderson, T. (2018). *How communities of inquiry drive teaching and learning in the digital age.* https://teachonline.ca/tools-trends/insights-online-learning/2018-02-27/how-communities-inquiry-drive-teaching-and-learning-digital-age

Arend, B. (2009). Encouraging critical thinking in online threaded discussions. *The Journal of Educators Online, 6*(1). http://doi.org/10.9743/JEO.2009.1.1

Bandman, E. L., & Bandman, B. (1994). *Critical thinking in nursing* (2nd ed.). Appleton & Lange.

Booth, T. L., Emerson, C. J., Hackney, M. G., & Souter, S. (2016). Preparation of academic nurse educators. *Nurse Education in Practice, 19*, 54–57. http://dx.doi.org/10.1016/j.nepr.2016.04.006

Boston, W., Diaz, S., Gibson, A., Ice, P., Richardson, J., & Swan, K. (2009). An exploration of the relationship between indicators of the community of inquiry framework and retention in online programs. *Journal of Asynchronous Learning Network, 13*(3), 67–83. http://doi.org/10.24059/olj.v14i1.1636

Bozkurt, A., Akgun-Ozbek, E., Yilmazel, S., Erdogdu, E., Ucar, H., Guler, E., … Aydin, C. (2015). Trends in distance education research: A content analysis of journals 2009–2013. *International Review of Research in Open and Distributed Learning, 16*(1), 330–363. http://doi.org/10.19173/irrodl.v16i1.1953

Breen, H. (2013). Virtual collaboration in the online education setting: A concept analysis. *Nursing Forum, 48*(4), 262–270. http://doi.org/10.1111/nuf.12034

Candela, L. (2020). Theoretical foundations of teaching and learning. In D. M. Billings & J. A. Halstead (Eds.), *Teaching in nursing: A guide for faculty* (6th ed., pp. 247–269). Elsevier.

Cormier, D., & Siemens, G. (2010). Through the open door: Open courses as research, learning, and engagement. *EDUCAUSE Review, 45*(40), 30–39.

Edwards, M., Perry, B., & Janzen, K. (2011). The making of an exemplary online educator. *Distance Education, 32*(1), 101–118.

Frayer, L. (2014). A multi-case study of student perceptions of online course design elements and success. *International Journal for the Scholarship of Teaching and Learning, 8*(1), Article 13. http://doi.org/0.20429/ijsotl.2014.080113

Garrison, D. (2007). Online community of inquiry review: Social, cognitive, and teaching presence issues. *Journal of Asynchronous Learning Networks, 11*(1), 61–72. http://doi.org/10.24059/olj.v11i1.1737

Garrison, D., Anderson, T., & Archer, W. (2010). The first decade of the community of inquiry framework: A retrospective. *The Internet and Higher Education, 13*, 5–9. http://doi.org/10.1016/j.iheduc.2009.10.003

Garrison, D. R., & Anderson, T. (2003). *E-learning in the 21st century: A framework for research and practice.* Routledge/Falmer. http://doi.org/10.4324/9780203166093

Garrison, D. R., Anderson, T., & Archer, W. (1999). Critical inquiry in a text-based environment: Computer conferencing in higher education. *The Internet and Higher Education, 2*, 87–105.

Getzlaf, B., Perry, B., Toffner, G., Lamarche, K., & Edwards, M. (2009). Effective instructor feedback: Perceptions of online graduate students. *Journal of Educators Online, 6*(2). http://doi.org/10.9743/JEO.2009.2.1

Giddens, J. (2020). Demystifying concept-based and competency-based approaches. *Journal of Nursing Education, 59*(3), 123–124. http://doi.org/10.3928/01484834-20200220-01

Harasim, L. (2017). *Learning theory and online technologies.* Routledge.

Kearney-Nunnery, R. (Ed.). (2020). *Advancing your career: Concept of professional nursing.* F. A. Davis.

Kingsley, P. (2011). The Socratic dialogue in asynchronous online discussions: Is constructivism redundant? *Campus-Wide Information Systems, 28*(5)320–330. http://doi.org/10.1108/10650 741111181599

Kyong-Jee, K., & Bonk, C. J. (2006). The future of online teaching and learning in higher education: The survey says… *EDUCAUSE Quarterly, 29*(4), 22–30.

Liu, Y. (2019). Using reflections and questioning to engage and challenge online graduate learners in education. *Research and Practice in Technology Enhanced Learning, 14*(3), Article 3. http://doi.org/10.1186/s41039-019-0098-z

Mandernach, B. J. (2018). Strategies to maximize the impact of feedback and streamline your time. *Journal of Educators Online, 15*(3). https://www.thejeo.com/archive/archive/2018_153/mandernachpdf

Merriam, S. (2001). Andragogy and self-directed learning: Pillars of adult learning theory. *New Directions for Adult and Continuing Education, 89*, 3–14. http://doi.org/10.1002/ace.3

Oyler, D. R., & Romanelli, F. (2014). The fact of ignorance: Revisiting the Socratic method as a tool for teaching critical thinking. *American Journal of Pharmaceutical Education, 78*(7), 144.

Palloff, R. M., & Pratt, K. (Eds.). (2007). *Building online learning communities: Effective strategies for the virtual classroom.* Jossey-Bass.

Paz, J., & Pereira, A. (2015). *Regulation of learning as distributed teaching presence in the community of inquiry framework.* Presentation at the Technology, Colleges, and Community Online Conference 2015: The Future Is Now, Honolulu, HI.

Sadaf, A., & Olesova, L. (2017) Enhancing cognitive presence in online case discussions with questions based on the practical inquiry model. *American Journal of Distance Education, 31*(1), 56–69. http://doi.org/10.1080/08923647.2017.1267525

Shackelford, J., & Maxwell, M. (2012). Sense of community in graduate online education: Contribution of learner to learner interaction. *International Review of Research in Open and Distance Learning, 13*, 228–249. http://doi.org/10.19173/irrodl.v13i4.1339

Shea, P. (2006). A study of students' sense of learning community in online environments. *Online Learning, 10*(1). http://doi.org/10.24059/olj.v10i1.1774

Shea, P., & Bidjerano, T. (2010). Learning presence: Towards a theory of self-efficacy, self-regulation, and the development of communities of inquiry in online and blended learning environments. *Computers & Education, 55*(4), 1721–1731. https://doi.org/10.1016/j.compedu.2010.07.017

Smith, T. C. (2005). Fifty-one competencies for online instruction. *The Journal of Educators Online, 2*(2). http://doi.org/10.9743/JEO.2005.2.2

Stavredes, T. (2011). *Effective online teaching: Foundations and strategies for student success.* Jossey-Bass

Swan, K., Garrison, D. R., & Richardson, J. (2009). A constructivist approach to online learning: The community of inquiry framework. In C. R. Payne (Ed.), *Information technology and constructivism in higher education: Progressive learning frameworks* (pp. 43–57). IGI Global.

Vygotsky, L. (1997). Interaction between learning and development. In M. Gauvain & M. Cole (Eds.), *Readings on the development of children* (Vol. 2, pp. 29–36). W. H. Freeman and Company. (Reprinted from *Mind and society*, pp. 79–91, by L. Vygotsky, 1978, Cambridge University Press.)

Weimer, M. (2013). *Learner-centered teaching* (2nd ed.). John Wiley & Sons.

Learning Through Writing in Online Classrooms

Melissa Robinson and Henny Breen

"Over the last two years in the RN to BSN program, my writing skills have significantly improved. At the beginning of the program, I found it challenging to participate in forums and write papers and it was very time consuming. Over the course of the program, my writing has become much more efficient and I feel more confident. This is an important feat because it translates into my ability to think clearly and concisely as well."

Online RN-to-BSN student (anonymous)

Overview

This chapter addresses opportunities for learning through writing in online nursing education. Strategies that can be used to teach information literacy across all levels of nursing education are discussed, including the importance of collaboration between nurse faculty and distance librarians. Writing across the nursing curriculum, technical aspects of professional writing, and examples of writing assignments in online nursing programs are addressed.

Effective writing is essential for nursing practice and for career progression within the healthcare system. A priority outcome for nursing education programs is for graduates to communicate their ideas in writing in an organized, logical, and persuasive manner (Oermann, 2013). Nurses use written communication with team members and across disciplines to document patient care, to create teaching materials for patients and staff, to develop policies and procedures, and to write for publication (Troxler, Vann, & Oermann, 2011). As a result of continual online engagement through reading and writing, online education programs provide the opportunity for students to significantly develop their information literacy and writing skills.

Information Literacy

Information literacy is defined as the ability to formulate questions, search for, find, evaluate, get, and use scholarly information responsibly (Association of College and Research Libraries, 2000), which is fundamental to online nursing education. Flood, Gasiewicz, and Delpier (2010) emphasized the importance of including information literacy across the curriculum so that it can become a part of nursing practice. Additionally, information literacy education has become a core activity in academic libraries across the country that aim to promote information literacy as a way to ensure student success as a lifelong learner (Xiao, 2010).

In a previous article written with our distance librarian, we shared strategies for teaching information literacy to online registered nurse (RN)–bachelor of science in nursing (BSN) students that enhanced students' confidence in searching online for scholarly information on evidence-based practice (McCulley & Jones, 2014). The intentional placement of activities focused on information literacy at the beginning of the program can prepare online students for meaningful writing experiences throughout the curriculum. Four strategies that could be considered to implement in an online program are (a) collaboration between librarians and nursing faculty; (b) embedded librarians; (c) research guides and tutorials; and (d) student-centered learning, including authentic (real-life) activities.

Collaboration Between Librarians and Nursing Faculty

Collaboration between librarians and nursing faculty in online programs is recommended to help students develop the information literacy skills they need to conduct research at all levels of nursing education. Collaboration takes full advantage of the support from both disciplines to improve student outcomes, to ensure that information literacy outcomes are integrated into course learning outcomes, and to build student confidence with the research process (Arguelles, 2012; Kvenild & Calkins, 2011; Schutt & Hightower, 2009). Collaborative strategies could include working together on the development of research guides and tutorials, shared facilitation of interactive course discussions, and codevelopment of information literacy assignments. Ultimately, successful collaboration between librarians and nurse faculty can lead to strong connections between nursing practice and the evidence on which it is based (McCulley & Jones, 2014).

Embedded Librarians

A primary role for health sciences librarians includes the "distribution of knowledge and ideas, including teaching and facilitating access to knowledge," which has changed dramatically in recent years as a result of the explosion of the information universe and educational technology (Cooper & Crum, 2013, p. 275). Embedded librarianship brings both the library and the librarian, virtually, to online students in their learning environment (e.g., work, school, community). The embedded librarian needs to have online teaching expertise and be comfortable working with online students in the learning management system (LMS), by phone, and using a variety of audio- and video-conferencing tools. One of the main advantages of embedding the librarian in the first two courses of the program is that it helps students gain familiarity and comfort with contacting the librarian for questions and support. The teaching strategies used by the librarian may include posting a personal introduction to the class, sharing reminders about library resources in announcements, and facilitating chat sessions to address questions about the library. Having a librarian who is proactive, as evidenced by offering tips and reminding students about specific tutorials and research requirements for upcoming assignments, facilitates student success (McCulley & Jones, 2014). Having a regular presence in the online classroom demonstrates best practices and allows the librarian to serve students most effectively.

Research Guides and Tutorials

LMSs allow links to library pages and research guides to provide students with access to resources in the online classroom. A unique library class page or research guide designed for a specific course can provide convenient access to CINAHL, PubMed, and Google Scholar, in addition to providing a way to contact the librarian for support, which enhances students' information literacy skills (McCulley & Jones, 2014; Turnbull, Royal, & Purnell, 2011). Personalizing a library guide by posting frequently asked questions and contact information for the librarian and other support persons is helpful to students. Reeb and Gibbons (2004) found that including a picture of the librarian in the library guide increased the number of times students reached out to make contact with the librarian.

Tutorials that are integrated within library pages and course guides can also help improve students' information literacy skills. Videos can be powerful learning tools when students have opportunities to engage with them (Nilson & Goodson, 2018). Short videos can be designed to address the most frequently asked questions and to create a reference bank of materials for students. For example, tutorials such as "how to obtain a full-text article from the library" or "how to narrow your search results when performing library research" are relevant to student learning. We have found that students frequently comment on the value of brief, informative videos that help them refine their skills in the moment and provide reminders on the process of using library resources. Several resources can be used to create video tutorials, including tools in the LMS, such as Kaltura videos, or free external tools such as Jing, YouTube, and Zoom. To enhance engagement, it is important to avoid complex technology with high technical requirements.

Student-Centered Learning

In addition to being embedded in the online classroom and providing instruction for using online resources, distance librarians can be integrated into specific courses to provide direct instruction on activities related to issues students encounter in nursing practice. Authentic student-centered (real-life) assignments that are problem based and utilize course-integrated library instruction have a positive effect on information literacy learning outcomes (Diekema, Holliday, & Leary, 2011; Fox & Doherty, 2012). With the replacement of teaching-centered pedagogy with student-centered pedagogy, online nursing students benefit from using real clinical problems that stimulate their growth as critical thinkers, problem-solvers, communicators, and collaborators (Hickey, Forbes, & Greenfield, 2010). Distance librarians can facilitate the development of the skills students need to find and apply the most current evidence to practice problems.

Table 10-1 Problem-Based Practice Activity

Once you have studied the resources in the module on evidence-based practice and participated in the library search strategies and tools:

1. Reflect on a clinical issue or problem from practice that you would like to investigate.
   Here are a few examples to get started on brainstorming:
   - Fall prevention in long-term-care settings
   - Best practices for managing wounds
   - Family presence during codes
   - Visitation policies in critical care
   - Medication safety
   - Other quality and safety issues

You may use one of these examples, but you must be able to apply it to a real practice experience, or you can choose another topic that works better for you.

2. Search for your chosen topic in the **CINAHL database**.
   - Be sure to follow the handout in the module on crafting a search statement: form a question, identify concepts, choose key words, and so forth.
3. Find one article that addresses the situation and answer the following questions about the search and your article:
   - What is your research question?
   - What key words did you search? List any synonyms or related words that you identified as possible search terms even if they did not yield the best results.
   - What recommendations for best practice does the article give? How do these recommendations compare to your real-life practice?
4. Lastly, craft a full citation in American Psychological Association (APA) style for the article that you have used for this activity.

In an assignment designed in collaboration with nursing faculty, our distance librarian engaged students in the iterative process of finding the relevant scholarly information that they needed to address a real-life clinical problem (McCulley & Jones, 2014). In addition to finding evidence to address the current practice issue chosen for the assignment, the goal is for students to develop lifelong skills in research and writing. An example problem-based practice activity is included in **Table 10-1**.

Writing Across the Curriculum in Nursing Education

When identifying goals and outcomes for writing across the curriculum, it is important to emphasize the application of evidence to nursing practice and writing expectations that progress as the student moves through the program. The American Association of Colleges of Nursing (AACN, 2008) suggests that BSN graduates should be prepared to find and use evidence to inform their practice and that "professional nursing practice at all levels is grounded in the ethical translation of current evidence into practice" (p. 15). As nurses advance their education, the expectations for integrating scholarship into nursing practice grow. The AACN Essentials for baccalaureate and graduate programs can serve as a guide for faculty when planning for writing across the curriculum in online programs. **Table 10-2**

Table 10-2 AACN Essentials for Writing and Scholarship Outcomes

AACN Essentials	Knowledge, Skills	Sample Activities, Assessments
Baccalaureate Education, Essential III (AACN, 2008) *Scholarship for Evidence-Based Practice*	"Professional nursing practice is grounded in the translation of current evidence in one's practice" (p. 3)	Collaborative group discussions Critical reflection activities Case studies Annotative bibliographies Analysis activities Advocacy/Debate activities Professional development Papers
Master's Education, Essential IV (AACN, 2011) *Translating and Integrating Scholarship Into Practice*	"Examines policies and seeks evidence for every aspect of practice, thereby translating current evidence and identifying gaps where evidence is lacking" (p. 15) "Apply research outcomes within the practice setting, resolve practice problems (individually or as a member of the healthcare team), and disseminate results both within the setting and in wider venues in order to advance clinical practice" (p. 15)	Collaborative group discussions Process-improvement reports Quality-assurance projects Policy (practice) development Policy (public) statements
Doctoral Education, Essential III (AACN, 2006) *Clinical Scholarship and Analytical Methods for Evidence-Based Practice*	"Scholarship and research are the hallmarks of doctoral education ... application involves the translation of research into practice and the dissemination and integration of new knowledge. Nursing practice epitomizes the scholarship of application through its position where the sciences, human caring, and human needs meet and new understandings emerge." (p. 11)	Collaborative group discussions Research reports Dissertation studies Grant writing Writing for publication

The Essentials of Baccalaureate Education for Professional Nursing Practice, American Association of Colleges of Nursing, 2008.
The Essentials of Master's Education in Nursing, American Association of Colleges of Nursing, 2011.
The Essentials of Doctoral Education for Advanced Nursing Practice, American Association of Colleges of Nursing, 2006.

includes a sample of course activities and assessments that can be used to facilitate the development of essential writing competencies in baccalaureate and graduate nursing education programs.

Institutional-Level Policies

Nursing programs may have institutional-level goals or outcomes related to writing for the discipline or for degree attainment. These could be addressed through policies related to course requirements, institutional assessment practices, or governance structures that ensure quality oversight. It is important that online programs are included in the same processes and that online students are provided with the resources needed to be successful in meeting the expectations for writing in the online classroom. Some examples of these types of structures include the following:

- Specific courses designated as major writing-intensive courses
- Policies addressing academic integrity and plagiarism
- Discipline-specific writing and format requirements (e.g., American Psychological Association [APA] format)
- Writing task force created to address a new policy or procedure
- Writing policies assigned to curriculum or evaluation committees for oversight within the nursing program or institution
- Procedures for decision making related to support needs for students (e.g., writing center, tutoring support, peer mentorship for writing, remediation)
- Online course expectations or "netiquette"

Technical Aspects of Writing for the Discipline

As students enter online nursing programs, it is important for them to understand the value and importance of discipline-specific writing to the profession of nursing. Online faculty can articulate the ways that nurses utilize their writing skills in documentation, reports, and policy development and when communicating with accuracy and confidence in their written communications. As nurses continue their education, the ability to write scholarly papers, evidence-based project reports, and clinical practice studies becomes paramount to their own professional development and to the advancement of the nursing profession (Oermann, 2013).

It is not uncommon for nursing students to enter online programs with limited development of their writing skills because of the emphasis on testing and clinical education in previous prelicensure programs. The research and writing requirements of advanced education programs can also create anxiety for students who enter online programs. To minimize student anxiety and enhance learning, online faculty can demonstrate a commitment to supporting students' ability to gain experience with scholarly writing, and they can model the use of scholarly writing in the online classroom. This can be achieved by developing opportunities for students to practice their skills in writing evidence-based discussions and written assignments, providing resources in the online classroom to support writing, and delivering meaningful feedback that addresses the content and technical aspects of students' writing. Students also benefit from experiencing the iterative process of writing, which includes idea generation, reading and research, writing, editing, feedback, and revision, across the curriculum.

Mechanics

APA style is the most commonly used style among natural scientists, social scientists, educators, and nurses because of the value placed on new research and current findings. Like other citation styles, APA emphasizes clarity of font style, font size, spacing, and paragraph structure (APA, 2020). The focus of online coursework that requires APA format should be on communicating ideas clearly and applying evidence in written form.

It is not uncommon for faculty to place a heavy focus of assessment and grading on the correct use of APA format, as opposed to the content of the writing or the quality of the writing itself (Oermann, 2013). This creates frustration for students, who feel that faculty are less concerned with the ideas they have presented in their work than the technical aspects of APA format. One way to address this is to create specific course activities and assessments that help students develop their knowledge and skills in using APA format. In the first couple of weeks in an online RN-to-BSN transition course, we have used a group discussion to help students become familiar with the competencies in the AACN Baccalaureate Essentials and another discussion to cover the importance of evidence-based practice. Both discussions help students build their knowledge of the expectations for professional writing in the online program and in the nursing profession. To build their skills in using APA format, we have developed an online APA quiz and an APA formatting assignment (**Table 10-3**).

Table 10-3 Sample APA Formatting Assignment

Purpose: The purpose of this assignment is to help the student develop knowledge and skills in the use of APA format, which is required for professional writing in the nursing profession. This assignment affects your ability to meet the following course outcome: *Demonstrate discipline-specific writing.*

Instructions: Study the assigned resources in the learning module and familiarize yourself with the resources in the APA folder (Course Content). The resources and the required APA manual will support your success with APA and professional writing throughout the program.

1. **Word Document:** Create a 3-page Word document for this APA formatting assignment.
   __/1 Submit as a *.doc or .docx* file only.
   Create the template that will be used for the upcoming Professional Practice Paper.

2. **Title Page:** Create a title page with the following elements:
   __/1 An accurate running head using a short version of the title of the paper
   Create a full title for the Professional Practice Paper; use the short version for the running head.

   __/1 Correct placement of the three elements required for the title page
   __/1 Accurate use of font and typeface
   __/1 Accurate placement of page numbers
   __/1 Accurate page layout (margins)

(continues)

Table 10-3 Sample APA Formatting Assignment   *(continued)*

3. **Page 2:** Create an accurate running head that begins on page 2 (Hint: different from the running head on the title page) and a set of APA headings for the Professional Practice Paper on page 2, including Level 1 and Level 2 headings.
    *Please note the difference between the header and headings.
    __/2 An accurate running head for page 2 of the document
    __/1 Correct placement of title of paper on page 2
    __/3 Accurate Level 1 and Level 2 APA headings

4. **Page 3:** Create a reference page with the following elements:
    __/1 Accurate heading for the reference page
    *Choose four items (two journal articles and two web sources) in the "Professional Practice Paper Resources" folder.
    __/6 An accurate, complete reference for two web sources
    __/6 An accurate, complete reference for two journal articles
    __/25 = TOTAL POINTS

Once students have built their confidence with the use of APA format, they will be prepared to further develop their writing skills as they move through the online program. Grading rubrics can be used to help faculty design assessments that emphasize the content of the paper while they continue to support student development with the mechanics of professional writing. In this way, students can grow to understand the value of both components of their development. An example of a grading rubric for an introductory writing assignment in an online RN-to-BSN transition course is included in **Table 10-4**. The rubric illustrates the point allocation applied to the content of the paper and the mechanics. As online nursing students advance to higher levels of education, such as graduate programs, faculty may place a stronger emphasis on writing development that prepares students to contribute to the scholarship of nursing.

Academic Integrity

Academic integrity and preventing plagiarism are key areas of focus when students are communicating their ideas in writing. The availability of the internet has provided access to unlimited online resources, resulting in an increased threat of cheating, plagiarism, and sharing of assignments and discussion responses in online education (McAfooes, 2016; Starnes-Vottero, 2011). Plagiarism includes lifting information (text or graphics) from an original source without quotation marks, reference, or acknowledgment, as well as paraphrasing without reference to or acknowledgment of the original source (Bender, 2012).

There are several things that online faculty can do to create a culture of academic honesty and integrity. It is important to educate students about the institution's definition of academic integrity and the consequences of violations in the academic integrity policy (see an example policy in **Table 10-5**). There are also multiple opportunities to model academic integrity by (a) citing sources for all images, videos, audio clips, and websites; (b) ensuring that all course materials comply with

Table 10-4 Introductory Writing Assignment: Online RN-to-BSN Transition Course

Grading Rubric: Professional Practice Paper Required Criteria	Points 100	Comments
Introduction ▪ Introduce the reader to the main idea of your paper. ▪ Create an interesting introduction to capture the attention of the reader. ▪ Develop a very specific purpose for the paper.	10	
Personal Definition of Nursing ▪ Describe the meaningful components of your professional identity (who you are as a nurse). ▪ Examine your personal and professional values. ▪ Develop your personal philosophy of nursing.	20	
Mentorship in Nursing ▪ Describe the importance of mentorship in nursing. ▪ Reflect on your professional experiences with mentorship in education and/or practice. ▪ Examine the values you have developed as a result of mentoring relationships. ▪ Identify your goals for seeking mentorship and mentoring others as part of professional practice.	20	
Goal Setting ▪ Identify what motivates you, personally and professionally; include both internal and external motivating factors. ▪ Discuss your goals for professional advancement in the next 5 years and the next 10 years. ▪ Describe how you will overcome any challenges that you anticipate in meeting your goals.	20	
Conclusion ▪ Summarize the main points of your paper. ▪ No new information should be introduced.	10	
Mechanics—Required APA Format ▪ Accurate grammar, spelling, and punctuation ▪ An organized paper with accurate use of Level 1 and Level 2 APA headings ▪ Accurate APA format for title and reference page, in-text citations, headings, page numbers, spacing, and font (typeface) ▪ First person is acceptable for this paper. ▪ Five references are required for this paper (minimum). ▪ No use of direct (exact) quotations in the paper ▪ The length of the paper should be 5–7 pages, not including the title and reference pages ▪ *No abstract is required for this paper.*	20	

Table 10-5 Institutional Policy on Academic Integrity

Linfield College operates under the assumption that all students are honest and ethical in the way they conduct their personal and scholastic lives. Academic work is evaluated on the assumption that the work presented is the student's own, unless designated otherwise. Anything less is unacceptable and is considered a violation of academic integrity. Furthermore, a breach of academic integrity will have concrete consequences that may include failing a particular course or even dismissal from the college. Violations of academic integrity include but are not limited to the following:

- **Cheating:** Using or attempting to use unauthorized sources, materials, information, or study aids in any submitted academic work.
- **Plagiarism:** Submission of academic work that includes material copied or paraphrased from published or unpublished sources without proper documentation. This includes self-plagiarism, the submission of work created by the student for another class, unless he or she receives consent from both instructors.
- **Fabrication:** Deliberate falsification or invention of any information, data, or citation in academic work.
- **Facilitating Academic Dishonesty:** Knowingly helping or attempting to help another to violate the college's policy on academic integrity.

Academic Integrity, Linfield College, 2019.

online copyright guidelines; and (c) letting students know the specific expectations for academic integrity in the course (Nilson & Goodson, 2018). Additional strategies that online faculty may consider to support academic integrity include the following:

- Include expectations for academic integrity, using specific examples, in the course syllabus.
- Provide links to campus policies, academic support, and writing resources in every online course.
- Be proactive in assisting students with learning how to cite published work.
- Develop an honesty statement that students submit to acknowledge the assignment as original work.
- Change or rotate online course assignments every semester.
- Advise students that faculty track and compare their work to the assignments of previous students.
- Create personalized assignments that require original work (e.g., interview assignments, practice-focused assignments, student-chosen topic papers).
- Develop course activities that teach students how to paraphrase and cite sources.
- Build in opportunities for students to complete larger assignments in a series of submissions to avoid completing work at the last minute.
- Develop policies that require students and faculty to use plagiarism detection tools (e.g., Turnitin), and prepare them to use the tools.

Types of Writing Students Do in Online Nursing Programs

In Table 10-2, we presented a few sample activities that can be created for students to develop competencies in writing and applying evidence to nursing practice in online baccalaureate and graduate programs. There are different requirements at each level of nursing education, and, in addition, students come into the online classroom with varying levels of experience and writing skills. The role of the faculty member begins with assessment of the student's writing skills and includes instruction, coaching, encouragement, assessment, and feedback. It is also important that faculty carefully consider the purpose or goal for writing assignments. Oermann (2013) has proposed four main purposes of writing assignments in online nursing programs: (a) enhance writing ability; (b) help students learn about concepts, theories, and other information; (c) foster students' critical thinking about a topic and develop higher-level thinking skills; and (d) explore feelings, beliefs, and values (p. 161).

Online course discussions provide students with meaningful opportunities to develop writing competencies and higher-level thinking skills. Discussion expectations and grading rubrics (also covered in Chapter 8) provide a great deal of structure and can address requirements for the application of evidence and APA format. As new ideas and evidence are discussed collaboratively in groups, there is a strong focus on the analysis and synthesis phases of learning (Billings & Halstead, 2016). Students, peers, and faculty share their perspectives and examples from their own experiences in clinical practice or in their families and communities, and students apply new knowledge to practice and build on the foundation of experiences. When students consistently participate in online discussions, we have seen them benefit from the "practice" of consistent writing. They demonstrate development with the process of writing while their critical and higher-level thinking also develop.

Best-Practice Recommendations for Online Programs

- Integrate information literacy activities into the online classroom to build a strong foundation for learning through writing and for the application of evidence-based practice in nursing.
- Collaborate with distance librarians to utilize cross-disciplinary strengths to foster students' confidence with evidence-based practice and nursing scholarship.
- Create policies and practices that will create a culture of academic honesty and integrity in the online classroom.
- Develop course discussions and assignments that enhance students' writing abilities, and develop students' critical and higher-order thinking skills.

References

American Association of Colleges of Nursing. (2008). The essentials of baccalaureate education for professional nursing practice. https://www.aacnnursing.org/Portals/42/Publications/Bacc Essentials08.pdf

American Association of Colleges of Nursing. (2006). The essentials of doctoral education for advanced nursing practice. https://www.aacnnursing.org/Portals/42/Publications/DNPEssentials.pdf

American Association of Colleges of Nursing. (2011). The essentials of master's education in nursing. https://www.aacnnursing.org/Portals/42/Publications/MastersEssentials11.pdf

American Psychological Association. (2020). *APA style.* https://apastyle.apa.org/?_ga=2.225359443 .855680682.1581349340-1040669385.1581349340

Arguelles, C. (2012). Program-integrated information literacy (PIIL) in a hospital's nursing department: A practical model. *Journal of Hospital Librarianship, 12*(2), 97–111.doi:10.1080/15 323269.2012.665717

Association of College and Research Libraries. (2000). *Information literacy competency standards for higher education.* https://alair.ala.org/bitstream/handle/11213/7668/ACRL%20Information%20 Literacy%20Competency%20Standards%20for%20Higher%20Education.pdf?sequence =1&isAllowed=y

Bender, T. (2012). *Discussion-based online teaching to enhance student learning: Theory, practice, and assessment.* Stylus.

Billings, D., & Halstead, J. (2016). *Teaching in nursing: A guide for faculty.* St. Louis, MO: Saunders.

Cooper, D., & Crum, J. (2013). New activities and changing roles of health sciences librarians: A systematic review, 1990–2012. *Journal of Medical Library Association, 101*(4), 268–277. http:// dx.doi.org/10.3163/1536-5050.101.4.008

Diekema, A. R., Holliday, W., & Leary, H. (2011). Re-framing information literacy: Problem-based learning as informed learning. *Library and Information Science Research, 33*(4), 261–268.

Flood, L. S., Gasiewicz, N., & Delpier, T. (2010). Integrating information literacy across a BSN curriculum. *Journal of Nursing Education, 49*(2), 101–104. http://doi.org/10.3928/01484834 -20091023-01

Fox, B. E., & Doherty, J. J. (2012). Design to learn, learn to design: Using backward design for information literacy instruction. *Communications in Information Literacy, 5*(2), 144–155. http:// doi.org/10.7548/cil.v5i2.163

Hickey, M. T., Forbes, M., & Greenfield, S. (2010). Integrating the Institute of Medicine competencies in baccalaureate curricular revisions: Process and strategies. *Journal of Professional Nursing, 26*(4), 214–222. http://doi.org/10.1016/j.profnurs.2010.03.001

Kvenild, C., & Calkins, K. (2011). Embedded librarians: Moving beyond one-shot instruction. Association of College and Research Libraries.

Linfield College. (2019). Academic integrity. https://www.linfield.edu/catalog/academic-policies -and-procedures-all-campuses/other-policies-and-procedures/academic-integrity.html

McAfooes, J. (2016). Teaching and learning in online learning communities. In D. Billings & J. Halstead (Eds.), *Teaching in nursing: A guide for faculty* (pp. 357–384). Elsevier.

McCulley, C., & Jones, M. (2014). Fostering RN-to-BSN students' confidence in searching for scholarly information on evidence-based practice. *The Journal of Continuing Education in Nursing, 45*(1), 22–27. http://doi.org/10.3928/00220124-20131223-01

Nilson, L. B., & Goodson, L. A. (2018). *Online teaching at its best: Merging instructional design with teaching and learning research.* Jossey-Bass.

Oermann, M. (2013). Enhancing writing in online education. In K. Frith & D. Clark (Eds.), *Distance education in nursing* (pp. 145–162). Springer.

Reeb, B., & Gibbons, S. (2004). Students, librarians, and subject guides: Improving a poor rate of return. *Portal: Libraries and the Academy, 4*(1), 123–130.

Schutt, M., & Hightower, B. (2009). Enhancing RN-to-BSN students' information literacy skills through the use of instructional technology. *Journal of Nursing Education, 48*(2), 101–105.

Starnes-Vottero, B. (2011). E-learning assessment. In T. Bristol & J. Zerwekh (Eds.), *Essentials of e-learning for nurse educators* (pp. 165–179). F. A. Davis.

Turnbull, B., Royal, B., & Purnell, M. (2011). Using an interdisciplinary partnership to develop nursing students' information literacy skills: An evaluation. *Contemporary Nurse: A Journal for the Australian Nursing Profession*, *38*(1/2), 122–129.

Troxler, H., Jacobson Vann, J. C., & Oermann, M. H. (2011). How baccalaureate nursing programs teach writing. *Nursing Forum*, *46*(4), 280–288. https://dx.doi.org/10.1111/j.1744-6198.2011.00242.x VIEW ITEM

Xiao, J. (2010). Integrating information literacy into Blackboard: Librarian-faculty collaboration for successful student learning. *Library Management*, *31*(8/9), 654–668. http://doi.org/10.1108/01435121011093423

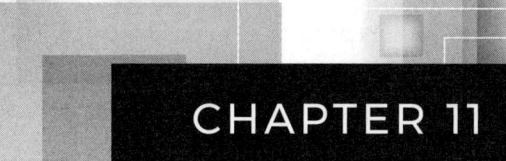

CHAPTER 11

Experiential Learning in Online Nursing Programs

Henny Breen and Melissa Robinson

Overview

Experiential learning is an essential component of learning in nursing education, and online nursing education programs are no exception. Experiential learning theory is built on six propositions, as discussed in Chapter 2. Prior to reading this chapter, it is recommended that the reader review these propositions. Kolb's (2015) theory of experiential learning helps explain how experience is transformed into learning through a holistic perspective that combines experience, perception, cognition, and behavior.

This chapter provides an overview of experiential learning, including simulation and the popular experiential learning cycle developed by Kolb that many educators use. Experiential learning in online programs across the curriculum is discussed. Examples are provided for ways that experiential learning can be integrated to provide opportunities for online students to achieve deep conceptual learning.

Experiential Learning Overview

Experiential learning is important to all nursing education, prelicensure and postlicensure, including online programs, because it bridges the gap between theory and practice. How students perceive and practice nursing is influenced by their personal and professional experiences (Hartley, 2010). Experiential learning is built on six propositions: (1) a process rather than an outcome; (2) grounded in ongoing experience; (3) driven by working through conflicting perceptions through iterations that involve reflection, action, feeling, and thinking; (4) a holistic process of adaptation that integrates thinking, feeling, perceiving, and behaving; (5) involves ongoing transaction between the student and the environment as new experiences are assimilated into existing concepts; and (6) the process of creating knowledge (Kolb, 1984; Kolb & Kolb, 2013). Another way of describing experiential learning is to think of it as providing learning experiences within one or more of the three domains of learning: psychomotor, affective, and cognitive learning. It is important to understand how the domains are related to each other through experiential learning.

Psychomotor learning is the relationship between cognition and physical movement and is the most commonly used in developing skill competencies, such as the administration of an intravenous (IV) infusion or changing a dressing. However, the cognitive domain is an integral part of developing skill competencies because the student needs to learn the theory and principles that guide the skills. Further, the affective domain is an integral part, given that students need to appreciate the need to assess the patient's emotional response to any procedure.

Within prelicensure nursing education, experiential learning mostly involves the development of clinical skills to enable students to provide direct nursing care. It is often limited to real-world settings. However, the need to replicate the clinical environment is increasingly necessary to provide safety as students practice clinical skills. Clinical simulation within a simulation laboratory addresses this need and is also becoming increasingly important as clinical sites are becoming more difficult to obtain.

Simulation

Simulation is an evidence-based teaching strategy that facilitates experiential learning to allow students to learn and practice psychomotor skills and foster critical thinking and clinical reasoning. There are several different types of simulations. When discussing simulation, it is important to address the learning domain, tool, and environmental realism (Forneris, 2020; Forneris et al., 2015). Tools and environmental realism are further categorized into low, medium, and high fidelity. The types of fidelity are on a continuum, depending on how close they are to reality. For example, case studies are considered low fidelity, whereas virtual reality, such as Second Life or standardized patient actors, is considered high fidelity (Forneris, 2020).

Simulation is an exciting and growing modality that uses technology to give students varied experiences that address the different learning domains and provide varying degrees of environmental realism experiences. Examples include virtual skill-based platforms, virtual communities, generic web-based interactive patient simulation systems, digital standardized patients, and platforms that use avatars. **Table 11-1** includes examples of virtual platforms that can be used for simulation in online programs.

Simulations as Experiential Learning

Huun (2018) reviewed several different virtual simulations using a framework based on Quality Matters (QM). Quality Matters developed a rubric that is used to ensure that an online course design meets specific standards based on best practices. Please refer to Chapter 6 for more information on Quality Matters and online nursing programs. The work examined by Huun (2018) was focused on simulation experiences that met the outcome requirements for the development of the clinical skills of prelicensure nursing students. Simulation was based on the theory of deliberate practice, which suggests that expertise is developed through repeated practice with

Table 11-1 Virtual Platforms for Simulation in Online Programs

Platform	Environmental Realism
CathSim	*Intravascular catheterization simulator* Three-dimensional (3D) interactive graphical interface for realism
The Neighborhood	*Virtual community* Unfolding stories of several characters representing community and nurse members that are enhanced with pictures, video clips, medical records, and newspaper clippings
Web-SP	*Generic web-based interactive patient simulation system* A virtual patient system in which faculty can create cases to help students meet specific learning outcomes
Shadow Health	*Digital standardized patients* Students can perform exams and practice documentation through the use of a virtual patient, for example, Tina, who responds based on how she is treated or the questions she is asked by the student. The student can use this at any time, day or night.
Second Life	A virtual world in which the users interact in real time with other users using an avatar, a 3D version of themselves

feedback. Simulation provides the opportunity for students to repeat an activity to gain mastery of specific skills (Forneris, 2020).

The focus of many simulation activities tends to be on the learning outcomes. However, experiential learning is built on the premise that it is a process rather than an outcome. A focus on how one learns is important for building confidence and the willingness to take on new challenges. There is a growing body of research regarding the use of Second Life and the use of avatars for creating experiences that help students gain an appreciation for process issues, such as inclusivity, diversity, and cultural awareness (Tiffany & Hoglund, 2016). However, for online students attending programs that are primarily asynchronous, it can be challenging to rely on synchronous activities.

We believe that using less expensive simulation tools, such as the Neighborhood, a virtual community, can be just as effective. In an article published in the *Journal of Continuing Education*, we described how we used the Neighborhood to engage students in thinking about social justice and health policy, as well as teaching concepts such as community, leadership, advocacy, collaboration, and vulnerable populations (Breen & Jones, 2015). Three different learning activities using the Neighborhood virtual community were developed: (1) a clinical reasoning assignment, (2) a disaster nursing case study, and (3) a coalition planning document that addressed homelessness among veterans. To share a detailed description of each virtual learning activity, we have included the article as an appendix in this chapter. The disaster nursing case study was used for a research study and is found in Chapter 15. The advantages of using this type of virtual simulation include the relatively lower cost to the school and student and the ability to adapt the virtual community to meet the learning needs of the student.

Synchronous Versus Asynchronous Simulation

The value of synchronous simulation has been well established, whereas asynchronous simulation is currently in its infancy and requires more research. Yeh et al. (2019) studied an asynchronous online simulation they developed using deliberate practice for the development of interprofessional communication to report critical incidents among prelicensure nursing students. The researchers found that an asynchronous simulation intervention based on deliberate practice opportunities resulted in a statistically significant group difference in performance and confidence levels in reporting skills using the situation, background, assessment, and recommendation (SBAR) format. The activity involved the student recording an SBAR report after listening to a professionally recorded audio story. Real-time feedback included the use of a self-assessment checklist and responding to self-reflective questions, followed by recording an SBAR report based on the feedback. Students then listened to an example of an effective SBAR report by expert clinicians. This was followed by individual feedback about their performance within 48 hours. This is a promising study regarding the use of asynchronous online simulation among prelicensure students.

Simulation is one of several ways to facilitate experiential learning. Although experiential learning in online education is not well understood or developed (Huun, 2018), we have created several strategies, keeping in mind the experiential learning cycle by Kolb and Kolb (2018).

Experiential Learning Cycle by Kolb and Kolb

Kolb and Kolb (2018) developed the very popular four-stage experiential learning cycle of experiencing, reflecting, thinking, and acting, which is the most widely used concept in experiential learning theory (see **Figure 11-1**).

Based on the experiences of others using the cycle, Kolb and Kolb (2018) identified eight important insights, of which we discuss four that we have found relevant to our experience in teaching online students. Some of the insights are very similar to what was discussed earlier in the experiential learning overview and in Chapter 2. However, it bears repeating, given the significance of being able to apply the theory to the development of meaningful experiential learning activities for students.

Learning Is an Endlessly Recurring Cycle, Not a Linear Process

The learning cycle is an endless exchange between the learner's work and the external environment. Learners receive information through concrete experience and transform it through reflection and thinking and then transform it again through their actions. Thus, they are both receivers and creators of information. As they spiral through the cycle over and over, their depth of understanding and skills deepen.

Kolb and Kolb (2018) suggest organizing the course or program as a series of learning cycles that expands in complexity and application. This is similar to the concept of scaffolding, which is based on Vygotsky's (1978/1997) concept of the zone of proximal development (ZPD), as discussed in Chapter 2. Scaffolding, or the ZPD, is the process of a more knowledgeable peer or adult supporting the learner in constructing knowledge until the support is no longer needed. It is a collaborative process in which the instructor develops learning activities that support students in developing to their fullest potential (Harasim, 2017). An example of scaffolding conceptual learning with experiential learning strategies in an online program is provided in **Table 11-2**. Within nursing, the ZPD could also be conceptualized as mentoring. Faculty in online postlicensure programs often see themselves as mentors as they work collaboratively with students.

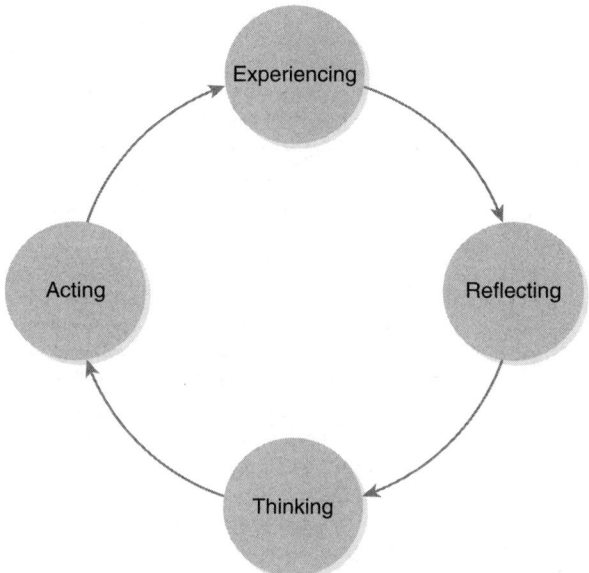

Figure 11-1 Kolb and Kolb four-stage experiential learning cycle

Data from Kolb, A.Y., & Kolb, D.A. (2018). Eight important things to know about The Experiential Learning Cycle. *Australian Educational Leader, 40*(3), 8–14. Retrieved from https://learningfromexperience.com/research-library/eight-important -things-to-know-about-the-experiential-learning-cycle/

Table 11-2 Online RN-to-BSN Program: Semester 1

Curricular Concepts: *Assessment, Community, Vulnerable Populations*	
Phase of the Learning Cycle	**Learning Activities**
Knowledge Building *Community Assessment*	The students learn how to conduct a community assessment. Students are provided with essential information for understanding their own community and for thinking critically about the strengths, challenges, assets, and deficits in the community.

(continues)

Table 11-2 Online RN-to-BSN Program: Semester 1 *(continued)*

Curricular Concepts: *Assessment, Community, Vulnerable Populations*

Phase of the Learning Cycle	Learning Activities
Experiencing *Windshield Survey*	Students drive or walk around their community to observe the physical environment and look for signs of economic development, environmental strengths and concerns, educational systems, safety and transportation options, health and social support systems, housing and recreation, communication, and culture.
Reflecting *Self-Reflection and Collaborative Reflection*	Students are asked to reflect on their findings and write a summary that is shared with the class on the discussion board. Often, they approach this assignment with preconceived notions about what they will find, which are quickly challenged. They often think that their community does not lack any resources. Examples of reflective comments: ■ "It was definitely eye opening." ■ One student reported not feeling safe in some areas because they were not as "nice" as the area where she lived, which challenged her thinking about poverty and race. ■ One student noticed that a major contributor to the economy was an abundance of wineries, which had the student thinking about the risks of drinking and driving. ■ One student noticed the number of gas stations and convenience stores that sell both alcohol and cigarettes, vaping devices, and chewing tobacco, all of which contribute to poor health. ■ One student noticed a lack of parks where children could play in the community.
Nursing Practice	Many students whose experience is limited to acute care begin to understand nursing practice as inclusive of the community.

Experiencing Is Necessary for Learning

For an experience to truly result in critical reflection, it needs to be a jarring experience that disrupts students' normal way of being in the world—something that challenges their beliefs and behaviors. Field trips, role-plays, and other experiential exercises where students are actually experiencing as opposed to completing an exercise can provide this kind of experience (Kolb & Kolb, 2018). Creating this kind of jarring experience can be challenging. We provide examples of what we have used in our registered nurse–bachelor of science in nursing (RN-to-BSN) program later in the chapter. It is important to note that what is "jarring" for one student may not be for another. Therefore, offering a variety of different experiences is recommended.

As faculty, we have found it helpful to reflect on our own experiences that led to significant learning that changed our perceptions. We have slowly and steadily advanced our education and worked in various settings as nurses. This has provided us with a wealth of experiences to draw on. Further, collaborating with other educators can result in creative and inexpensive ideas for experiential learning that can lead to the kind of jarring experience that is needed to advance learning and change students' perspectives to lead to a change in how they practice nursing.

The Brain Is Built for Experiential Learning

Exciting research by James Zull (2002, 2011) and discussed by Kolb and Kolb (2018) shows that learning can be understood in neurological terms. Modification, growth, and pruning of neurons, synapses, and neuronal networks result from learning through experience. Learning actually "physically changes the brain[,] and educating is the art of changing the brain" (Kolb & Kolb, 2018, p. 10). Zull (2002, 2011) found that the learning cycle naturally arises from the structure of the brain. Concrete experience comes through the sensory cortex; reflective observation involves the integrative cortex; the frontal cortex is involved in creating new, abstract concepts; and active testing involves the motor brain (see **Figure 11-2**).

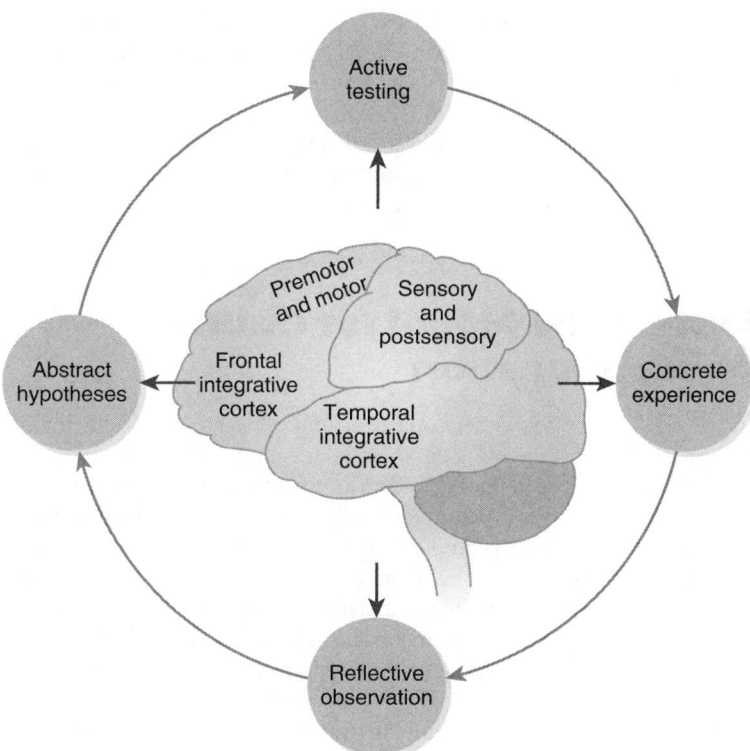

Figure 11-2 The experiential learning cycle and the cerebral cortex

Data from Kolb, A.Y., & Kolb, D.A. (2018). Eight important things to know about The Experiential Learning Cycle. *Australian Educational Leader, 40*(3), 8–14. Retrieved from https://learningfromexperience.com/research-library/eight-important-things-to-know-about-the-experiential-learning-cycle/

The importance of giving time for reflection in order to process thoughts and feelings cannot be understated. Asynchronous online learning inherently gives students the time they need for reflection.

The Dialectic Poles of the Learning Cycle Are What Motivates Learning

Students strive to understand new information through concrete experience (CE) or abstract conceptualization (AC) and, at the same time, are transformed through reflective observation (RO) or active experimentation (AE). Some students grasp new experiences through their senses by immersing themselves in concrete reality (CE), whereas others learn new information through symbolic representation or abstract conceptualization by thinking and analyzing (AC). In processing the experience, some students like to carefully watch others who are involved in the experience and reflect on what happens (RO), whereas others like to jump right in and start doing things (AE). Each student has elements of each learning style. However, they tend to have a preferred style they gravitate toward because it comes easier to them and feels more natural. However, Kolb (2015) found that the most complete and effective learning takes place when the student is challenged to learn from the perspective of every learning style. It is what motivates learning. When one pole dominates, learning is inhibited. For example, rigid beliefs can leave the student closed to new experiences, whereas total immersion in an experience can cloud clear thinking (Kolb & Kolb, 2018).

Learning experiences that engage the dialectic polarities of the cycle promote learning. This can be done by adding systematic reflection and conceptual analysis to a concrete experience (Kolb & Kolb, 2018). For example, when students engage in a concrete experience such as service learning, time for reflection needs to be integrated. When students are asked to reflect on their nursing practice when processing new knowledge in collaborative discussions, they put themselves back in the practice experience.

Adapting the Model for Online Nursing Education

The insights related to the experiential learning cycle are important to consider when planning and implementing experiential learning within the online program. Experiential learning can be embedded throughout an online program, with the intent of advancing learning within not only the cognitive domain but also the affective domain in order to promote action or change in practice. Integration of experiential learning theory and the domains of learning assists the faculty member in planning for experiences that facilitate higher-level learning. For example, cognitive learning deals with the intellectual side, such as knowledge building, whereas affective learning reaches the student's emotions and beliefs. Working through inherent conflicts between and within these domains facilitates the personal and professional growth that extends into nursing practice. We believe it is this integration of cognitive and affective learning that leads to change in practice. However, further research needs to be done in order to examine the impact of experiential learning in online programs on practice. At this point, we know what students tell us and how their thinking about nursing practice has changed.

Several factors need to be considered when planning for experiential learning, such as the student population and where the learning will take place, within the online classroom or outside the classroom in a clinical or community setting. Planning also involves scaffolding the learning experiences so that understanding deepens and skills develop progressively as students move through the program. Intentionally aligning online learning experiences across the curriculum, as opposed to within standalone courses, is a high-impact practice that creates a more holistic, comprehensive experience for students (Linder & Hayes, 2018).

As with conceptual learning, one of the goals is for students to be able to generalize new knowledge and apply it in different settings and circumstances. As they gain confidence and experience, students no longer need a mentor. In fact, the student may become the mentor.

Given what we have learned from designing experiential learning activities in an online program, we propose an adapted model for postlicensure online teaching and learning. In keeping with Kolb and Kolb's (2018) theory, our model emphasizes that learning is a process. The cycle is one in which nurses' perceptions of their practice evolve with new knowledge and experiences as they engage in ongoing self-reflection and collaborative reflection.

Figure 11-3 illustrates an adapted model for experiential learning in nursing education. To further illustrate the learning that occurs, we have used three

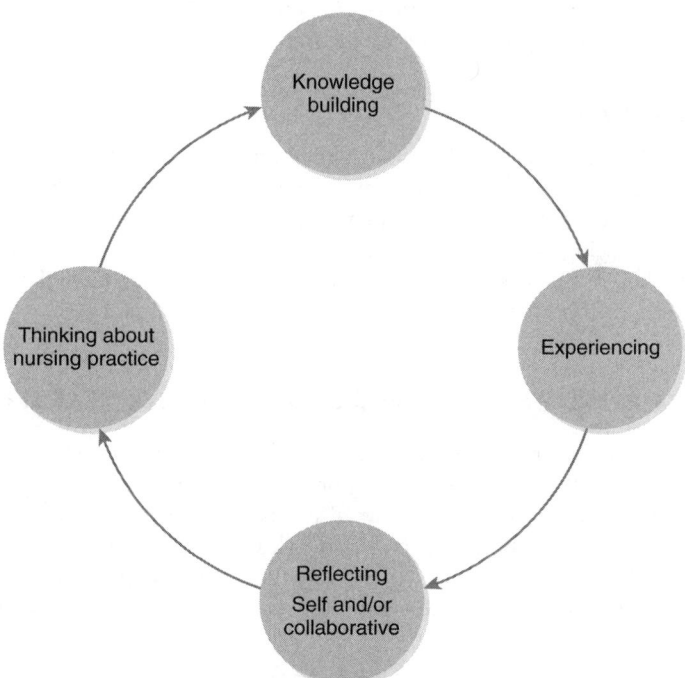

Figure 11-3 Online experiential learning

Data from Kolb, A.Y., & Kolb, D.A. (2018). Eight important things to know about The Experiential Learning Cycle. *Australian Educational Leader, 40*(3), 8–14. Retrieved from https://learningfromexperience.com/research-library/eight-important-things-to-know-about-the-experiential-learning-cycle/

different experiential learning strategies applied sequentially across three semesters (Tables 11-2–11-4) of the curriculum to promote higher-level thinking, challenge assumptions, and construct new knowledge related to the concepts of assessment, community, and vulnerability. The descriptions also demonstrate how scaffolding or the ZPD can be applied in online education.

Semester 1

Identifying key concepts helps in determining which concepts are important to reinforce using experiential learning strategies. Our program has an emphasis on community and vulnerability, which is why it is important to introduce these concepts early in the program and scaffold the learning as students progress through the program. The experiential learning strategy highlighted in Table 11-2 has students beginning to think about nursing beyond the acute care of an individual, expanding to assessment and vulnerability in the community, during the first semester.

Semester 2

In the second semester, the same concepts of assessment and vulnerability are addressed at a deeper level through the lens of diversity among patients and staff in the workplace. Assessment and vulnerability are important considerations when addressing inclusivity, equity, and immigration experiences. Deepening self-awareness through self-reflection is key to developing cultural humility (Foronda, Baptiste, Reinholdt, & Ousman, 2016). **Table 11-3** demonstrates how the concepts are taught at a deeper level through a scaffolding approach to the learning experience.

Semester 3

As students move to the third semester, they are introduced to the concepts of assessment and vulnerability at the level of population health (**Table 11-4**). The expectations for students increase in relation to professional communication, working in groups, and using evidence to make decisions. The progression of the curriculum and scaffolding of the learning activities are reinforced through activities designed to help students continue to develop as leaders in their community.

Other Experiential Learning Strategies

Most students in postlicensure programs have previous work experience and are working while in the program. In addition to the experiential learning activities offered in their educational program, we also consider their work in the profession as experiential learning. Best practice for adult learning is to facilitate collaborative reflection and application to their current and future nursing practice. The following are some strategies that we have used, with positive feedback from students.

Arts and Literature Activity

Using arts and literature can be an effective teaching strategy for evoking emotional responses, generating discussion, and enhancing clinical decision making

Table 11-3 Online RN-to-BSN Program: Semester 2

Curricular Concepts: *Assessment, Community, Vulnerable Populations*

Phase of the Learning Cycle	Learning Activities
Knowledge Building *Culture Assessment*	Students are introduced to a couple of different cultural assessments.
Experiencing *Conducting a Cultural* *Self-Assessment*	Using a Cultural Assessment Tool such as Purnell's (2000) Domains of Cultural Competence or Giger and Davidhizar's (2002) Transcultural Assessment Model, students complete their own cultural assessment.
Reflecting *Self-Reflection and* *Collaborative Reflection*	Students share their personal cultural self-assessment on the discussion board. Many Caucasian American students are very challenged to think of themselves as having a cultural identity and struggle with this. In sharing their cultural history, values, and beliefs, respect and understanding of differences are appreciated. Insight is gained by sharing the challenges faced by immigrant students.

It is not necessary to go through all the phases in order. Sometimes, it is important to repeat a phase or phases before moving on. This is a two-part experience in which self-reflection moves to a deeper level as students assess their own communication skills in conducting a cultural assessment.

Experiencing *Conducting a Cultural* *Assessment of a Colleague*	Using Purnell's (2000) Cultural Assessment Tool or Giger and Davidhizar's (2002) Transcultural Assessment Model, students conduct an interview of someone from a different culture to experience conducting a cultural assessment using therapeutic communication and learning about the challenges in their community or workplace.
Reflecting *Self-Reflection*	Students write a paper highlighting their findings and compare their beliefs and values to those of a colleague. They are required to look up one evidence-based strategy in working with someone of a different culture. Students reflect on their own communication style in conducting the interview. In their papers, they are asked to identify their own cultural identity to provide context for the reader. Many of the Caucasian American students fail to do this, which reinforces how challenging it is for them to understand their own White privilege, whereas students of other ethnic backgrounds have no problem completing this part of the assignment. Failure

(continues)

Table 11-3 Online RN-to-BSN Program: Semester 2   *(continued)*

Curricular Concepts: *Assessment, Community, Vulnerable Populations*

Phase of the Learning Cycle	Learning Activities
	to identify their own culture demonstrates a lack of cultural humility, which requires self-reflection, openness, self-awareness, and supportive interactions to foster the ability to be other-oriented in relation to aspects of cultural identity (Foronda et al., 2016). *Note:* It is critical to provide feedback regarding this when evaluating the paper.
Nursing Practice	Caucasian students often express surprise that the person they ask to meet with is willing to share. They learn that all they need to do is express interest and engage in a meaningful conversation in which they actively listen. Once they interview someone of a different culture, they realize they didn't really know the person they have worked with for years and start to gain deeper insight into their own culture and their understanding of someone else. Some students gained a deeper appreciation related to immigration because they often interviewed someone who immigrated from another country, such as the Philippines, Russia, Mexico, Ukraine, or Bosnia, to name a few. Their preconceived notions were challenged. As one student wrote, "It made me rethink how I communicate with my patients[,] and I wondered if I was as open minded as I had hoped I had become over time." They also expressed increased comfort in working with colleagues of a different ethnicity, which was also applied to their patients. This has implications for working with a diverse workforce in health care.

Table 11-4 Online RN-to-BSN Program: Semester 3

Curricular Concepts: *Assessment, Community, Vulnerable Populations*

Phase of the Learning Cycle	Learning Activities
Knowledge Building *Social Determinants of Health (SDOH)*	Students are introduced to the social determinants of health (SDOH) as a framework for the online population health course. They complete learning activities throughout the course that address economic stability, education, social and community context, health and access to health care, the neighborhood and built environment, and global health and epidemiology.

Curricular Concepts: *Assessment, Community, Vulnerable Populations*	
Phase of the Learning Cycle	**Learning Activities**
Experiencing *Advocacy Proposal With Group Discussion and Debate Activity*	Students develop an advocacy proposal that addresses a current health or social issue that is affecting a specific vulnerable population in the local, national, or global community. Students are required to gather assessment (epidemiologic) data that reflects the scope of the problem affecting the population, discuss the short- and long-term health effects, and propose a policy-level solution to address the problem. Students are required to design the one-page advocacy proposal in a way that it could be presented to a specific audience (e.g., grant committee, tribal council, school board) that is in a position to make decisions or allocate resources to address the issue. In assigned small groups in the online classroom, students present their proposals to their group members. Their group members, serving as members of the intended audience, are required to develop an opposing view (evidence based), which is addressed through collaborative discussion. Goals include developing skills in the assessment of vulnerable populations and persuasive, effective communication that uses evidence to support their positions.
Reflecting *Self-Reflection and Collaborative Reflection*	Students report that the experience with this activity allows them to articulate the needs of a specific vulnerable population that they have a passion for serving (e.g., homeless teens, veterans, adults with disabilities). They report growth in their awareness of the social and health issues affecting the group after performing research to inform their advocacy. In their groups, they recognize the challenges of being persuasive in their advocacy as well as providing an opposing view to important issues. An important outcome they report after participating in the online activity is growth in their ability to communicate effectively.
Nursing Practice	An important outcome from this activity includes moving from a community-level perspective on assessment and vulnerability to a population-level perspective. Students report developing a broader view of issues affecting vulnerable populations.

(Herrman, 2006). An additional benefit of using visual arts in the online classroom includes appealing to visual learners. We have used arts and literature in a variety of online courses, including a population health course when teaching about epidemiology and disease outbreak investigation. Components of the assignment are included in **Table 11-5**.

Table 11-5 Using Arts and Literature for Online Experiential Learning

Purpose	Explore a variety of biographical, historical, political, and popular culture events and perspectives that may influence health behaviors, decision making, health outcomes, and the overall well-being of the public through **critical analysis** and **dialogue**.
Instructions	Go to the Arts & Literature Activity on the Discussion Board. This activity will require meaningful and active participation during the required time frame as well as evidence that you have read the novel and watched the movie.
Critical Analysis	■ Post a one-paragraph review of the book *Vaccinated: One Man's Quest to Defeat the World's Deadliest Diseases* by Dr. Paul Offit. ■ Post a one-paragraph review of the movie *Contagion* (motion picture, 2011). Think critically about the concepts from the course that are revealed in the book and movie: epidemiology, disease outbreak, global travel/globalization, vaccinations, roles of healthcare professionals and epidemiologists, the role of the Centers for Disease Control and Prevention (CDC) and other major public health organizations, and other issues that may have occurred to you.
Critical Reflection	■ Share your thoughts, any new awareness, or links to the course material or global health caused by the review of this literature and cinema. ■ Did the material change or support your views on vaccinations or disease outbreak?
Generate Discussion	■ Use details from the book and/or movie to develop one vaccine-related discussion question or topic that will advance the discussion.
Apply Literature	■ Integrate at least two pieces of scientific literature supporting your position or advancing the discussion related to vaccinations.
Collaborate With Peers	Post at least two replies to your peers: ■ Thoughtfully analyze the issues, ask questions, and expand on the discussion. ■ Respectfully debate the various perspectives and views on the issues. ■ Be sure to respond to all comments that involve you.

Interviews

In addition to the interview assignment mentioned Table 11-3, we have used interviews to enhance higher-level thinking about interprofessional communication and leadership. Interprofessional communication and collaboration are critical to patient safety. Developing experiences that enhance interprofessional communication can be challenging in a school that does not have other health-related schools, such as a health sciences educational institution. More and more schools are providing educational experiences in which students from different disciplines share in coursework. In our program with working nurses, we have them interview different members of the healthcare team using a simple guided-interview process. They reflect on the findings and share the results of the interview and their thoughts about it with the class on the discussion board.

Through this activity, they have gained insight into how nurse-centric they were and how they focused mostly on their communication with physicians, other nurses, nurse's aides, and possibly social workers. This had more to do with how they could help the nurse in meeting the patient's needs. Prior to this assignment, they did not give a lot of thought to how much other health-related professionals, such as pharmacists, lab technicians, physical therapists, and occupational therapists, cared about the patient and how much they wanted to work with the nurses and have nurses value their contribution. Once they took the time to engage with them in a meaningful way, many students expressed a desire to collaborate more with other professionals in order to improve patient care.

In a leadership class, students have been assigned to interview a manager about many of the concepts discussed in the class, such as patient safety, just culture, disaster planning, holding staff accountable, leadership style, and facilitating change, to name a few. Students are asked to interview in depth on no more than three topics. This experience has not only helped students gain a deeper appreciation of leadership and the management role but also allowed students to gain a deeper understanding of the organizations they work for.

Small-Group Work Using a Case Study

Using a comprehensive case study, students work in small groups of three to four students to write a scholarly paper addressing several questions related to the case study. This group project is required in the third semester, and students are given the following instructions:

> The goal of this assignment is to engage in some cooperative but mostly collaborative work. *Cooperative* work refers to dividing up the work in order to complete a part of the final product independently. *Collaborative* work is based on working together to produce the final product. Many minds on the same issue will produce better results. This means that every group member needs to be involved in every part of the assignment. You can have leads on different parts, but everyone needs to become familiar with all the concepts related to this assignment. This means providing feedback and adding to the topic and not merely agreeing with what someone else wrote.

The case study is very comprehensive; it chronicles the development of a nurse leader and her experiences as a nurse manager through two different organizations. The topics include leadership style, mentoring, major change in which two units merge, conflict, incivility, social media, patient safety, a close call in which a patient nearly dies, and "Just Culture," to name a few.

Students express that this group assignment was very challenging for them, but they learned a great deal about themselves and teamwork. As one student stated:

> I have to say working on the group paper challenged me the most and taught me the most about teamwork in this class. I felt it was the most involved and demanding lesson in that it involved constant touching base and communication throughout the entire process. Also, all the learning will help me be a better communicator and collaborator in my role as a PACU nurse.

In this assignment, there is an opportunity to assess the students not only on the outcome of their work but also on their ability to collaborate.

Service Learning

A highlight of our online RN-to-BSN program is service learning. As part of their capstone course, students participate in a service-learning experience that allows students to serve the needs of the community while addressing academic requirements (Trail Ross, 2012). Service learning requires time to reflect on the complexity involved in the service issue, the context in which the experience takes place, the social meaning of the population served, and the link to program concepts (Gillis & MacLellan, 2010).

Shortly after our School of Nursing revised the baccalaureate program to a concept-based curriculum, we started to "think differently" about experiential learning for online RN-to-BSN students. Until that point, postlicensure students had participated in a traditional leadership clinical experience in an area of nursing practice that they identified as a professional goal or interest. Because many of them were already experienced registered nurses, their impression of the experience was that it was a "shadow" experience. Although they were not allowed to work directly with their managers or on units where they worked, many of them still identified a nurse manager whom they respected or a manager who was willing to work with them in their facilities.

As we considered a revision to experiential learning, several things were going on both locally and nationally, including the passage of the Affordable Care Act (ACA), which provided access to health care for millions of Americans. At the same time, patients were spending less time in the hospital, and the care of patients with chronic conditions was becoming increasingly challenging. We believed that we had a responsibility to address these issues in our curriculum while encouraging postlicensure students to meet their individual leadership goals in a less traditional, *required* community-based experience.

Students participate in service learning with a vulnerable population of their choice in their own communities or in an international community. They are required to work with their faculty and a community organization to set up the experience with a specific vulnerable population. As they develop and carry out the experience, they have the opportunity to bridge the gap between theory and practice in a way that works for them. Further, the goal for students in developing their own service-learning experience under the guidance of faculty is to develop confidence in their leadership skills.

Evaluation of Service Learning

By conducting an evaluation study, we found that students did, in fact, gain confidence as they began to recognize how much they were appreciated and respected as nurses. They developed their leadership skills as they worked independently in the community organization, assessing the learning needs of the population they were working with to provide education and nursing care (Breen & Robinson, 2016).

Students identified that their understanding of vulnerable populations changed as a result of the experience; for some it changed dramatically, as noted in the following student quote: "I have been more than undereducated and not aware of the struggles of people [living] in my community. I have been very self-absorbed with my own needs to be aware of others." Other students identified how the experience changed their practice. For example, another student stated:

> This experience has forever changed how I will work with vulnerable families, individuals, and groups. I am planning on completing my FNP [Family Nurse Practitioner] … this opportunity has shown me the real need for more primary care practitioners in my community and I am now planning on going into primary care after my masters. I have also applied for an on-call position in the free medical clinic so that I can continue the work I started with my service-learning project.

In researching the impact of service learning, we found that students demonstrated higher-level thinking by linking concepts learned earlier in the curriculum through ongoing reflection on their experience. Further, they reported applying this new learning to their nursing practice (Breen & Robinson, 2016). We built on this study by evaluating not only the student learning but also the impact on the community organizations the students worked with. The findings were remarkable. Four primary themes emerged related to the impact: (1) increased access to health support and education for the population, (2) improved involvement of the community members in health activities as a result of the credibility and qualifications of the student, (3) higher quality of care and services based on the expertise of the students, and (4) increased trust and confidence in the organization based on effective and therapeutic communication with clients (Breen & Robinson, 2019). The published research study can be found in Chapter 16.

Summary

Experiential learning is an ongoing process in which students discover new knowledge about themselves, their environment, and their nursing practice through direct experiences and focused reflections. Many different types of experiential learning were discussed in this chapter, from simulations to service learning. The importance of careful planning and scaffolding of the experiences was emphasized.

Best-Practice Recommendations for Online Teaching

- Experiential learning is an important component of all nursing education, including online education.
- Experiential learning is a process. It is important to attend to both the process and the learning outcomes. Attending to the process helps to instill lifelong learning through ongoing reflection.
- High-cost simulation is not required to provide effective experiential learning.
- Scaffolding concepts using experiential learning takes planning and creativity. Working collaboratively with other faculty to align learning experiences across the curriculum improves creativity and has a high impact on student learning.
- Community-based experiential learning activities, such as service learning, provide online nursing students with opportunities to serve vulnerable groups in their own communities while developing higher-level skills in advocacy, community engagement, leadership, and more.

References

Breen, H., & Jones, M. (2015). Experiential learning: Using virtual simulation in an online RN-to-BSN program. *The Journal of Continuing Education in Nursing, 46*(1), 27–33.

Breen, H., & Robinson, M. (2019). Academic partnerships: Social determinants of health addressed through service-learning. *International Journal of Nursing Education Scholarship, 16*(1). http://doi.org/10.1515/ijnes-2019-0062

Breen, H., & Robinson, M. (2016). Service learning enhances conceptual learning in a RN to BSN program. *International Journal for Innovation Education and Research, 4*(10), 197–210. https://ijier.net/index.php/ijier/article/view/609

Forneris, S. G. (2020). Teaching and learning using simulations In D. M. Billings & J. A. Halstead (Eds.), *Teaching in nursing: A guide for faculty* (6th ed., pp. 353 – 373). Elsevier.

Forneris, S. G., Neal, D. O., Tiffany, J., Kuehn, M. B., Blazovich, L. M., & Snerillo, M. (2015). Enhancing clinical reasoning through simulation debriefing: A multisite study. *Nursing Education Perspectives, 36*(5), 304–310. https://doi.org/10.5480/15-1672

Foronda, C., Baptiste, D. L., Reinholdt, M. M., & Ousman, K. (2016). Cultural humility: A concept analysis. *Journal of Transcultural Nursing, 27*(3), 210–217. http://doi.org/10.1177/1043659615592677

Gillis, A., & MacLellan, M. (2010). Service learning with vulnerable populations: Review of the literature. *International Journal of Nursing Education Scholarship, 7*(1), 1–27. http://doi.org/10.2202/1548-923X.2041

Giger, J.N., & Davidhizar, R. (2002). The Giger and Davidhizar Transcultural Assessment Model, *Journal of Transcultural Nursing, 13*(3). doi:10.1177/10459602013003004

Harasim, L. (2017). *Learning theory and online technologies* (2nd ed.). Routledge.

Hartley, M. P. (2010). Experiential learning using Kolb's cycle of learning. *Journal of Nursing Education, 49*(2), 120. https://doi.org/10.3928/01484834-20100119-02

Herman, J. (2006). Using film clips to enhance nursing education. *Nurse Educator 31*(6). DOI: 10.1097/00006223-200611000-00010

Huun, K. (2018). Virtual simulation in online nursing education: Align with quality matters. *Clinical Simulation in Nursing, 22*, 26–31. https://doi.org/10.1016/j.ecns.2018.07.002

Kolb, D. A. (1984). *Experiential learning: Experience as the source of learning and development.* Prentice-Hall.

Kolb, D. A. (2015). *Experiential learning: Experience as the source of learning and development* (2nd ed.). Pearson Education.

Kolb, A., Kolb, D.A. (2013). *The Kolb Learning Style Inventory 4.0: A comprehensive guide to the theory, psychometrics, research on validity and educational applications.* Experience Based Learning Systems. Inc. https://learningfromexperience.com/research-library/the-kolb-learning-style-inventory-4-0/

Kolb, A. Y., & Kolb, D. A. (2018). Eight important things to know about the experiential learning cycle. *Australian Educational Leader, 40*(3), 8–14.

Linder, K. E., & Hayes, C. M. (2018). *High-impact practices in online education: Research and best practices.* Stylus.

Purnell, L. (2000). A description of the Purnell model for cultural competence. *Journal of Transcultural Nursing, 11*(1), 40–46.

Tiffany, J. M., & Hoglund, B. A. (2016). Using virtual simulation to teach inclusivity: A case study. *Clinical Simulation in Nursing, 12*(4), 115–122. https://doi.org/10.1016/j.ecns.2015.11.003

Trail Ross, M. E. (2012). Linking classroom learning to the community through service learning. *Journal of Community Health Nursing, 29,* 53–60.

Vygotsky, L. (1997). Interaction between learning and development. In M. Gauvain & M. Cole (Eds.), *Readings on the development of children* (Vol. 2, pp. 29–36). W. H. Freeman and Company. (Reprinted from *Mind and society*, pp. 79–91, by L. Vygotsky, 1978, Cambridge University Press.)

Yeh, V. J. H., Sherwood, G., Durham, C. F., Kardong-Edgren, S., Schwartz, T. A., & Beeber, L. S. (2019). Online simulation-based mastery learning with deliberate practice: Developing interprofessional communication skill. *Clinical Simulation in Nursing, 32*(C), 27–38. https://doi.org/10.1016/j.ecns.2019.04.005

Zull, J. (2002). *The art of changing the brain.* Stylus.

Zull, J. (2011). *From brain to mind: Using neuroscience to guide change in education.* Stylus.

Appendix

Experiential Learning: Using Virtual Simulation in an Online RN-to-BSN Program

Henny Breen and Melissa Jones*

Abstract

This article highlights the innovative experiential learning used by an online RN-to-BSN program through the use of simulation that takes place in an online classroom. Three experiential learning activities using a virtual community are described. These learning activities engage the students in thinking about social justice and health policy, as well as teaching concepts that include community, leadership, influence, advocacy, networking, collaboration, and vulnerable populations. These concepts are critical to the learning needs of diploma and associate degree-prepared nurses who wish to continue their education to be better prepared to meet the complex needs of today's health care environment.

Background

The demands of the current health care environment require nurses to have a broader knowledge base that goes beyond technological competence to include abilities in leadership, health policy, system improvement, research and evidence-based practice, teamwork, and collaboration (Institute of Medicine [IOM], 2010; Smith, 2010). In addition to this broad-based knowledge, competency in specific content areas such as public health with a greater orientation to community-based primary care and an emphasis on health promotion are required (IOM, 2010).

Breen, H., & Jones, M. (2015). Experiential learning: Using virtual simulation in an online RN-to-BSN program. *Journal of Continuing Education in Nursing, 46*(1), 27–33.

In response to this need, a small liberal arts college in the northwestern United States developed an online RN-to-baccalaureate nursing (BSN) program that is community- and concept-based, emphasizing leadership, health promotion, illness prevention and treatment, and social justice through a learner-centered approach to nursing education. In recent years, several schools of nursing have adopted concept-based curricula as a framework that is well-supported in the literature. The advantages of this approach to nursing education include a more streamlined approach to managing content, a student-centered approach to teaching, and enhanced critical thinking on behalf of students (Giddens et al., 2008; Giddens & Morton, 2010). A learner-centered approach to education is a framework that provides the opportunity for students to engage in discourse about complex issues that emerge in higher education (Dolence, 2003). This approach is integral to the online program as students engage in collaborative written discourse in all of the courses.

RN-to-BSN programs build on diploma and associate degree in nursing (ADN) programs with coursework that facilitates professional development and a better understanding of the cultural, political, economic, and social issues that impact patients and health care delivery. Online education is recognized as offering the flexibility needed for practicing diploma and ADN-prepared RNs to return to school to earn their BSN (IOM, 2010). As a result, online learning in nursing education has been evolving at a rapid pace (Billings & Halstead, 2009). Providing experiences that enhance this learning is critical to the nurses' career development as they continue their education. Many schools of nursing report challenges involved in securing clinical teaching sites for their nursing students driving the need for innovative teaching strategies that meet student needs for experiential learning. This article highlights the innovative experiential learning used by an online RN-to-BSN program through the use of simulation that takes place in an online classroom.

RN to BSN Program

Approximately 150 RNs enter the online program each year, and a total of 324 nurses graduated with their BSN between 2010 and 2013. The majority of nurses who attend the program are employed in nursing and bring a variety of personal and professional experiences to the online classroom as they continue their education to meet the demands of the current health care environment. To enhance students' continuing education, the faculty who teach in the RN-to-BSN program are committed to a constructivist pedagogy based on constructivist-learning theory. Constructivist-learning theory suggests that learning is an active process in which learners make meaning of new information and construct new knowledge through experience and reflection on that experience (Harasim, 2012; Jahng, Nielsen, & Chan, 2010). This is vital in a program in which much of the learning occurs through students engaging with the course content by reflecting on new knowledge and integrating it with their previous knowledge, nursing practice, and personal experiences.

In addition, equally vital to learners enrolled in the online RN-to-BSN program is collaborative learning as much of the learning is enhanced through collaborative written discourse. Collaborative learning is an active process in which learners make meaning of new information and construct new knowledge with a group of knowledgeable peers rather than constructing new knowledge alone (Guilar & Loring, 2008; Jahng et al., 2010).

A unique feature of this program is the final course, Integrated Experiential Learning (IEL), as it integrates all of the previous learning in the program using three main strategies to meet students' learning needs. These strategies are:

- Clinical experience with a preceptor who is a nurse leader.
- Professional development activities that are negotiated between the student and instructor.
- Three experiential learning activities using a virtual community.

The three virtual learning activities use collaborative learning theory to guide students' engagement in the activity along with other theoretical orientations or strategies.

The IEL Course

Three learning activities using the virtual community, The Neighborhood™ developed by Jean Giddens, are highlighted with emphasis on the learning outcomes and students' evaluation of their own learning. The Neighborhood features unfolding stories of several characters representing community and nurse members. The stories are enhanced with pictures, video clips, medical records, and newspaper clippings (Giddens, 2010).

Students enrolled in the IEL course are required to become familiar with the virtual community throughout the course and to complete an orientation scavenger hunt for The Neighborhood to participate in the learning activities. The three learning activities in the IEL course include a clinical reasoning assignment, a disaster nursing case study, and a coalition planning document. All three learning activities are intended to meet the higher level learning requirements of leadership, health policy, system improvement, research and evidence-based practice, teamwork, and collaboration for BSN graduates.

Clinical Reasoning

An activity using clinical reasoning was chosen for students to demonstrate higher-order thinking in providing nursing care. Clinical reasoning is influenced by the nurse's attitude, preconceptions, philosophical perspective, and ability to think critically. Thus, clinical reasoning requires the nurse to master higher-order thinking skills that can be achieved through the development of critical and reflective thinking that requires the self-regulation of cognitive and metacognitive thinking in nursing practice (Kuiper & Pesut, 2004). Throughout the program, students are challenged to develop these skills through the use of collaborative discussion, reflective practice journal writing, and written assignments. This is consistent with constructivist pedagogy and collaborative learning as learning occurs individually through interactions with others in which the learners share, construct, and reconstruct their ideas and beliefs (Chikotas, 2008).

Students were provided with an overview of the Outcome-Present State Test (OPT) model of clinical reasoning used by the school of nursing. The OPT model of clinical reasoning is a third-generation nursing process meta-model. The OPT model is designed to assist students in planning and evaluating their nursing care by building on prior knowledge in an iterative fashion to further develop their nursing thinking skills (Bartlett et al., 2008; Kautz et al., 2009). The authors of the model, Pesut and Herman, based the model on Bandura's self-efficacy learning theory, which postulates that students' problem solving skills improve if they see that their actions make a positive difference (as cited in Kautz et al., 2009). As students understand how nursing diagnoses, nursing actions, and making judgments about the care they provide makes a difference in moving patients from their current state to a desired outcome, the students' ability to clinically reason improves (Kautz et al., 2009).

Clinical Reasoning Activity. Students were required to use the model in addressing the needs of one member or family of their choice from the virtual community. As the students worked on developing their individual plan, they had the option to collaborate with each other to learn from each other's expertise as practicing nurses. This learning activity highlights both their cognitive and metacognitive thinking by articulating their reasoning that includes patterns, filters, and assumptions as they write the client story gleaned from The Neighborhood.

Students then developed two nursing diagnoses, specific nursing and collaborative actions, which required other health care providers within the virtual community, to meet the client's needs, and identify potential risks from these actions. The students followed this model using nursing judgment to assess patient outcomes. Following the development of their plan for the virtual community member, students reflected on their learning, including how they used evidence-based strategies and ethical reasoning to provide nursing care.

Disaster Nursing

Disaster nursing was chosen as an exemplar activity for teaching concepts in the IEL course that included community, collaboration, leadership, and vulnerable populations. The IEL course provides an opportunity to engage more fully in the previously learned concepts by using experiential learning activities such as a simulated disaster. A problem-based learning (PBL) approach was used in the development and delivery of the simulated disaster experience.

PBL is a strategy that has been used to enhance collaboration among students while recognizing the prior knowledge and experiences of adult learners (Chikotas, 2008). Adult students appreciate a relevant approach to education that is immediately applicable to their life and work. In nursing education, PBL provides practical and effective learning experiences such as case studies, problem solving exercises, and service-learning experiences (American Association of Colleges of Nursing [AACN] & Association of American Medical Colleges, 2010).

In an experimental study that compared PBL and conventional teaching in an undergraduate nursing program, Lin, Lu, Chung, and Yang (2010) identified PBL as an organized, student-centered educational strategy. The results demonstrated evidence of learning effectiveness for both groups; however, the PBL group was found to be more effective. Students who participated in PBL reported higher satisfaction with skills in self-motivation and critical thinking compared to the group who participated in conventional teaching (Lin et al., 2010). The researchers also found that the distance between the students' developmental level and their potential was supported by engaging in a socially interactive process of problem solving that was influenced by the skills and abilities of each student. When developing the disaster nursing activity, the previous knowledge and experience of the RN-to-BSN students was considered. In addition, opportunities for interaction and peer collaboration were purposely integrated.

Disaster Learning Activity. To prepare for their work during the disaster in the virtual community, students were required to complete all of their reading assignments for The Neighborhood. At the start of this activity, an announcement was placed in the course to notify students that a disaster had occurred in the virtual community. For example, the following announcement was used to alert students to a simulated earthquake:

> Earthquake Strikes the Neighborhood
>
> A magnitude 6.8 earthquake struck The Neighborhood Community early this morning. Residents are warned to stay away from buildings that appear loosened from the initial earthquake due to the risk posed by aftershocks. Many of the residents of The Neighborhood have been displaced from their homes. Your work assignment today is working as a community/public health nurse, and you are to report immediately to The Neighborhood to care for the residents and assist your colleagues in addressing this disaster. Please let me know if you have any questions. Have fun!

To supplement The Neighborhood, video clips of past earthquakes were posted to give the students a visual picture of the disaster. Resources regarding disaster nursing were provided, such as peer-reviewed articles about the nurse's role in disasters and the International Council of Nursing's (2009) *ICN Framework of Disaster Nursing Competencies*. The students were instructed to role-play being a community health nurse and to collaborate with each other in providing care to the families who were impacted by the disaster.

As the students engaged in their roles, several themes and topics began to surface. Some of the topics included communication issues, such as cell phone batteries dying and access to ham radios; missing or displaced people; resources such as the role of the Red Cross, Federal Emergency Management Agency, and the Coast Guard; triage and transportation including START (simple triage and rapid transport); challenges regarding access to resources such as electricity, generators, or oxygen supply for a patient with chronic obstructive pulmonary disease; where to set up a safe shelter; damage to the community hospital; stress and loss; and the need for debriefing and support for their nurse colleagues as they cared for others. In their role as community health nurse, the students also engaged with other community partners such as teachers, law enforcement, physicians and other health care providers, and volunteers.

Following the role-play activity, students engaged in a more formal discussion in which they researched and shared information about leadership in a disaster; recovery and rehabilitation; ethical, legal, and accountability issues; and an assessment of the virtual community in terms of the resources needed to care for the community during a disaster. The following question, with an explanatory prelude, also was used to generate discussion:

> *Prelude:* Hurricane Katrina was one of the deadliest storms to ever reach the shores of the United States (Priest & Bahl, 2008). This storm devastated New Orleans and left its hospitals in utter chaos. Hospitals were

barely able to provide staff to provide minimal care and those who were available worked under the most extreme circumstances (Priest & Bahl, 2008). Following the devastation, a doctor and two nurses were arrested for concerns related to alleged "euthanasia" of patients at Memorial Medical Center (see newspaper article in the learning module).

Question: Describe the details of this situation; be sure to include the impact on patients, hospital personnel, and the community. Analyze the key ethical, legal, and accountability issues that the nurse should be aware of during a disaster.

In addition to the role-play, this activity was implemented by requiring students to develop a nursing action plan for one individual or family in The Neighborhood. The individuals and families chosen for this activity faced specific vulnerabilities, for example, an elderly couple who were displaced from their home as a result of the disaster. In this particular example, students used their action plan to identify how they would prioritize the needs of the elderly couple. Examples of their planning included how they would connect the couple with family members who could take them in, how they would obtain necessary medications, how they would meet their physical health needs, and how they could ensure their immediate safety in the community.

Through addressing the vulnerabilities of individuals in the community during a disaster, students developed additional interest and even formed bonds with the characters. The emotional engagement in the activity was expected to heighten the memory of the learned material (Zull, 2004). In addition, the context diversity that was achieved through engaging in multiple communication and interactive modes during the disaster allowed students to benefit from lived experience rather than reading an isolated case study (Carlson-Sabelli, Giddens, Fogg, & Fiedler, 2011).

Coalition Building

Coalition building for homeless veterans was chosen as an exemplar activity for engaging the students in thinking about social justice and health policy as well as teaching concepts in the IEL course that included community, leadership, influence, advocacy, networking, collaboration, and vulnerable populations. Sullivan (2004) defined a coalition as "an alliance of people or groups with similar goals who join to achieve their objectives" (p. 90). For this activity, smaller groups of three to five students were chosen because smaller groups provide the time and space available for learners to express their ideas (Boettcher & Conrad, 2010). In addition, small groups allow each student to contribute substantially to the final product. Faculty also are able to assess the students' leadership skills when they collaborate in small groups to produce a final product as decisions need to be made about how students will work together (Breen, 2014).

For this activity, homeless veterans were chosen as an exemplar to meet the Joining Forces pledge taken by Linfield-Good Samaritan School of Nursing in 2013. The pledge was taken to join the AACN, the Department of Veteran Affairs, the American Nurses Association, the National League for Nursing, the National Organization for Associate Degree Nursing, and other stakeholders that urged nursing schools across the United States to support the national initiative led by First Lady Michelle Obama and Dr. Jill Biden. By pledging their support, nursing schools agreed to enhance the education and preparation of the nation's nurses to care for veterans, service members, and their families (AACN, 2014).

Planning Document for a Community Coalition Activity. To prepare for the activity, students in an early learning module discussed how they could influence community change through the use of coalitions. They initially discussed an issue that was important to them and how they would start a coalition to address the issue using their influence as RNs. The students were provided with information about evidence-based practices for coalition building and examples of successful coalitions. Being able to choose an issue that was important to them engaged the students because it had special meaning.

Information about homeless veterans was provided along with a review about coalition building and planning steps for the development of a coalition. The students worked in a wiki to facilitate collaboration among the group members. Working in a wiki permitted group members to contribute and modify the document, and changes and additions were tracked ("Wikis," 2013). The students in the small groups were instructed to develop a planning document for a community coalition in The Neighborhood for an underserved population, namely homeless veterans. The planning steps for the community coalition were an adaptation of a quality improvement process. The steps included (Folse, 2014):

- Identifying the values of the community.
- Creating a vision statement.
- Identifying the needs of the stakeholders.
- Collecting data from The Neighborhood to measure the current status of services for homeless veterans and to identify assets and physical elements of the community that could be used.
- Establishing measurable outcomes and quality indicators, as well as how the data would be collected and evaluated for each outcome or indicator.
- Developing a plan to implement and meet the outcomes.

Student Evaluation

The students were asked to provide feedback about the virtual learning activities. Students were asked to identify when they felt the most engaged or interested in the activity, what concepts they will apply to their practice, and how their work with vulnerable populations was or was not influenced by their involvement in the learning activity. Student feedback was evaluated for evidence of meeting the learning goals of each activity.

Clinical Reasoning

The goal of the clinical reasoning activity was to provide an opportunity for students to demonstrate higher-order thinking in providing nursing care, thereby increasing confidence that their actions would move patients from their current state to a desired outcome. The following student comments reflect greater confidence and higher-order thinking in developing a plan:

- This provided me with an opportunity to. . .reflect on potential outcomes, interventions, and rationales behind the care. This assignment provided me an opportunity to put thought and rationale into the care plan versus clicking on premade categories and interventions that is used in developing care plans in most EMRs [electronic medical records].

- I have already begun watching patients' faces closely as their family talks to me, or as they talk to their families. In two situations already what I have seen has caused me to go back to the patient when the family has gone and ask them [the patient] to clarify the plan just to make sure I have it right. In both cases, I got the "I know what he [or] she said, but. . ." response. Even in situations where a spouse is clearly the official spokesperson for the patient, that patient may still have other ideas about how it is really going to be.
- I will continue to seek evidence-based and best practice knowledge to guide my decision making in clinical practice.

The students also gained a renewed and deeper appreciation for patients in the context of their social situation, as indicated by the following statements:

- Each patient had medical problems and social issues. Social issues such as living conditions, work environment, and lack of social support are an important part of one's health. I can apply the importance of assessing my patient's social issues to my nursing practice. Acceptance of what the patient's own needs are as being the most important to address, instead of assuming we know what they will need [or what] would help most. Collaboration is the key to success and satisfaction.
- The stories of the characters in The Neighborhood community were detailed, and the factors that make people vulnerable were discussed. For example, the character I worked on had many factors such as having a chronic disease, having disabilities, losing health insurance, losing a job, and being poor. It was interesting to learn how each problem contributed to other problems such as losing a job caused the character to lose health insurance and be poor.
- Be more compassionate of patients and their families. Realize that the glimpse I get to see during my short time with them in the OR [operating room] is just a fraction of the entire picture of their lives. I therefore have no right to judge in any way, shape, or form that which is different from what I would choose for myself.

Disaster Nursing

The primary goals of the disaster nursing activity were for the students to apply the concepts of community, collaboration, leadership, and vulnerable populations. The concepts of community, collaboration, and leadership are evident in the following student comments:

- I plan on putting together a disaster preparedness kit for my family, and it has made me do a lot of thinking about my own community and what our vulnerabilities would be in a disaster.
- It made me think about being more involved on a local level and maybe volunteering for the Medical Reserve Corp.
- I think this has increased my awareness of the importance of community involvement, networking, and political involvement in coalitions for disaster preparation.

- The virtual role-playing made me think about my leadership role in this scenario. . .I was able to picture myself in the disaster and that helped me think and learn. I also learned from my other group members.

The students gained a deeper appreciation for vulnerable populations through the disaster nursing activity as reflected in the following comments:

- I saw new vulnerabilities in everyone and new strengths too. Stable people became needy when faced with illness, injury, or the death of a loved one, and "vulnerable" people showed that they had skills to offer and the willingness to do so to help others. This underscores the creativity required when planning for disaster response—the helper [and] helpee may change places!
- The disaster plan case study taught me that nurses play a great role in disaster relief and taking care of the vulnerable populations in times of disaster. It is important for nurses to have critical thinking skills, communication skills, assessment skills, and technical skills.
- For the vulnerable population, even a minor disaster in society can mean devastation to those without resources. These troubles can be compounded exponentially in this group, and having an impact on society and the individual for years.

In addition, many of the students commented on the need to be better prepared for a disaster. For example, one student commented, "I plan on putting together a disaster preparedness kit for my family." Another student commented, "Understanding of the challenges in large-scale situations has encouraged me to encourage others to make efforts toward basic preparedness needs, such as canned food and water."

Coalition Building

The goal of this learning activity was to have students think about social justice and health policy using homeless veterans as the exemplar as well as the concepts of community, leadership, influence, advocacy, networking, collaboration, and vulnerable populations. The following comments reflect the students' perceptions that the goals of this activity were met:

- It was a great learning experience to collaborate with other nurses to provide help for the homeless veteran population. . .and [it] provided a great teamwork opportunity.
- I have new knowledge how to set up a coalition and delegate sections of work. Also, I have learned how to collaborate with team members, with focus on change in the community to help individuals.
- I have learned quite a bit about coalitions. . . One experience is that coalitions need to have goals related to all members not just from one person's perspective—each member may have a different interest in how to help the community.
- I am able to be a productive coalition member by researching, interviewing, and creating plans to help vulnerable populations. In addition, I realize becoming knowledgeable of vulnerable individuals within a community requires research, interviews, surveys, etc., to know how to approach an effective plan.
- It has increased my awareness of local coalitions and what they provide for the community members who may be at risk. I have learned to explore more of the

community resources and how important networking can be in providing care to at-risk individuals.

- Research on this coalition project opened my eyes to the staggering statistics about homeless veterans. Even in my work at the Veterans Hospital, I did not know many of the facts that came to light.

Conclusion And Recommendations

The three learning strategies using a virtual community were developed to meet the experiential learning needs of diploma and ADN-prepared RNs who were continuing their education to advance their career. The primary goal of the activities was for the students to demonstrate a broader knowledge base, which goes beyond technological competence, to include abilities in leadership, health policy, system improvement, research and evidence-based practice, teamwork, collaboration, and a greater orientation toward community-based care (IOM, 2010; Smith, 2010). Evaluation of the activities confirms that the goals were met and are recommended for use in other online programs.

Based on student and faculty experience throughout several semesters, several recommendations are suggested. First, different types of disasters are more prevalent in different regions of the country and world. In the northwestern United States, concerns about a major earthquake are more prevalent. In other parts of the country, hurricanes, tornadoes, and flooding are more of a concern. The simulated disaster could be changed to reflect the community that most of the students reside in. Other potential disasters could include technical or man-made disasters such as famine, industrial accidents, or chemical weapons. Second, the exemplar of homeless veterans was chosen in response to the school of nursing's Joining Forces pledge. Other exemplars could be used, or students could choose their own social issue based on what is important to the group members. Third, the use of role-playing is an effective teaching strategy that engages students in the context of real-life scenarios. Finally, the use of the virtual community is an effective learning strategy that uses technology to support learning and practice in nursing. The virtual community is recommended for engaging other student populations, such as traditional BSN students, in exploring complex concepts.

References

American Association of Colleges of Nursing. (2014). *Support joining forces*. Retrieved from http://www.aacn.nche.edu/joining-forces

American Association of Colleges of Nursing, & Association of American Medical Colleges. (2010). *Lifelong learning in medicine and nursing: Final conference report*. Retrieved from http://www.aacn.nche.edu/education-resources/MacyReport.pdf

Bartlett, R., Bland, A., Rossen, E., Kautz, D., Benfield, S., & Carnevale, T. (2008). Evaluation of the Outcome-Present State Test Model as a way to teach clinical reasoning. *Journal of Nursing Education, 47*, 337-344.

Billings, D.M., & Halstead, J.A. (2009). *Teaching in nursing: A guide for faculty* (3rd ed.). St. Louis, MO: Saunders-Elsevier.

Boettcher, J.V., & Conrad, R.M. (2010). *The online teaching survival guide: Simple and practical pedagogical tips*. San Francisco, CA: Jossey-Bass.

Breen, H. (2014). Assessing online collaborative discourse. *Nursing Forum.* Advance online publication. doi:10.1111/nuf.12091

Carlson-Sabelli, L.L., Giddens, J.F., Fogg, L., & Fiedler, R.A. (2011). Challenges and benefits of using a virtual community to explore nursing concepts among nursing students. *International Journal of Nursing Scholarship, 8*(1), 1-14.

Chikotas, N.E. (2008). Theoretical links: Supporting the use of problem-based learning in the education of the nurse practitioner. *Nursing Education Perspectives, 29,* 359-362.

Dolence, M.G. (2003). The learner-centered curriculum model: A structured framework for technology planning. *EDUCAUSE: Center for Applied Research Bulletin, 2003*(17), 1-12. Retrieved from https://net.educause.edu/ir/library/pdf/erb0317.pdf

Folse, V.N. (2014). Managing quality and risk. In P.S. Yoder-Wise (Ed.), *Leading and managing in nursing* (pp. 389-409). St. Louis, MO: Elsevier.

Giddens, J. (2010). *The Neighborhood: Faculty navigation guide.* Boston, MA: Pearson.

Giddens, J., Brady, D., Brown, P., Wright, M., Smith, D., & Harris, J. (2008). A new curriculum for a new era of nursing education. *Nursing Education Perspectives, 29,* 200-204.

Giddens, J.F., & Morton, N. (2010). Report card: An evaluation of a concept-based curriculum. *Nursing Education Perspectives, 31,* 372-377.

Guilar, J., & Loring, A. (2008). Dialogue and community in online learning: Lessons from Royal Roads University. *Journal of Distance Education, 22*(3), 19-40.

Harasim, L. (2012). *Learning theory and online technologies.* New York, NY: Routledge.

Institute of Medicine. (2010). *The future of nursing: Leading change, advancing health.* Washington, DC: National Academies Press. Retrieved from http://thefutureofnursing.org/IOM-Report

International Council of Nurses. (2009). *ICN framework of disaster nursing competencies.* Geneva, Switzerland: Author.

Jahng, N., Nielsen, W.S., & Chan, E.K.H. (2010). Collaborative learning in an online course: A comparison of communication patterns in small and whole group activities. *Journal of Distance Education, 24*(2), 39-58.

Kautz, D., Kuiper, R.A., Bartlett, R., Buck, R., Williams, R., & Knight-Brown, P. (2009). Building evidence for the development of clinical reasoning using a rating tool with the Outcome-Present-State-Test (OPT) Model. *Southern Online Journal of Nursing Research, 9*(1). Retrieved from http://www.resourcecenter.net/images/SNRS/Files/SOJNR_articles2/Vol09Num01Art15.html

Kuiper, R.A., & Pesut, D.J. (2004). Promoting cognitive and metacognitive reflective reasoning skills in nursing practice: Self-regulated learning theory. *Journal of Advanced Nursing, 45,* 381-391. doi:10.1046/j.1365-2648.2003.02921.x

Lin, C.F., Lu, M.S., Chung, C.C., & Yang, C.M. (2010). A comparison of problem-based learning and conventional teaching in nursing ethics education. *Nursing Ethics, 17,* 373-382. doi:10.1177/0969733009355380

Priest, C., & Bahl, M. (2008). Nursing during catastrophic disaster: A case study from New Orleans. *Journal of Nursing Law, 12,* 157-164.

Smith, T.G. (2010). A policy perspective on the entry into practice issue. *The Online Journal of Issues in Nursing, 15*(1). doi:10.3912/ OJIN.Vol15No01PPT01

Sullivan, E.J. (2004). *Becoming influential: A guide for nurses.* Upper Saddle River, NJ: Pearson.

Wikis. (2013). Retrieved from https://help.blackboard.com/en-us/Learn/9.1_SP_10_and_SP_11/Instructor/050_Course_Tools/Wikis

Zull, J.E. (2004). The art of the changing brain. *Education Leadership, 62*(1), 68-72.

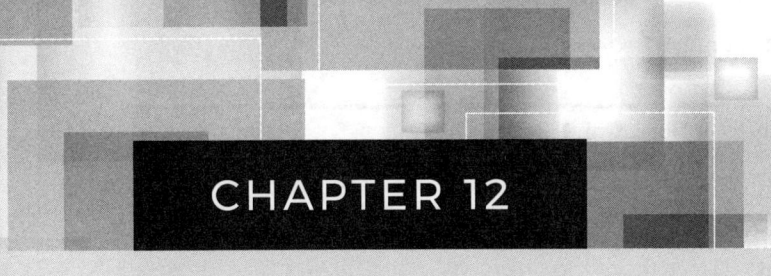

CHAPTER 12

Narrative Pedagogy

Henny Breen and Melissa Robinson

Overview

Narrative pedagogy is a research-based pedagogy developed within the discipline of nursing that arose out of the common *lived experiences* of students, teachers, and clinicians in nursing education. It complements our philosophy of constructivism and fits well with collaborative and reflective learning that guides our teaching practice, which is why we chose to highlight this pedagogy as a separate chapter. We continue to be in the process of reflection and collaboration about narrative pedagogy and how it applies to our practice. This chapter provides a brief overview of narrative pedagogy and some examples from the literature and our teaching practice.

Narrative Pedagogy

Narrative pedagogy is among the other innovations in teaching and learning that arose out of the need to reform nursing education from a more behaviorist approach that is teacher centered to an approach that is learner centered. Narrative pedagogy is grounded in the work of pragmatism theory, in which educational experiences must be meaningful to the learner in order for the learner to construct and reconstruct past and future experiences (Nehls, 1995). A pragmatic approach, such as adult learning theory, is not new to teaching practice. However, nursing was in the throes of needing educational reform, and narrative pedagogy was one alternative approach to teaching and learning.

Nehls (1995) identified that narrative pedagogy is not only based on pragmatism but also several other theoretical frameworks for understanding human behavior—for example, the hypothesis that humans think in narrative, meaning they make sense of phenomena by storytelling. Thus, "narrative pedagogy evolves from and creates the lived experiences of teacher, clinicians, and students" (Nehls,

---

Table 12-1 Strengths of Narrative Pedagogy

Nehls (1995) identified the following strengths of narrative pedagogy:

- Uses real-life situations, which engages students and faculty in the learning process in a different way from other simulated learning activities
- Facilitates thinking
- Encourages reflective thinking
- Links theory and practice
- Helps students appreciate how practical knowledge develops over time, as reflected by the stories of inexperienced nurses compared to those who are experienced
- Encourages cooperation, concern, and care among the students and faculty, with the possibility of being translated to students being able to demonstrate caring behaviors in their nursing practice

Nehls, N. (1995). Narrative pedagogy: Rethinking nursing education. *Journal of Nursing Education, 34*(5).

1995, p. 205). It is based on the assumption that teachers are learners and learners are teachers, reflecting reciprocity within the community of learners. **Table 12-1** provides a summary of how Nehls (1995) described the strengths of narrative pedagogy through her discussion of how narrative can be used as a means for reforming nursing education.

Interpretative Approach

Narrative pedagogy is an approach to teaching and learning that involves an interpretative phenomenological method to interpreting the shared experiences of students, teachers, and clinicians in the context of nursing (Andrews et al., 2001). Narrative pedagogy represents a shift to alternative interpretative pedagogies. As stated earlier, it is among other innovations in teaching and learning that arose out of the need to reform nursing education from a more teacher-centered, behaviorist approach to a learner-centered approach, such as critical, feminist, phenomenological, and postmodern pedagogies.

Nancy Diekelmann (2001) advanced nursing education through her 12-year study using an interpretative phenomenological hermeneutical methodology. Hermeneutical analysis is an interpretive process used to bring understanding to the *lived experience.* The reader is encouraged to review the literature for more details about this research methodology. Her work was at the forefront of nursing education reform. In fact, her study was initiated prior to the call for substantive curricular changes by significant organizations, such as the Institute of Medicine's Quality and Safety Education in Nursing and the Carnegie Foundation for the Advancement of Teaching's *Educating Nurses* (Taylor Sullivan, 2020).

The reader is encouraged to carefully review Diekelmann's (2001) impactful study, "Narrative Pedagogy: Heideggerian Hermeneutical Analyses of Lived Experiences of Students, Teachers, and Clinicians," in which Diekelmann presents narrative pedagogy. It is based on Diekelmann's earlier work, in which she conceptualized the nursing curriculum as caring, dialogue, and practice (Nehls, 1995). Her findings resulted in identifying the following patterns or practices as they emerged in her study, which she titled the "Concernful Practices of Schooling Learning Teaching" (Diekelmann, 2001, p. 57):

- *Gathering:* bringing in and calling forth
- *Creating places:* keeping open a future of possibilities
- *Assembling:* constructing and cultivating
- *Staying:* knowing and connecting
- *Caring:* engendering community
- *Interpreting:* unlearning and becoming
- *Presencing:* attending and being open
- *Preserving reading, writing, thinking, and dialogue*
- *Questioning:* meaning and making visible

Diekelmann (2001) identified that these patterns describe the common, shared experiences of teachers, students, and clinicians as they gather for learning and provide a new language for nursing education. They are not methods or strategies for teaching but, rather, describe how teachers, students, and clinicians experience teaching and learning. They reveal the need to explore assumptions based on traditional teaching that is teacher centered. Narrative pedagogy is a discipline-specific pedagogical approach that emphasizes creating respectful and interpretative learning communities that call attention to the Concernful Practices of Schooling Learning Teaching (Ironside, 2006).

The Concernful Practices of Schooling Learning Teaching

Although narrative pedagogy is an approach to reforming education that is site specific and not generalized from school to school, the processes of narrative pedagogy are transferrable through the language of concernful practices (Andrews et al., 2001; Ironside, 2014). The concernful practices provide for a learning environment in which creative and valuable dialogue can exist between clinicians, faculty, and students. This requires faculty to understand the nine themes of the concernful practices as well as develop skills in how to apply them when teaching (Candela, 2020). Narrative pedagogy is more than storytelling. Students and faculty often share stories that involve describing an experience they have had as a nurse. However, narrative pedagogy requires understanding the context, drawing attention to what stood out, what was noticed, and how it was interpreted within a community of learners.

Faculty who have a constructivist approach to teaching will find these concernful practices a good fit within their repertoire of teaching practices. Since Diekelmann's original research that gave birth to the phenomenon of narrative pedagogy in nursing, there have been a number of studies looking at what teaching and learning would look like when using the concernful practices.

Gathering: Welcoming and Calling Forth

How faculty gather students into a course, welcoming them into the learning environment, is a different way of thinking about common practices such as orienting students and describing the ground rules, learning outcomes, and expectations for the course. The concernful practices are reflective of a community, meaning that students also gather and demonstrate welcoming of faculty by their interest and participation in class. Faculty and students engage in a learning community that fosters thinking collaboratively while holding current perspectives, understanding, and assumptions as open to being problematic (Ironside, 2015).

Interpreting: Unlearning and Becoming

Between 2002 and 2005, Pamela Ironside (2006) used the same methodology of interpretative hermeneutic phenomenology to complete three studies that included over 20 schools of nursing, representing associate degree, baccalaureate, and graduate programs in the United States and Canada. She found that the same concernful practices as identified by Diekelmann (2001) emerged as patterns. However, she focused her attention on *interpreting: unlearning and becoming*, which she described as a common practice when faculty use narrative pedagogy. She referred to this as *learning and practicing interpretative thinking.*

Learning and practicing interpretative thinking is a process in which both students and faculty unlearn limited ways of thinking that often occur in nursing practice and didactic teaching. In the process of interpretative thinking, students broaden their thinking by challenging their assumptions as they think through situations from different perspectives, leading to different interpretations. This adds complexity to their understanding, which influences their nursing practice (Ironside, 2006). At the same time, faculty, in the same way, expand their thinking about pedagogy, which influences their teaching (Ironside, 2015).

Andrews et al. (2001) also found that faculty members began to challenge their assumptions of what it meant to teach based on conventional pedagogy by incorporating concerns of inclusiveness, cooperation, collaboration, and multiple ways of knowing. Shifting the emphasis from doing it right to exploring meaning and significance helped students think contextually. Narrative pedagogy defines learning by the context in which it exists. For example, we have found that students' interpretation of nonadherence or compliance with treatment recommendations changed depending on how they understood the specific circumstances of the patient.

Inviting: Waiting and Letting Be

Ironside (2014) also used hermeneutic phenomenology to conduct a 10-year study focusing on the concernful practice of *inviting: waiting and letting be.* She found that two themes were present:

1. *Inviting:* Cocreating transformative experiences
2. *Waiting and letting be:* Thinking time and keeping my mouth shut

Inviting students to learn with faculty does not mean abdication of authority or responsibility as the faculty with expertise. Inviting students to share their experiences about a phenomenon, such as the impact of caring for patients with a chronic illness, is much different than asking students what they would like to discuss or learn, which is asking them to make decisions about the course. Inviting students to share their experiences also enables them to consider experiences from different perspectives. *Inviting* is a teaching practice regardless of the instructional strategies used. The significance of a strategy is related to how it is experienced (Ironside, 2014). For example, the strategy may be to assign students to view a video, which only becomes significant learning when students are invited to share their thoughts and feelings within a learning community so that multiple perspectives are considered.

Waiting and letting be provides an opportunity for transformative learning. In the face-to-face classroom, it requires the ability to be comfortable with silence as students and faculty process and think about what they want to say. Waiting is not empty but an indication of deep engagement. It supports the struggle to understand and the process of how the community of learners listens and responds (Ironside, 2014). There is an element of the unknown because it is not clear what direction the discussion will take, which may be uncomfortable for faculty new to using narrative pedagogy. This kind of waiting is built into asynchronous online classrooms and is considered one of the many advantages. Regardless of the modality, faculty need to consider when and how they should enter into the discussion, as discussed in Chapter 9.

Listening: Knowing and Connecting

Faculty and student *presence* in an online learning environment is critical to the success of the online course. Ironside (2015) found that some faculty described how the concernful practices provided the means to becoming a supportive presence to students. For example, the tone used when writing to students was important as attention shifted to language. We have found this to be consistent with our experience as well. For example, students will often describe how they felt when a question about where to find something they overlooked in the instructions was responded to. Merely copying and pasting the instructions or advising them to review the instructions led to feelings of incompetence and could inhibit students' desire to ask more questions. However, responding in a nonjudgmental tone, noting that other students had the same question, or validating that it can be difficult to take in a lot of information in a new learning environment, followed by explaining where to find the information, exemplifies *listening: knowing and connecting* in a way that promotes openness because the faculty member is listening to the meaning behind the question.

The Use of Narrative Pedagogy in Online Classrooms

Narrative pedagogy is often used to complement other methods of teaching because it helps students reflect on the emotional experience or human response to illness and health and facilitates learning about complex topics (Fitzpatrick, 2017, 2018). Developing a curriculum for online programs that includes narratives or storytelling helps students move from cognitive to affective learning. We have used virtual communities, different art forms, and experiential storytelling to facilitate deep learning among our students.

Virtual Communities

A virtual community is an online teaching application that features a fictional community or a number of different communities in a region with multiple intersecting stories, including unfolding stories of the characters in the community. These unfolding stories are narrated through video, audio, images, and written materials (Giddens, Fogg, & Carlsen-Savelli, 2010). Consistent with our experience in using a virtual community, Walsh and van Soeren (2012) found that students think the stories are realistic and enable them to be exposed to conditions that they may not have the opportunity to experience as students. It is important to note that a virtual community is different from a virtual world, such as Second Life or Shadow Health. Virtual world applications are populated by avatars that cannot capture subtle nonverbal communication, thereby failing to meet the "true complexity of how communities function" (Walsh & van Soeren, 2012, p. 45).

Walsh and van Soeren (2012) found that virtual communities combined with narrative pedagogy provided an effective way for students from different healthcare and social care professions to work together with real stories. We found the virtual community effective for applying critical reasoning skills to community members' health needs, learning about disaster response, and coalition building, as discussed in the Appendix of Chapter 11. The virtual community supported the learning based on the narrative of the characters within the context provided by the faculty. Further, students added to the narrative in the disaster response context by inserting themselves as nurses within the community. By manipulating the context, the narrative can be altered, which in turn affects how the story is perceived and understood. Virtual communities can be adapted for prelicensure and postlicensure students in both face-to-face and online classrooms.

Art Forms: Literature, Cinema, Podcasts, Music

By using various art forms that draw upon the liberal arts education, we can facilitate students in developing sensitivity to promote caring in a cultural context, guided by their evolving ethical knowledge. This can be developed by having students read, listen to, and view narratives that illustrate illness, health, and healing as powerful enhancements to understanding the many different experiences faced by the people they will work with in their career (Saucier Lundy & Janes, 2016). Different art forms provide an opportunity for students to move beyond theoretical knowledge to explore what it means to have a chronic illness, suffer a major loss, or live in poverty, for example. As they enter another's world through the art form, they connect the narrative with their own lives and make interpretations based on their own personal and professional experiences (Saucier Lundy & Janes, 2016). In sharing with others, students' sensitivity and empathy are enhanced by different interpretations based on the different life experiences of the students in the class.

The use of cinema to teach family assessment was found to increase awareness of diversity in addition to increasing knowledge related to opportunities for health promotion in families (Smith & Jones, 2015). Personal and nursing practice experiences, along with theoretical knowledge, informed students' understanding of families. To enhance this learning, students were assigned to watch a movie that represented many aspects of cultural diversity and depicted family interactions and functions that addressed a number of different concepts, such as grief, poverty, racism, and mental health issues, to name a few. This approach enabled students to observe family interactions over time, and they gained a deeper appreciation of family dynamics and different perspectives, which affected their competency in assessing families (Smith & Jones, 2015).

Table 12-2 provides some suggestions of art forms that we have found effective for integrating narrative pedagogy in our teaching practice.

Table 12-2 Examples of Using Art Forms to Integrate Narrative Pedagogy in Online Classes

Example	Description
YouTube videos	"Being Mortal: Medicine and What Matters in the End" by Atul Gawande (2017) "Qualities of a Nurse—Therapeutic Communication for Nurses" Uses music, pictures, and words "Gladys Wilson and Naomi Feil" Communicating with an elderly person with dementia "Empathy: The Human Connection to Patient Care" Uses music, pictures, and word
TED Talk	"Transparency, Compassion, and Truth in Medical Errors: Leilani Schweitzer" Leilani Schweitzer's son died after a series of medical mistakes. She discusses the importance of transparency and how truth and compassion are essential for healing.
Cinema	*Erin Brockovich* (Universal Pictures, 2000) An unemployed single mother becomes a legal assistant and almost single-handedly brings down a California power company accused of polluting a city's water supply. Based on a true story. *Paper Tigers* (KPJR Films, 2015) Chronicles a year in the life of Lincoln High School in Walla Walla, Washington. Students have a history of truancy, behavioral problems, and substance abuse. After Lincoln's principal is exposed to research about the effects of adverse childhood experiences (ACEs), he decides to radically change the school's approach to discipline. With the aid of diary camera footage, the film follows six students, from getting into fights to grappling with traumatic events in their lives and being on the cusp of dropping out. They find healing, support, and academic promise at Lincoln High.

(continues)

Table 12-2 **Examples of Using Art Forms to Integrate Narrative Pedagogy in Online Classes** *(continued)*

Example	Description
	Precious (Lionsgate, 2009) The story of a young girl raised in poverty who survived physical, sexual, and verbal abuse as she grew up. Concepts revealed in the film include socioeconomics/poverty, single parenting, abuse, obesity, education, teen pregnancy, HIV, birth defects, and more.
	The Kids Are All Right (Gilbert Films, 2010) The story of a diverse same-sex couple and their family is chronicled. Concepts revealed in the film include sexual orientation, alcoholism, same-sex marriage, family conflict, coping, infidelity, adolescent development, and more.
Novels	*Bad Blood: The Tuskegee Syphilis Experiment* by James H. Jones (1993) An account of the experiment performed on unknowing African American sharecroppers; illustrates how the U.S. Public Health Service allowed syphilis to progress, without treatment, while research was performed. The novel illustrates how such a tragedy occurred.
	Do They Hear You When You Cry? by Fauziya Kassindja (1998) Nonfiction work about a young woman who sought political asylum to avoid female genital mutilation.
	Half the Sky: Turning Oppression into Opportunity for Women Worldwide by Nicholas D. Kristof and Sheryl WuDunn (2010) A factual odyssey through Africa and Asia to meet extraordinary women who are struggling, including a Cambodian teenager sold into sex slavery and an Ethiopian woman who suffered devastating injuries in childbirth. Through their stories, the authors show how a little help can transform the lives of women and girls abroad, engage females as a rich economic resource across the globe, and ultimately fight global poverty.
	Heat Wave: A Social Autopsy of Disaster in Chicago by Eric Klinenberg (2002, 2015) Following the heatwave of 1995 in Chicago, the author investigated why so many people died alone in their homes, why some neighborhoods experienced greater mortality than others, how city government responded to the crisis, how public health officials responded, and more. He uncovered unsettling forms of social breakdown that affected the most vulnerable in the community and contributed to high mortality rates.
	If You Poison Us: Uranium and Native Americans by Peter H. Eichstaedt (1994) A true account of the devastating health consequences affecting Native American miners and millers on the Navajo Reservation, where some of the richest deposits of uranium were found, which fueled the Cold War. For nearly three decades, state and federal agencies neglected to warn the miners or impose safety measures in the mines, despite growing evidence of the risks.

Example	Description
	The Glass Castle: A Memoir by Jeanette Walls (2005) A powerful memoir about growing up in a dysfunctional family that often lived in poverty, with experiences that required the children to fend for themselves among the chaos and challenges of alcoholism and mental health issues.
	The Spirit Catches You and You Fall Down by Anne Fadiman (1997) A powerful account of a Hmong family in California that addresses difficulties in communicating across barriers of mistrust, religion, and healing beliefs and practices.
	There Are No Children Here: The Story of Growing Up in the Other America by Alex Kotlowitz (1992) This is the moving and powerful account of two remarkable boys struggling to survive in Chicago's Henry Horner Homes, a public housing complex disfigured by crime and neglect.

The following examples, not listed in Table 12-2, are highlighted in order to include student responses to illustrate the value of using different art forms.

Documentary: **The Invisible War**

One film we use is *The Invisible War*, written and directed by Kirby Dick, which is a very impactful documentary about the rape of women in the military (Ziering, King Barklow, & Dick, 2012). One student responded, "I had a strong emotional response to the video *The Invisible War*. In my current practice I care for Veteran patients and this video is helpful for me to gain a deeper understanding of their experiences." We were cautioned by our students to warn future students of the difficulty in viewing this documentary, given the emotional response it evoked in many of our students. As faculty, this was a reminder about the need to be aware that powerful narratives such as this may not be an uncommon experience and could trigger painful memories as students initially relate the narratives to their personal experiences.

Book: **I'm Here: Compassionate Communication in Patient Care**

The book *I'm Here: Compassionate Communication in Patient Care* by Marcus Engel (2010) is very popular among students. They reflect on the personal narrative of Marcus's experience as a patient following a devasting accident at 18 years of age in which he was left blind and every bone in his face was broken, among other devasting injuries and burns to his body. He had approximately 300 hours of surgery as a result of the accident, in which he and his father, who was killed, were hit by a drunk driver (Engel, 2010). This a very powerful personal narrative from the patient's experience that students describe as changing their nursing practice immediately as they reflect on what the author writes. As they are reading, they feel a great deal of emotion as they reflect on his experiences. It changes even the simplest of actions, such as introducing themselves to the patient, as their perception of what they formerly viewed as merely a formality shifts to an act with deep meaning.

The following are some student quotes from the collaborative reflections posted on the discussion board about their experience in reading this novel. The quotes demonstrate how students connect the author's experience and that of other students to their own practice.

- "I am embarrassed to say that introducing myself to other patients that see me only once or twice did not occur as often as it should have. This book made re- alize that there are many nursing skills that I need to brush up on, such as this."
- "Reading *I'm Here* by Marcus Engel has left me completely confused about what kind of nurse I am, and I'm if I'm even a good one."
- "This book was amazing[;] being able to hear from the patient's perspective was life changing. Barb is my idol; she is so smooth with her delivery of informa- tion. She never showed disappointment in Marcus; she understood he was out of his element and in pain.... I channeled my inner Barb the other day when I walked into my patient's room after getting shift report and found her sitting on the floor. I calmly, but briskly, walked over to her and asked her if she was okay, and calmly asked my fellow nurse to go grab help. I asked her where she was going, and assured her that we would help her go to the bathroom as soon as we got her off the floor. It was not perfect, but I definitely keep Barb in mind when I'm at work."
- "Throughout each chapter of *I'm Here*, I caught myself reflecting upon my own nursing interactions with my patients thinking, 'Have I ever treated a patient like this? Have I been asking permission before performing tasks? Have I ever told someone they had a nasty wound?' This book was an excellent read that allowed me to have more self-awareness of my strengths and weaknesses."
- "Reflecting on my practice while I read this book, definitely reminded me to be more aware of the patient's perspective. It can be all too easy to get busy and try to rush through and unfortunately not provide the best individualized care. I know I can slow down and be more descriptive in my practice by talking the patient through the tasks more, even if I want to assume they are very familiar with the process."
- "I need stories like these because though I am a mother, wife, sister and I care about how others feel, I get tied up in the heavy work flow current preoccupied with med pass times and documentation time limits, etc. I am empathetic as an in- dividual[,] but when I get in this role[,] it is easy to become jaded by all the noise."
- "This book is a grounding example of the extent to which therapeutic com- munication and emotional intelligence plays out in the patient experience; the things that we say and do have a major impact on the lives of these individuals, their experience and perception of the effectiveness of healthcare."
- "Marcus's statement that if you are helping the family members, you are helping the patient really hit home with me. I'll be honest, sometimes I just tune family members out, especially when they start telling me about their health problems."
- "Your discussion about the patients' families discussing their own problems jogged my memory a bit. We have used information gleaned from casual con- versations with families in patient rooms to provide insight during care confer- ences regarding discharge plans."

Book: **When Breath Becomes Air**

The autobiographical novel *When Breath Becomes Air* (2016), written by 36-year-old neurosurgeon Paul Kalanithi, chronicles his life trajectory following a diagnosis of stage IV lung cancer. One moment he was a resident physician; the next, he was a patient struggling to live. He explores the relationship between a doctor and patient while reflecting on the challenge of facing death. As a husband, son, and young father, he wrestled with life's most challenging questions while confronting his own mortality. Paul Kalanithi died while working on his book, yet his words live on in his book: "I began to realize that coming face to face with my own mortality, in a sense, had changed nothing and everything." He wrote, "seven words from Samuel Beckett began to repeat in my head: 'I can't go on. I'll go on" (Kalanithi, 2016). Students have responded to the book and Paul's narrative from a variety of perspectives, as follows.

The personal impact on the reader in existential terms:

- "What ultimately drew me to this book was the fact that it is not only a personal account of coming to terms with death and the process of dying, but it presents an idea of what it means to live and what makes life worth living."
- "One of the questions presented at the very beginning of the book was 'what makes life worth living in the face of death?' This particular question, along with a few others, was addressed throughout the book, as Dr. Kalanithi struggles to find his own answers. As for me, I can only interpret his work and develop my own."
- "In the many judgement calls Paul had to make throughout his medical career regarding a patient's quality of life as well as his personal journey through terminal illness, this question really stood out to me and made me think. I realized how extremely personal this is to every single individual and how each unique perspective should be respected and valued."

The impact on the reader as a provider:

- "To me, his doctor did a skillful job of preserving hope without giving a false sense of it, which is a difficult and fine line to walk."
- "I feel the author has done a great service for all medical professionals who read his work, as it helps us all to gain a fresh view from not only a patient's perspectives, but also from the other perspectives he presents, helping us to see patients as more than their illness, in a more personal, human and holistic way."

Students also placed themselves in Paul's shoes and considered how they would approach the topic of death with their own family members, including their children, or considered their own legacy:

- "I am certain though that I don't want my child to be excluded from the realities of death. My current conversation with him explains that 'Death is where everything that is not you falls away.' The legacy I would want to leave, may not be a book…but it could be a book of poems that I love, a CD, some art work. And ultimately I would want my death story to be my gift to my children and their children. I would want a death full of life."
- "I *hated* this story in the same way that I would hate anything that causes me to feel vulnerable, question my legacy, or realign my perspective on the time I have remaining in this life. The *hate* that makes me uncomfortable, and with being uncomfortable forcing me to grow as a person. Dr. Kalanithi's story will be one that I listen to several more times in my life, probably at time that I need to re-align my perspective on life and work."

Experiential Storytelling

Experiential storytelling is often built into online classes because students are encouraged to share experiences they have had to illustrate the concepts and theories they are learning. This provides nurses with the opportunity to reflect on their experiences and share with each other. Students also value hearing stories from faculty. Hearing one story often moves other nurses to remember their own experiences, providing more opportunities to share what meaning they have assigned to the experience. **Table 12-3** provides some examples of students sharing stories from two different online elective courses. In the Trauma-Informed Care course, the students' stories illustrate how looking through a trauma lens changes their perspective on patient behavior. In the Palliative Care course, students share stories about "transitions of care" and aging in their own families. Reflecting on their own personal experiences and that of other students facilitates developing greater empathy and understanding of the experiences of others.

Table 12-3 Storytelling by Students

Trauma-Informed Care. *Students are asked to share experiences with patients and how looking through a trauma-informed lens changed their perspective.*
I currently have a client who I will call Sara, who is bipolar and a borderline. She has a history of multiple ACEs and sexual trauma as a young adult, which could explain her borderline personality disorder. Sara seeks connections with people but lacks the trust and social skills. Sara is easily triggered by loud noises, and there are currently loud peers on the unit. When the milieu becomes loud, Sara will come out of her room, go stand in the middle of the milieu and scream at her peers that they "don't care" about her and that they are "triggering" her. The popcorn effect then takes place, one client yelling and becoming dysregulated after another. The milieu becomes chaotic, and I forget the real problem. Sara needs skills to help her to deal with the triggers. The sounds that take her back to when her trauma took place. The chaos of the milieu overshadows her pain and struggle in the moment. I need to remember to go back and have conversations with her after she is re-regulated.

    I currently have a pediatric patient who has been severely neglected[,] and I've noticed that the child is able to pick up on the cues that we, the nurses, give as we are finishing our treatments or assessments and ready ourselves to leave the room. The child's behavior changes[,] and the child will cry inappropriately or complain of abdominal pain, anything to keep us from leaving the room. This child has very few family visitors due to active investigations and is often left alone in the room despite our best efforts to have a staff member or volunteer sit with the child. With this child, I have learned to make sure to set very clear boundaries and to also be clear as to when I will be back in the room; I do my very best to stick to my word. I feel this is building a trusting relationship where the child understands the boundaries and is able to trust that they will not be left alone for long with the hope that this will alleviate some anxiety for this patient.

    Student name, your experience with the patient who liked to hoard her things reminded me of a similar patient I took care of a few times. He would always ask for an extra blanket or pillow and then try to sneak it into his bag to take home with him. He was also very needy but would only communicate his needs to certain staff members and not others, which placed a higher burden on people who he liked to keep up with his demands. This patient was very difficult to take care of[,] and I felt burned out from having him for only 3 days. Similar to you[,] we would often talk about this patient in terms of his disease processes or the difficult to understand aspects of his personality, but I don't remember any of us ever asking if the patient had been through something traumatic that had caused this behavior. Your post made me think about this as a potential barrier to his care, and we could have possibly identified something before his discharge that could have helped him be more successful in managing himself at home.

Palliative Care Nursing. *After reading* Being Mortal: Medicine and What Matters in the End *by Atul Gawande (2014) and considering the transitions in life that patients experience as they age, have a change in their level of function, or experience a terminal or debilitating illness, students are asked to reflect on their experiences in their own families or when caring for patients and families.*

This book enlightened me as I read about so many of the issues our elderly population face as they age. The book made me reflect on many elderly relatives or people I know who are gradually losing their independence. Like Alice Hobson, my grandfather mistook the gas pedal for the brake, but he drove into the front of a Sheri's Restaurant. Learning how to promote independence among the elderly population is so important in allowing the individual to express their self-worth.

After reading the book, my concern is that the conversations about wishes do not occur in a timely manner, and people might place their loved ones in a nursing home without taking time to identify what key aspects promote independence. How can nurses play a role in encouraging loved ones of patients [to] establish conversations before the aging process?

One point Dr. Gawande made that really impacted me was that as a society we focus on safety for the elderly rather than focus on living. We can make them safe by keeping them in a facility, in a wheelchair, but we are not focusing on giving their life meaning and a purpose.

It was amazing to me that during these studies and discussions, seeing the impact of even having discussions with patients on their plans, in terms of longevity, quality of life, and costs. From this, I could relate to what Dr. Gawande said, "Death may be the enemy but it is also the natural order of things. I knew these truths abstractly, but I didn't know them concretely—that they could be truths not just for everyone but also for this person right in front of me, for this person I was responsible for" (Gawande, 2014, p. 8).

One recurring theme was societal acknowledgement of the inevitability of death and embracing what life the elderly have yet to live. No one wants to talk about death, and it does seem that important conversations such as this are often overlooked in busy fast-paced facilities. And when these conversations do arise, are they clear and completely transparent in what the patient and family should expect? This theme highly resonates with me and has already impacted my practice. I talk with patients and families to try understanding what matters to them during their care, and find what seem like small ways to promote their independence and autonomy that might end up being a significant matter to them.

Faculty Storytelling

When faculty share stories from practice, it should be done purposefully to facilitate deep learning. **Table 12-4** is an example used by faculty to facilitate learning about how to engage in reflective practice using Gibbs's model of reflection (Gibbs,

Table 12-4 **Faculty Storytelling to Illustrate Reflective Practice**

Use Gibbs's model of reflection to examine one situation from your practice in relation to one of the following relevant concepts: boundaries, caring, empowerment, trust, empathy, mutuality, and/or veracity, as discussed in Chapters 10 and 11 in your text. This can be challenging and may feel risky, however being open is how we learn. I am responding first to provide you with an example from my own practice.

Description: As a fairly new psychiatric nurse working on an inpatient unit, I had a 16-year-old girl I had been working with for about a year. She had been severely abused and cut herself when highly stressed. I had a very good working relationship with her. She had been given a pass, but there was no one to take her out, so I did at the end of my shift. I took her to pick up my two young children (5- and 7-year-old girls at the time), and we spent about an hour at the park. After this time, I took her back to the unit, and I later learned she started cutting herself.

Feelings: Initially I felt bad for her because she had no one to take her out. When I found out that she started cutting herself when she got back to the unit, I felt hurt, betrayed, and confused because I thought she had enjoyed herself while out. She seemed to really enjoy her time on the pass. I also felt bad for the staff who had to deal with her acting-out behavior after I dropped her off.

Evaluation: In hindsight, I realize I did have some qualms about taking her out, but I ignored them because I wanted to give her this "special" experience between the two of us. I also thought meeting my children would be fun. I also did not discuss that I would be the one taking her out with her child/adolescent psychiatrist who gave her a pass. The fact that I was not open about this should have been a clear message to me that there was a part of me that was uncomfortable with this. In looking more deeply at my motivation, I felt good about being seen as "special" by this patient, and my ego was stroked by the very misguided thinking that I was that one nurse who understood her better than any other nurse.

Analysis: The patient felt the immense pain of abandonment and betrayal by her mother, who did not protect her from serious abuse, when she saw me as a mother with my children rather than her nurse. I thought about what happened and really "got" how important it is to maintain the nurse–patient relationship and how important boundaries are, in a way I had not before. I think this is a boundary issue because I was meeting outside of the nurse–patient relationship. I lost emotional objectivity because I did not have enough self-awareness to understand my own motivations in crossing the boundary from a therapeutic relationship to one that was more social in nature.

Conclusion: I was grateful for the excellent mentoring that helped me understand the dynamics of this situation, and it improved my emotional intelligence as I developed deeper empathy—a deeper understanding of what the patient was thinking and feeling. This happened years ago, and it still stays with me because the learning was so meaningful. It is one of those experiences that changed my practice.

Action Plan: My action plan at the time was to pay attention to the little voice in my head that says to be careful. My motto became, *when in doubt, don't do it.* If you don't want to share what you plan to do, don't do it because that is keeping a secret, which is very unhealthy in mental health nursing.

1998). Reflective practice is the foundation for analyzing real experiences (Fitzpatrick, 2017). This particular example was used to facilitate students' sharing of experiences that might be difficult to share.

Table 12-5 is another example of faculty sharing a story to illustrate the concepts of suffering and crisis. One of the major purposes of sharing this particular story is to highlight understanding human behavior in a severe crisis and responding to the meaning of the behavior while at the same time maintaining safety for self, the patient, and family.

Table 12-5 Faculty Storytelling: Suffering and Families in Crisis

As we examine the concept of suffering this week, I would like to share an experience that I had caring for a hospice patient and her family several years ago. This patient was truly suffering with significant end-of-life symptoms, and the family was in crisis.

At the time, I was working at night for a hospice and palliative care program and was called out to assist a family who was in crisis. During this particular night, I was called to the home of a middle-aged female patient in the end stages of ovarian cancer. She was being cared for by her husband, who was very stressed over the phone and felt that he could no longer manage her symptoms.

The couple lived in a rural area. It was the middle of winter, and there was a ton of snow and ice on the road. When I attempted to get up the hill to their home, my car would not make it. Since it wasn't too far, I gathered my phone and supply bag and walked up the hill. I did not hesitate to walk up the hill because I knew that there was a patient suffering who needed immediate support and care. When I got to the door of the home, I immediately realized that I had placed myself at a safety risk by leaving my car.

When the patient's husband opened the door, he was holding a bottle of morphine and said, "If you don't give her all of this morphine now to end her suffering, I will end it another way." When I asked him what he meant, he went on to say that he had a gun and he would "put her down" like people who put down their animals when they are suffering.

I stayed in the doorway and told him that I could see that he was in distress, and I could hear his wife's breathing, which was also distressed. I told him that I would not be giving her the entire vial of morphine and that I would not be able to help him end her life. I also told him that if I didn't feel safe, I would need to leave and would not be able to help his wife. I was firm and clear with him, and I was also willing to leave the home if I needed to.

He stated he understood my role, which was that I was there to help relieve her symptoms and support him, not to end her life. He calmed down and promised that his gun was in plain view at the bedside so that I would be able to see it. Before I entered the home, I told him that I needed to call for additional help. He agreed to this and listened while I called for assistance from the hospice chaplain. Once he heard me describe his presentation in an honest and direct way, I believe he realized how desperate he had become. I told him that I believed that he did not want his wife to die, but rather, he just wanted her suffering to end. He agreed, and I entered the home to help them.

(continues)

Table 12-5 **Faculty Storytelling: Suffering and Families in Crisis**   *(continued)*

I asked him to join me at her bedside while I cared for her. She was awake, alert, but unable to talk because her breathing was so rapid and distressed. With her eyes, it seemed like she was begging me for help. I reassured her that I was there to help her and her husband and went to work to get her comfortable.

Over the past 24 hours, she had been unable to swallow her long-acting morphine or her short-acting breakthrough morphine tabs. She was no longer responsive verbally and had not been swallowing food or fluids. She had also been incontinent of urine, and her bed was soaked. She was febrile, pale, and tachycardic; had extreme dyspnea; and had mottling in her cold legs.

As I gave her liquid morphine and lorazepam to help her to breathe and relax, I explained all of the changes that she was experiencing to her and her husband. Once she started to breathe easier, I bathed her, performed oral care, and positioned her on her side to facilitate her breathing.

When the chaplain arrived, he asked the husband to join him in the next room. As he worked with him to listen to his concerns and provide support, I stayed with the patient and assured her that we would help her husband. I told her that I suspected that they had a difficult day and that as her symptoms escalated, so did their stress level. I assured her that we would stay with them until she was comfortable and he felt stronger. She whispered "thank you" and began to relax. After some time with the chaplain, they both came into the room with the patient. With encouragement, he was able to talk to his wife in a calm and loving manner. He apologized for not handling her decline with grace and said that he didn't think he could face losing her. He told his wife that she had been brave and fought this cancer for so long. He told her that he would follow her lead and be brave for her now.

He sat quietly with her and told her all of the ways that she had made him happy. He told her what a wonderful mother she was to their children and what an incredibly strong and supportive wife she had been to him. Because she couldn't talk, he reminisced and shared all of their favorite memories and stories. As he spoke, she relaxed more and more. As she relaxed, he held her and then lay beside her in bed. Over the next few hours, she required less medication and died peacefully in his arms.

When faculty invite students to participate in collaborative discussions using experience-based storytelling, it not only strengthens the learning community, but it also facilitates the development of reflective and critical thinking skills, along with empathy and contextual sensitivity. Stories tend to be remembered because they make the reader or listener feel something.

Summary

Narrative pedagogy, like experiential learning, bridges theory to practice because it reaches the affective level of learning. It came out of nursing research linking nursing science, practice, and education. We continue to be in the process of reflection and collaboration about narrative pedagogy and how it applies to our practice. When students and faculty collaborate through narration, we believe the art and science of nursing merge in a way that cultivates the evolving profession of nursing science without losing our and our patients' humanity.

Best-Practice Recommendations for Online Teaching

- Consider using narratives to complement other methods of teaching because narratives help students reflect on the emotional experience or human response to illness and health and facilitate learning about complex topics.
- Be purposeful in how narrative pedagogy is used. Because it is more than sharing stories, consider how to develop specific teaching strategies and experiences for students that use narrative pedagogy.
- Use narrative pedagogy to develop approaches that deepen understanding by encouraging interpretative thinking and a spirit of inquiry to seek evidence-based best practices (Fitzpatrick, 2017, 2018).
- Facilitate understanding of the context of the narrative, drawing attention to what stood out, what was noticed, and how it was interpreted within a community of learners.
- Implement narrative pedagogy when applying theory to practice to help students reach the affective level of learning.
- Use narrative pedagogy to help shift teaching from a teacher-centered, behaviorist approach to a learner-centered, constructivist approach.

References

Andrews, C. A., Ironside, P. M., Nosek, C., Sims, S. L., Swenson, M. M., Yeoman, C., ... Diekelmann, N. (2001). Enacting narrative pedagogy: The lived experiences of students and teachers. *Nursing and Health Care Perspectives, 22*(5), 252.

Candela, L. (2020). Theoretical foundations of teaching and learning. In D. M. Billings & J. A. Halstead (Eds.), *Teaching in nursing: A guide for faculty* (6th ed., pp. 247–269). Elsevier.

Diekelmann, N. (2001). Narrative pedagogy: Heideggerian hermeneutical analyses of lived experiences of students, teachers, and clinicians. *Advances in Nursing Science, 23*(3), 53–71.

Engel, M. (2010). *I'm here: Compassionate communication in patient care.* Ella Press.

Fitzpatrick, J. J. (2017). Narrative nursing: Applications in practice, education, and research [Editorial]. *Applied Nursing Research, 37.* http://doi.org/10.1016/j.apnr.2017.08.005

Fitzpatrick, J. J. (2018). Teaching through storytelling: Narrative nursing [Editorial]. *Nursing Education Perspectives, 39*(2), 60. http://doi.org/10.1097/01.NEP.0000000000000298

Gibbs, G. (1988). *Learning by doing: A guide to teaching and learning methods.* Oxford Brookes University.

Giddens, J., Fogg, L., & Carlsen-Sabelli, L. (2010). Learning and engagement with a virtual community by undergraduate nursing students. *Nursing Outlook, 58*(5), 261–267.

Ironside, P. M. (2006). Using narrative pedagogy: Learning and practicing interpretive thinking. *Journal of Advanced Nursing, 55*(4), 478–486.

Ironside, P. M. (2014). Enabling narrative pedagogy: Inviting, waiting, and letting be. *Nursing Education Perspectives, 35*(4), 212–218.

Ironside, P. M. (2015). Narrative pedagogy: Transforming nursing education through 15 years of research in nursing education. *Nursing Education Perspectives, 36*(2), 83–88. http://doi.org/10.5480/13-1102

Kalanithi, P. (2016). *When breath becomes air.* Random House.

Nehls, N. (1995). Narrative pedagogy: Rethinking nursing education. *Journal of Nursing Education, 34*(5), 204–210.

Saucier Lundy, K., & Janes, S. (2016). *Community health nursing: Caring for the public's health* (3rd ed.). Jones & Bartlett.

Smith, P., & Jones, M. (2016). Evaluating an online family assessment activity: A focus on diversity and health promotion. *Nursing Forum, 51*(3), 204–210.

Taylor Sullivan, D. (2020). An introduction to curriculum development. In D. M. Billings & J. A. Halstead (Eds.), *Teaching in nursing: A guide for faculty* (6th ed., pp. 103–134). Elsevier.

Walsh, M., & van Soeren, M. (2012). Interprofessional learning and virtual communities: An opportunity for the future. *Journal of Interprofessional Care, 26*, 43–48. http://doi.org/10.3109/13561820.2011.620187

Ziering, A., King Barklow, T. (Producers), & Dick, K. (Director). (2012). *The invisible war.* Cinedigm Corp. http://www.documentarytube.com/videos/the-invisible-war

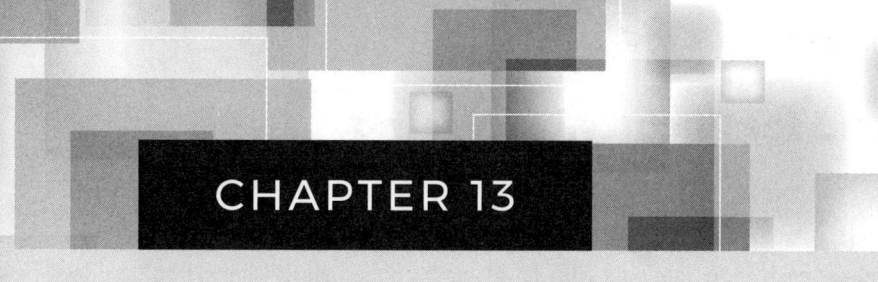

Faculty Role in Academia

Melissa Robinson and Henny Breen

Overview

This chapter addresses how faculty members in online education can fit into traditional roles within academic institutions. We discuss what nursing faculty who make the transition from traditional face-to-face teaching to online teaching can do to demonstrate readiness, preparation, competency, and ongoing professional development. We include reflections on our teaching philosophies and exemplars of the work we have done to develop a scholarship of online teaching through collaboration and mentorship consistent with Boyer's (1990) model.

Nurses in Academia

We recognize nursing education as an area of advanced nursing practice and online teaching as a specialty practice in nursing education. Specialty areas in nursing education are varied and include administrative leadership, clinical teaching, simulation, online education, and more. Nursing education also crosses multiple levels of nursing practice, including undergraduate (associate degree, baccalaureate, registered nurse–bachelor of science in nursing [RN-to-BSN]) and graduate (master's, doctoral, advanced practice) degree programs. Each requires nursing faculty to demonstrate readiness, preparation, competency, and ongoing professional development. In this chapter, we discuss how each of these elements can be applied to online teaching as a specialty practice. We also share our experience as online faculty moving through the ranks of academia. Lastly, we propose that collaboration in teaching and scholarship is an effective way to improve productivity and enhance satisfaction with the faculty role.

Demand for Faculty in Nursing

Competency and satisfaction in the faculty role in nursing have become more critical as the demand for registered nurses and higher levels of nursing education has increased. Overall, there is a shortage of qualified nurse faculty, which has resulted in a demand to teach more students with fewer faculty members (Fisher, 2016). According to the American Association of Colleges of Nursing (AACN, 2019) report on 2018–2019 enrollment and graduations in baccalaureate and graduate programs in nursing, nursing programs in the United States "turned away 75,029 qualified applicants from baccalaureate and graduate nursing programs in 2018 due to an insufficient number of faculty, clinical sites, classroom space, clinical preceptors, and budget constraints" (p. 1). In an annual survey, most nursing schools cited faculty shortages as a reason for not accepting all qualified applicants into baccalaureate programs (AACN, 2019). In 2018, nursing schools with baccalaureate and/or graduate programs cited a total of 1,715 faculty vacancies, and 90.7% of those were faculty positions that required or preferred a doctoral degree (AACN, 2019).

At the same time that the United States is experiencing a faculty shortage in nursing, online education continues to grow rapidly and is providing ample opportunities for students to access nursing education globally. As more faculty transition from traditional face-to-face teaching to teaching in online classrooms, they are challenged to develop new pedagogies, adopt new teaching strategies, and use technology to deliver high-quality education (Hampton et al., 2020). When nursing faculty are prepared for online teaching and feel successful, they are more likely to have higher levels of job satisfaction and thus may be more likely to stay in academia.

Readiness for Online Teaching

Taking an active approach to self-assessment of readiness for online teaching is an important first step. One of the most common concerns reported by faculty making the transition to online teaching is being prepared for the challenges of working with new forms of technology. Although this is a critical piece, we also recommend that faculty reflect on their teaching style and how comfortable they are moving from sharing knowledge and content in a traditional, face-to-face classroom to facilitating learning that occurs through collaborative learning experiences in the online classroom. It is important to use theory to guide online teaching pedagogy and use teaching strategies that place the student at the center of the learning experience, as described in earlier chapters. Each of these elements is an important consideration when making a successful transition to online teaching.

Preparation and Competency for Online Teaching

Faculty need training and support when transitioning to online teaching. When faculty first begin teaching online, they may be concerned that they don't have the skills to use the technology required to teach effectively and see the experience as threatening (Grant & Thornton, 2007; Johnson & Meehan, 2013). They may approach the transition with skepticism about the quality of online learning (Lin, Dyer, & Guo, 2012) or express concerns about losing the ability to establish strong individual connections with students. Faculty may underestimate the time it takes to transition a face-to-face course to the online classroom. They also may be apprehensive about the time needed to acquire online teaching skills (Horvitz, Beach, Anderson, & Xia, 2015) and have concerns about the lack of training available on their campuses for online design and teaching (Hunt et al., 2014).

The experience and expertise of faculty members in nursing education programs vary considerably. Faculty members in nursing are often hired with extensive expertise in specific nursing specialties but may have minimal or no teaching experience and no experience with online teaching (Blodgett, 2008). Some faculty members have attended formal nursing education programs and have experience with curriculum design and assessment, program evaluation, and teaching strategies and may also have formal education in distance education. There are also faculty who report learning to teach online by working individually to improve their knowledge and skills, sometimes through trial and error. Other faculty are fortunate to be mentored by more experienced online faculty and skilled instructional designers. Developing the skills to facilitate learning in the virtual classroom is the goal of becoming a competent online educator (Johnson & Meehan, 2013).

Competent Online Teaching

While online education has been growing in popularity and accessibility, many institutions have implemented orientation and preparation courses of their own, developed and taught by instructional design experts and online faculty. Institutional programs have the advantage of ensuring that faculty are oriented to the culture and philosophy of the institution and the expectations for online teaching. Other institutions may require previous experience in online teaching or have specific certification requirements to document preparation and competency prior to teaching online courses, each designed to increase the quality and integrity of the online education program.

Competent online educators have the knowledge and skills that enable them to effectively perform in their roles. Our approach to our own development, and to supporting others as they develop the competencies for quality online teaching, includes elements of professional development, mentorship, and collaboration. Mentorship, in particular, is critical to developing competence in online teaching that is a "complex combination of knowledge, skills, attitudes, and values displayed in the context of task performance" (Kerka, 1998, p. 6). We have developed a course lead model for online teaching that promotes skill development and helps faculty develop in their ability to support the unique needs of online students, in their role as facilitators of learning, and in their ability to achieve faculty presence in the classroom. Course leads are responsible for the orientation, mentoring, and evaluation of faculty assigned to the courses they lead.

Online Adjunct Faculty

Supporting online adjunct faculty, particularly in relation to online teaching, is an important role for the course lead. Adjunct faculty members are assigned to teach on a part-time or as-needed basis and are not on an academic track toward promotion and tenure. Adjunct faculty serve an important role in teaching in the online program but may struggle to adapt to the role unless they are provided with sufficient support and mentorship. Adjunct nursing faculty have content expertise that is needed in the online classroom, they are less expensive to the institution, and they strengthen program staffing models when enrollment fluctuates (Forbes, Hickey, & White, 2010). On the other hand, they may be difficult to retain because of their other work commitments, and it can be costly to continually hire and orient adjunct faculty.

In an effort to develop strategies to support the needs of adjunct faculty, increase their job satisfaction, and promote overall retention, Forbes et al. (2010) conducted a study to identify problems related to their teaching role. Adjunct faculty reported confusion related to role expectations, inconsistencies leading to role ambiguity, the need for resources and help with technology, and the need for a more adequate orientation. To address these challenges, the investigators recommended formalizing orientation efforts to allow inexperienced adjuncts to work closely with more experienced faculty to exchange ideas about best practices (Forbes et al., 2010). They also recommended a course coordinator model that aligns with the course lead model we have implemented for the online program. The coordinator or course lead is responsible for orienting the adjunct and providing mentorship, maintaining close contact throughout the semester, assisting with student issues as they arise, and connecting the adjunct to the resources needed to be successful. A compressive discussion of the course lead model is included in Chapter 5.

Orientation and mentorship are both important, yet distinctly different, and as a result of the course lead model, there is close integration between the two in our online program.

Orientation

Orientation includes orienting faculty to the online course, the online program, and the institution. The orientation is important for helping faculty understand a variety of cultural and governance structures with the institution as well as expectations for their role and responsibilities in the course they are teaching. Orientation is also important for getting faculty off to a strong start with working across departments to learn the support services available to staff, faculty, and students. A strong introduction to the campus community is an important way to make faculty feel welcome and begin to acclimate to their role.

Mentorship

Mentorship is essential for helping faculty grow in the role of a facilitator of learning and developing their confidence in supporting online students. The mentor supports faculty members as they develop their skills in best practices in online teaching and implementing strategies that support the success of online students. Mentors are in a privileged position to benefit from what mentees have to offer from their own experience while developing a meaningful relationship with a colleague. We have included components of orientation to the online program and mentorship for online teaching in **Table 13-1**. Mentorship for full-time faculty moving through the ranks of promotion and tenure and developing a scholarship of teaching is also discussed later in this chapter.

Table 13-1 Orientation to the Online Program and Mentorship for Online Teaching

Orientation to the Online Program

- Understanding program and institution governance structures
- Sharing information about the culture of the institution
- Understanding faculty rights, role, and responsibilities
- Understanding department policies and procedures
- Introductions to program support staff and departmental functions
- Sharing information about resources for student support (e.g., advising, financial aid, technology, learning management system [LMS], library)
- Connections to internal resources for teaching, research, and service opportunities

Mentorship for Online Teaching

- Understanding the teaching aspect of the faculty role
- Support for implementing best practices in online teaching
- Modeling for establishing presence in the online classroom
- Encouragement for ways to create meaningful connections with online students
- Advice for professional development opportunities and career growth
- Creating opportunities for professional networking and collegial relationships
- Support and coaching for student issues such as maintaining flexibility and holding students to expectations
- Classroom observations to share experiences and examples
- Sharing and recommending resources for professional development
- Providing a safe, nonjudgmental approach to providing feedback and answering questions
- Interrater reliability and support for course assessments
- Support for delivering high-quality, effective student feedback
- Problem solving for student issues, teaching challenges, and managing the workload

Table 13-2 provides an example of mentoring activities that we have found to be effective when working with online adjunct faculty. This particular example demonstrates the importance of working closely with adjunct faculty members to identify their learning needs in order to more effectively support them in their online teaching role. Each of the activities can be mutually beneficial for the mentor and mentee, which can lead to rewarding collaborative working relationships and improved outcomes for students.

Professional Development

Professional development in online teaching can contribute credibility to online education when institutions can demonstrate a commitment to sharing best practices, applying evidence to online teaching, and maintaining high standards of excellence in online education. Faculty satisfaction with online teaching can be enhanced significantly with ongoing, high-quality professional development. As a result of higher

Table 13-2 Examples of Mentoring Activities for Online Adjunct Faculty

Sarah was an experienced RN with a master's degree in nursing and some experience teaching in BSN, accelerated BSN, and RN-to-BSN programs. Her clinical and leadership background included community and population health, management of public health programs, and care of vulnerable populations. Early meetings with her revealed that she was an ideal choice for an adjunct role in the online population health course. She was a passionate advocate for vulnerable populations, a strong role model for postlicensure students, and a knowledgeable content expert. The learning needs she identified included becoming comfortable with the learning management system, understanding the layout of the course and expectations for her role as the facilitator, growing in her ability to provide feedback for grading and student development, as well as being able to balance the workload of teaching the online course while working in clinical practice full time. Mentoring for Sarah included the following:

- Provided Sarah with access to the mentor's online course she would be teaching during the semester before she was scheduled to teach, as an observer
- Conducted multiple meetings prior to the start of the semester and in the first weeks of the course to go over the design of the course, expectations for teaching, and strategies to support student success; shared tips for managing online teaching responsibilities and workload
- Shared graded discussions and assignments with Sarah to help her develop confidence in providing substantive, meaningful feedback to students; conducted interrater reliability on a regular basis to discuss grading practices and policies
- Solved problems and addressed student challenges collaboratively; as her confidence grew, she became more independent with each course that she taught.
- Included Sarah on team emails that modeled student support strategies and problem solving
- Discussed strategies that Sarah could implement to share her experiences as a nurse leader and model professional behaviors through continual faculty engagement in the online classroom
- Collaborated on ways to continually improve and update the course by developing new content and course activities

satisfaction and competency, the quality of their teaching improves, and students' satisfaction and achievement of outcomes are enhanced (Dietrich, 2015). Several scholars have described successful online teaching approaches that are mentioned here because of the importance of ongoing professional development, including quality teaching, course management, and student-support-related methods:

1. Specific strategies are being present, prompt, organized, respectful, creative, and encouraging to students (Stavredes, 2011).
2. To be effective, online instructors should create learning activities that promote interaction and build community (Nilson & Goodson, 2018).
3. Online teachers should employ strategies that allow students to make connections with them and help students experience the presence of the online teacher (Aspden & Helm, 2004).
4. Students value teachers who demonstrate respect for students, value what students express, are enthusiastic, are subject matter experts, have "fun" and

show humor, provide outside assistance, and promote their self-efficacy and self-esteem (Mowrer-Reynolds, 2008).
5. Ensure relevance—make connections, set meaningful goals, and build on student interests (Johnson, 2013).
6. Help students identify their learning needs and offer choices to students about topics and the sequence of their learning (Nilson & Goodson, 2018).

There are certainly many more qualities and characteristics that contribute to high-quality teaching and learning, which we have discussed in several chapters. In order to consider ways to build knowledge and develop the requisite skills that lead to high-quality online teaching, we have compiled a list of sample topics for ongoing professional development. The list in **Table 13-3** is a sample of topics rather than an exhaustive list.

Table 13-3 Sample Topics for Professional Development

- Fundamentals of Online Teaching and Learning
- Best Practices in Online Education
- Characteristics of Online Learners
- Role of the Online Instructor
- Principles of Effective Online Teaching
- Creating Instructor Presence
- Course Management Strategies
- Strategies for Promoting Learner Engagement
- Continual Faculty Engagement
- Planning for Instructional Design in Online Education
- Theoretical and Practical Considerations for Online Education
- Curriculum Development in Online Education
- Online Course Models for Successful Online Instruction
- Assessment and Evaluation in Online Education
- Teaching Strategies in Online Education
- Key Components of an Effective Online Course
- Developing the Online Learning Community
- Transitioning Face-to-Face Course Activities to Online Format
- Evidence-Based Online Teaching
- Myths of Online Teaching and Learning
- Social Media and Web 2.0 Tools
- Retention and Supporting the Success of Online Students
- Challenges Faced by the Online Learner
- Skills and Competencies That Help Online Learners Succeed
- Designing Authentic Learning Activities That Stimulate Engagement
- Designing Online Activities That Foster Active Learning
- Best Practices for Promoting Academic Honesty and Integrity in Online Courses
- Policy Development for Communication, Course Administration, and Management
- Strategies for Managing Groups in the Online Classroom
- Expectations for Communication in the Online Classroom
- Online Presence Versus Online Engagement
- Faculty Satisfaction and Workload Management
- Delivering Effective Student Feedback

Certification programs provide additional opportunities for professional development for nursing faculty. Faculty may complete professional development programs to achieve certification in nursing education or online education. Certification allows faculty to demonstrate their knowledge and mastery of online teaching (Quality Matters, 2020). In addition to skill development, certification provides faculty with recognition for their accomplishments while increasing the credibility of online education for students, the institution, and the discipline. Examples of certification programs in nursing education and online teaching are discussed in the following sections. **Table 13-4** includes resources for professional development, including certification and other opportunities. This is a sample of activities rather than an exhaustive list.

Certified Nurse Educator

Nurse educators have the opportunity to seek credentialing as a certified nurse educator (CNE) through the Academic Nurse Educator Certification Program of

Table 13-4 Professional Development for Online Teaching

Professional Certification	
Certified nurse educator (CNE)	National League for Nursing (NLN) http://www.nln.org/Certification-for-Nurse-Educators/cne
Certified online instructor (COI) Certified faculty developer (CFD)	Learning Resources Network (NLN) https://lern.org/events-education/faculty-training/ Certification course, faculty development, continuing education, publications, newsletters, and more
Professional certification in online education (PCOE) Distance teaching and learning badges and courses	University of Madison–Wisconsin, Continuing Studies Distance Teaching and Learning https://continuingstudies.wisc.edu/distance-teaching-learning/ Online professional development, an annual conference, and custom programs for distance-learning professionals
Teaching online certificate Peer reviewer course (PRC) Master reviewer certification (MRC) Online facilitator certification (IOFC) QM coach certification (QMCC)	Quality Matters https://www.qualitymatters.org/professional-development Online professional development, organizational resources, individual and organizational membership, QM-designated courses, webinars for continuing education, workshops, and more

Professional Certification	
Online teaching certificate (OTC) Advanced online teaching certificate	Online Learning Consortium https://onlinelearningconsortium.org/ Certificate programs, individual and organizational memberships, workshops, professional development opportunities, mastery development classes, and more
Faculty Focus: Higher ed teaching strategies from Magna Publications	Faculty Focus https://www.facultyfocus.com/ Newsletters, free resources, the Teaching Professor conferences, *Journal of Faculty Development* access, and more

the National League for Nursing (NLN). Although not specific to online teaching, certification in nursing education is a mark of distinction for nursing faculty. It establishes nursing education as a specialty area of practice and creates a means for faculty to demonstrate their expertise in the role (NLN, 2020).

As a role model in leadership and education, CNEs demonstrate a commitment to the highest standards of excellence to students, colleagues, and the academic and healthcare communities. The major practice-related content areas addressed in the CNE exam include the following: (1) facilitating learner development and socialization; (2) assessment and evaluation strategies; (3) curriculum design and evaluation of program outcomes; (4) continuous quality improvement in the academic nurse educator role; (5) engaging in scholarship, service, and leadership; (6) functioning as a change agent and leader; (7) engaging in the scholarship of teaching; and (8) functioning effectively within the institutional environment and academic community (NLN, 2020). The certification provides a comprehensive level of preparation for the role of the faculty member in nursing, which is encouraged for all nursing faculty, including those working in online programs. The CNE requires renewal every 5 years, which requires faculty to demonstrate ongoing professional development and competency.

Certified Online Instructor (COI)

The certified online instructor (COI) designation is a professional certification course available from the Learning Resources Network (LERN) for online faculty in higher education. A priority is given to faculty development for developing online courses and teaching online and hybrid courses. The COI certification course models best practices for online education, offers mentorship and training for faculty, and provides valuable feedback for decision making for online teachers and administrators (LERN, 2020). The certification course was developed by Dr. Mary Dereshiwsky and Dr. William Draves, leaders in the field of online education. The course includes an interdisciplinary, interactive online course experience conducted over several weeks. It also provides educators with an opportunity to have the online course they are teaching evaluated by the faculty and includes feedback and comments obtained directly from students. The COI designation demonstrates that the individual's knowledge about online teaching is benchmarked with a standard of achievement developed by the leading thinkers and practitioners in the field (LERN, 2020). The COI does not require periodic renewal; therefore, a plan for ongoing professional development is needed. After taking the COI course ourselves, we recognize that it is a valuable experience for learning the basic fundamentals of online education.

Quality Matters

There are a variety of certification opportunities available to faculty interested in advanced preparation in online course design through Quality Matters (QM). QM professional development is designed to help educators deliver quality online learning opportunities to multiple levels of learners, including those teaching in online or hybrid programs in higher education. Professional development opportunities are available to instructional designers, faculty, administrators, adjunct instructors, and more. Experienced online faculty may choose to serve as QM Peer Reviewers, which includes taking a certification course on the foundational principles of QM and the QM rubric, then applying their knowledge in the review of courses that seek QM designation. The reviewer course is an opportunity to further demonstrate preparation and leadership in online education. QM and the importance of continuous quality improvement in online education are further discussed in Chapter 6.

Scholarship in Nursing Education

In 2016, the AACN released *Advancing Healthcare Transformation: A New Era for Academic Nursing*, which advanced a new definition of "academic nursing":

> Academic nursing encompasses the integration of practice, education, and research within baccalaureate and graduate schools of nursing. Faculty engaged in academic nursing demonstrate a commitment to inquiry, generate new knowledge for the discipline, connect practice with education, and lead scholarly pursuits that improve health and health care. (p. 5)

Scholarship is critical to contribute to the body of knowledge that informs educational practices in academia. In addition to teaching and working with students, faculty in nursing education are called upon to advance the development of nursing education as a science (Oermann, DeGagne, & Cusatis Phillips, 2018). Nursing faculty engage in a variety of teaching practices that are guided by the application of the most recent, relevant evidence. Scholarship in nursing education also encompasses a broad set of contributions made by faculty that can be shared with others, including developing curricular models, teaching strategies, evaluation activities, and best educational practices. Conducting primary research and other forms of inquiry and writing for publication are also contributions made by faculty. In order for the work of nursing faculty to be considered scholarly, it should be peer reviewed, disseminated in some form, and critiqued in order for others to use that work for application in their setting (Oermann, 2018).

Boyer's Model of Scholarship

Boyer (1990) was the first to propose a framework for scholarship and the faculty role that emphasized teaching as a scholarly activity. He suggested that it is important to develop a balance between research and teaching when measuring the faculty member's success in academia (Fisher, 2016). His approach to scholarship depicted four overlapping and connected functions of scholarship: the scholarship of teaching, the scholarship of application, the scholarship of discovery, and the scholarship of integration.

Scholarship of Teaching

The scholarship of teaching "focuses on understanding, describing, explaining teaching-learning strategies, assessing their impact on learner outcomes, and disseminating results" (AACN, 2018, p. 7). Faculty in nursing may demonstrate the scholarship of teaching by applying theory to the practice of teaching, developing new teaching methodologies, updating curriculum models, or contributing to best practices within the discipline.

Scholarship of Application

The scholarship of application (practice) is "directly related to the need to address and solve specific practice issues, related to individual patients, organizations, and social problems" (AACN, 2018, p. 5). The scholarship of application is an essential underpinning for practice disciplines (Riley, Beal, Levi, & McCausland, 2002) that allows nursing faculty to demonstrate scholarship in a diverse range of practice settings that include teaching, clinical practice, and advanced practice in nursing. Nursing faculty demonstrate the scholarship of practice through the application of evidence to health interventions, by developing policy and practice protocols, and when developing innovative teaching and practice initiatives.

Scholarship of Discovery

The scholarship of discovery expands current knowledge and understanding in the field through primary empirical research, analysis of large data, theory development, methodological studies, and philosophical inquiry (AACN, 2018). Nursing faculty may demonstrate the scholarship of discovery through inquiry that emphasizes health promotion and illness prevention or through inquiry that advances the art and science of nursing education.

Scholarship of Integration

The scholarship of integration is defined as interdisciplinary inquiry that creates or combines knowledge into new insights through the interconnection of ideas and critical analysis (Boyer, 1990). In nursing education, faculty may engage in interdisciplinary work that takes place through other mediums for scholarship, such as discovery, teaching, or practice (application) (AACN, 2018).

Boyer's model has been embraced widely across many different disciplines in academia. In nursing, the AACN position statement entitled *Defining Scholarship for Academic Nursing* (2018) identifies a specific framework used in academia for making faculty promotion and tenure recommendations that utilizes the Boyer model.

Faculty Promotion and Tenure

Our institution has adopted the framework as a component of the "discipline-specific guidelines" for promotion and tenure in nursing. The guidelines provide a comprehensive definition of nursing scholarship that includes examples intended to (1) guide promotion and tenure decisions appropriate for the discipline of nursing, (2) delineate the scope of recognized scholarly activities in nursing, and (3) guide faculty members in developing a plan for their professional development and career trajectory. Please refer to the AACN's *Defining Scholarship for Academic Nursing: Task Force Consensus Position Statement* (2018).

Depending on the institution, faculty evaluation may take place within the department or school of nursing, or it may include evaluation outside of the department and within the larger institution. Having a discipline-specific guideline for nursing faculty has been particularly important for our own evaluations that have been completed outside of the school of nursing, by our liberal arts faculty colleagues. Even more critical to our promotion and tenure evaluations was the fact that we were the first two faculty members within the traditional institution to teach full time and exclusively in the online program. Our institution considers promotion as recognition of meritorious work in teaching, professional achievement, and service. It is expected that the level of scholarship, leadership, and responsibility of an individual faculty member will increase with experience and rank. Faculty may conduct different kinds of scholarship during different stages of their professional development. In nursing, professional diversity is encouraged, and it is not anticipated that any one faculty member would engage in all areas of scholarship as defined by Boyer's model. A significant depth of scholarship in one area or breadth of professional achievement across various areas of scholarship is highly encouraged, and it is incumbent on faculty members to describe their professional achievement. A component to our School of Nursing discipline-specific guidelines that outlines the requirement for promotion and tenure in nursing is included in **Table 13-5**.

Table 13-5 Sample Component of Discipline-Specific Promotion and Tenure Guidelines

Promotion to Associate Professor and Tenure
■ The associate professor must have evidence of a doctorate earned from a nationally accredited graduate institution.
■ Promotion to associate professor normally requires tenure status.
■ Tenure decisions inevitably rely on accomplishments to date; however, the granting of tenure is a future-oriented decision. It represents a confident prediction by the college that (a) the individual will continue to do outstanding work, and (b) there will be a significant degree of professional compatibility between the individual's contributions and the needs of the college.

- To establish merit, using the AACN's *Defining Scholarship for Academic Nursing: Task Force Consensus Position Statement* (2018), the candidate is expected to demonstrate professional achievement in one of the domains described earlier: scholarship of teaching, practice, discovery, or integration. This work should demonstrate professional achievement that goes beyond what was accomplished in the candidate's doctoral work.
- It is incumbent that candidates describe their plan for professional achievement as well as their achievement up to this point in time.
- Ultimately, candidates must also communicate their professional identity and philosophy of teaching, establish themselves as a competent academic, and articulate a rigorous career trajectory.

Promotion to Full Professor

- Promotion to full professor implies "special merit."
- To establish "special merit" in teaching and service, the candidate must provide evidence demonstrating continued excellence beyond that exhibited prior to promotion to associate professor, in teaching effectiveness and service to the college, the nursing profession, and/or the community.
- In terms of teaching effectiveness, faculty may have demonstrated a high degree of consistent expertise in teaching effectiveness by strong qualitative (student comments) and quantitative feedback on student evaluations of instructor or implemented measurable innovations in the classroom that demonstrate an increase in student learning. Feedback by colleagues who have observed and/or cotaught with the candidate document these results.
- In terms of service, the candidate must demonstrate leadership to benefit the college community (e.g., serving as the chairperson of major department and/or college committees) or leadership that benefits the local, state, national, or international healthcare community (e.g., serving on a committee of a state or national nursing organization or other health-related organizations or boards).
- To establish "special merit" in professional achievement, candidates must demonstrate how they have demonstrated an increased depth and achievement of scholarship in the area described in their promotion to associate professor and tenure narrative and/or further development of scholarship in one or more additional domains of professional achievement.
- Although the rate and form of professional achievement may change over time (e.g., become more diversified and demonstrate a significant integration of professional activities across one or more of the domains of scholarship), candidates must demonstrate greater recognition and deeper engagement in their area(s) of scholarship.
- For example, the candidate may have demonstrated leadership in developing an innovative nursing curriculum with colleagues, an increased number of invited presentations and/or peer-reviewed publications, influenced healthcare policy that led to improved healthcare delivery, collaborated with others to provide international learning experiences for students, and so on.
- It is the responsibility of candidates to document and articulate their achievements.
- Candidates may seek external letters that support their narrative and speak to their expertise and experiences.

Our Journey to the Scholarship of Teaching and Learning

Our journey to the scholarship of teaching and learning in a traditional liberal arts college has been somewhat unique. We thought it would be helpful to share our experience, as the first two tenure track faculty members in our institution who teach entirely online, in moving through the ranks of promotion and tenure. We were fortunate that our efforts to develop a scholarship of teaching aligned with the emphasis that our institution places on effective teaching. The AACN definition of scholarship in academic nursing and Boyer's model have provided a useful framework for articulating our scholarly practice in teaching, professional achievement, and service. The well-known "continuum of growth toward the scholarship of teaching" proposed by Weston and McAlpine (2001, p. 89) is a framework that resonates with our experience. In their work as faculty developers, they challenged the idea that teaching occurs in isolation, separate from the other work of faculty, such as research and practice, to suggest that the scholarship of teaching is actually integrated within the scholarship of discovery (Boyer's model). Thus, the path toward the scholarship of teaching and learning begins with good teaching, moves toward scholarly teaching, and then ultimately arrives at the scholarship of teaching and learning (Weston & McAlpine, 2001). In the following sections, we discuss the phases on the "continuum of growth," including (1) growth in teaching, (2) exchanging knowledge about teaching and learning, and (3) growth in the scholarship of teaching. We have also shared exemplars of scholarship that can be considered for each phase, specific to online teaching and learning.

Growth in Teaching

In the first phase, faculty start out with the intention of developing their own teaching through mechanisms of action, reflection, and ongoing improvement that become more formalized (McAlpine, Weston, Beauchamp, Wiseman, & Beauchamp, 1999). As they move through this phase, they experience growth in their knowledge of their teaching and their students' learning, thereby developing a sense of competence in their teaching. Some actions taken by faculty in this phase include reflecting on their teaching, engaging in professional development activities, evaluating their teaching to make improvements, and studying best practices (Weston & McAlpine, 2001). During this phase, faculty may be able to describe the theoretical rationale for their teaching and demonstrate their practical knowledge of teaching. When we engaged in discussions about what helped us develop knowledge about our own online teaching and our students' learning, we recognized how important it had been to collaborate with our peers, develop an ongoing commitment to self-reflection on our teaching, and continually refine our individual teaching philosophies.

Reflection on Teaching

As faculty, reflecting on our teaching helps us identify what works and what doesn't work in our courses. Evaluating instructional effectiveness may include conducting formal course evaluations or creating less formal opportunities to ask students to share their perspectives on course design, materials, time lines, and specific course activities (Hanna, Glowacki-Dudka, & Conceicao-Runlee, 2000). It is our responsibility to engage students in evaluation activities, not only to provide valuable feedback for reflection but also to demonstrate our commitment to student learning. When students are asked to reflect on their learning experiences, not only does it provide rich opportunities for faculty reflection, but it can also empower students to become experts in their own learning, increase their self-esteem and confidence, and increase their leadership in the classroom, even beyond what they might develop in a traditional classroom (Palloff & Pratt, 2004).

Stephen Brookfield (1995) asserted that without a reflective orientation, faculty members are leaving "an unseemly amount of trust in the role of chance" (p. 24). He suggested that faculty members become critically reflective through the application of adult learning principles and by using critical reflection for continuous personal and professional development. Critical reflection can help faculty (1) take informed actions that have a good chance of achieving the intended effect; (2) develop a rationale for practice that can be communicated to others; (3) develop resilience to the challenges and rewards of teaching; (4) energize the classroom by modeling critical thinking, openly questioning our own ideas, and inviting students to critique our efforts; and (5) learn the effects we are having on students (Brookfield, 1995).

In addition to the benefit of individual reflection, our institution has placed a strong emphasis on colleague appraisal as a component of faculty evaluation during the promotion and tenure academic track. Individually, our growth as faculty is influenced by the mentoring of more experienced faculty members during the formal process. We also benefit from feedback generated during collaborative teaching experiences and informally, when soliciting feedback on our teaching. Ultimately, our growth in teaching is influenced by the input of students and colleagues through the process of self-reflection.

Reflection on Teaching Philosophy

Institutions may require faculty to reflect on their teaching philosophy as part of the faculty evaluation process. Nurses, regardless of their role within nursing, benefit from reflecting on their philosophy of caring, nursing, or teaching. As they gain experience, their philosophy evolves and changes. The values, beliefs, and assumptions about nursing education held by faculty develop over time and are influenced by our experiences as learners, by our experiences as faculty, and by our students. This is an ongoing process that may also be influenced by the mission and philosophy of the institution and by influences in the community that are social, economic, or political.

Online nursing faculty experience a dynamic relationship between curricula, professional requirements, pedagogy, and technology (Koehler, Mishra, Hershey, & Peruski, 2004). This requires faculty to consider what they believe about online teaching and learning in the online classroom. In a study that examined the variables that affect nursing faculty self-efficacy and participation in online teaching, Robina and Anderson (2010) found that the years of general teaching experience did not correlate with online teaching efficacy. Although there may be some debate about this, high levels of online teaching effectiveness were associated with significant preparation, instructional design support, and experience teaching at least three online courses. The experienced faculty members who participated in the study reported that they had to rethink their philosophies of teaching and learning when moving from traditional face-to-face teaching to teaching in the online classroom (Robina & Anderson, 2010). We share our individual teaching philosophies in **Table 13-6** and **Table 13-7**.

For us, the process of becoming effective online faculty and scholars within our discipline was a developmental experience. This is an important reason why the "continuum" of the scholarship of teaching proposed by Weston and McAlpine (2001) resonated so closely with our experiences. As we developed and moved further along on the continuum, we felt we could demonstrate progress toward scholarship (Boyer's model). In **Table 13-8**, we include exemplars of scholarship from our own experiences that demonstrated our growth in online teaching.

Table 13-6 Online Faculty Reflection on Teaching Philosophy:
Dr. Henny Breen

My philosophy of teaching starts with understanding how my experiences have influenced how I learn and practice nursing. I believe learning evolves over a lifetime and is influenced by personal experience and engagement with others. Being able to critically reflect on new information and collaborate with others enables students to grow personally and professionally. I believe it is my responsibility to facilitate these types of learning experiences as they grapple with increasingly complex concepts. Students are inspired to lifelong learning when their ideas and experiences are shared, heard and respected. They are then able to respect other ideas, seek new information, and be open to considering how to apply new insights to their nursing practice.

Table 13-7 Online Faculty Reflection on Teaching Philosophy:
Dr. Melissa Robinson

My teaching philosophy includes theoretical components of constructivism. I believe in demonstrating respect for the diverse experiences and backgrounds of my students and helping them build on that foundation. I value collaborative teaching, evidence-based practices, experiential and "active" learning experiences, innovation, and opportunities for reflection and personal growth for students and teachers. I believe that learning is an interpersonal experience and that education should be individualized, student centered, and compassionate. My teaching practice is an extension of my nursing practice. It includes facilitation, mentoring, leadership, and commitment to the community. Gratitude, a strong sense of ethics, and responsibility energize and motivate me in nursing and education.

Table 13-8 Exemplars of Scholarship That Demonstrate Growth in Teaching (Phase One)

- Develop a personal process of self-reflection.
- Conduct course evaluations every semester in order to make course improvements.
- Create additional opportunities for students to provide feedback on specific course materials and activities and at different times during the semester (e.g., midterm).
- Participate in institutional faculty development workshops designed and taught by instructional designers or experienced online instructors.
- Apply scholarly evidence (best practices) to the practice of online teaching.
- Develop, implement, and evaluate an innovative online teaching strategy.
- Attend a professional conference for online teaching and learning.
- Take a certification course for online teaching; earn certification.
- Demonstrate validity of teaching through assessment by students, colleagues, and administrators.

Exchanging Knowledge About Teaching and Learning

During the second phase, faculty begin to take more responsibility for improving teaching within their department and more leadership roles within the institution related to teaching (Weston & McAlpine, 2001). They begin to engage with colleagues in collaboration to build a more complex understanding of pedagogy and knowledge of content for their discipline, which advances the integration of teaching overall (Weston & McAlpine, 2001). During this phase, faculty members may be participating in faculty governance, leading a departmental event or committee related to teaching and learning, or engaging in external service activities that serve the community or discipline. Throughout their careers, nursing faculty have been mentored and have mentored others. Earlier in this chapter, we discussed the importance of mentoring for online teaching. We also recommend formal mentorship for faculty members who are developing their scholarship of teaching and moving through the academic track.

Formal Mentorship Program

We recognize that mentorship occurs in a variety of forms and across the continuum of growth toward the scholarship of teaching; however, during the second phase, when faculty are better prepared to exchange knowledge about teaching and learning, mentorship becomes even more important. Faculty members in this phase may also be beginning to mentor others in their specialty area or within the discipline. Mentorship relies on an individualized, reciprocal relationship that helps the mentee develop personally and professionally. Ideally, mentors in nursing are credible and generous role models with effective communication and leadership abilities (Ellis, 2016).

Like many other nursing schools, we have found that high-quality mentoring is critical for addressing challenges with retaining faculty amid a critical shortage, having a high percentage of new and inexperienced faculty, and experiencing a lower number of tenured faculty due to high numbers of faculty retirements. In a review of the literature on mentoring in academia, Bland, Taylor, Shollen, Weber-Main, and Mulcahy (2009) found that mentoring programs not only have a higher incidence of faculty satisfaction, but faculty members also perform at higher levels related to their role as scholars. To address the challenges in our nursing school, a formal mentorship model was developed. A position summary for the faculty mentor is included in Appendix A. The components of the orientation and mentoring for full-time faculty members are included in a checklist in Appendix B.

Mentoring can help junior faculty acquire the key competencies and work relationships that improve career success and satisfaction, build their professional networks, and help them become socialized to the norms and culture of the department and institution (Bland et al., 2009; Fisher, 2016). High-quality mentoring relationships provide benefits for mentors as well. Mentors may experience increased personal and professional satisfaction, grow in their own knowledge and skills, and receive recognition through career advancement or promotion. Ultimately, a strong commitment to mentorship improves the success of individual faculty members and the department while strengthening the nursing profession. **Table 13-9** includes exemplars of scholarship from our own experiences that demonstrate the exchange of knowledge about online teaching and learning. Although nursing faculty move through the phases on the "continuum" at their own pace and as a result of their unique experiences, it was at

Table 13-9 Exemplars of Scholarship That Demonstrate Exchange of Knowledge (Phase Two)

- Serve as course lead for the online program; mentor online faculty (scholarship of teaching).
- Work collaboratively with online faculty to redesign experiential learning for online students (scholarship of teaching).
- Develop a collaborative teaching model for the online program with nursing faculty and distance librarians (scholarship of integration).
- Represent the online program on the department curriculum committee (scholarship of integration).
- Chair a task force designed to enhance enrollment and student success in the online program (scholarship of integration).
- Chair the work group assigned to develop a formal mentorship program (scholarship of integration).
- Engage in a formal peer-review role with Quality Matters to review online courses across the country (scholarship of practice).
- Seek an external review of online teaching and evaluation from a distance education expert (scholarship of teaching).

this phase that we felt that we were developing a scholarly practice in teaching. Therefore, we have demonstrated how each exemplar also applies to scholarship using Boyer's model.

Growth in the Scholarship of Teaching

In the final phase on the continuum toward the scholarship of teaching, faculty members are sharing their expertise within the institution and disseminating it widely within the discipline (Weston & McAlpine, 2001). Their scholarly knowledge about teaching and learning has significance for the field, and they are likely mentoring others within the discipline. Faculty members who demonstrate the scholarship of teaching may be conducting research on teaching and learning and publishing and presenting their scholarship in a variety of forms, and they have a comprehensive knowledge of best practices and the literature on teaching and learning (Weston & McAlpine, 2001). In **Table 13-10**, we provide exemplars of scholarship from our own experiences that demonstrate the scholarship of online teaching and how each exemplar aligns with Boyer's model.

Our growth as faculty members in online nursing education and our path through the promotion and tenure process have been supported by a commitment to ongoing professional development, supportive mentorship, experience

---

Table 13-10 Exemplars of Scholarship That Demonstrate Scholarship of Online Teaching (Phase Three)

- Disseminated peer-reviewed presentations on teaching strategies and innovations (scholarship of teaching)
- Conducted primary research on online teaching methodologies (scholarship of discovery)
- Applied theoretical approaches and used best practices to advance teaching (scholarship of teaching)
- Disseminated best practices, teaching strategies, and program development models in peer-reviewed journal articles within the discipline (scholarship of teaching, integration)
- Obtained funding for research on teaching and program evaluation (scholarship of discovery)
- Conducted interdisciplinary, collaborative research designed to advance health and health education in local and international communities (scholarship of discovery, integration)
- Developed a certificate program in collaboration with a nongovernmental agency for international service learning (scholarship of application)
- Mentored online faculty within the institution and externally to share knowledge and best practices (scholarship of teaching)
- Disseminated research findings or teaching practices at national and international conferences (scholarship of teaching, discovery)
- Facilitated faculty development activities to enhance online teaching within the institution and within the discipline (scholarship of teaching, application)

in online teaching, service opportunities, and leadership experiences within the institution and community. Our experience aligns closely with the literature that addresses the growth of faculty members and the scholarship of teaching; faculty are expected to move along a path of growth as teaching professionals, supported by rigorous experiences in professional development on their campuses and within their discipline (Bernstein & Ginsburg, 2009). We would add that our experience in moving to the scholarship of teaching and learning has been significantly influenced by *collaboration*, which aligns with our philosophy of online education.

Collaborative Scholarship

As a pillar of professional practice in nursing, collaboration allows all team members to contribute based on their strengths, thus enhancing the quality of the outcome. Collaboration also provides faculty with the opportunity to model collaboration for others and participate in the evaluation process (Johnson & Meehan, 2009). In nursing education, we are faced with balancing the need for scholarly activity with the challenges of heavy workloads, possible burnout, and risks related to recruitment and retention. Collaboration is an important way to promote faculty development while also reducing faculty burnout (Igbo, Landson, & Straker, 2019). Igbo et al. (2019) recommend that faculty seek out collaborators to dedicate meeting and writing time, commit to projects, and contribute to the function of the team by listening to the insights of others and sharing values, which can build trust while working together toward a common goal (Igbo et al., 2019). Further points on the promotion of collaboration among faculty members to enhance scholarly productivity include the following:

- Collaboration promotes engagement and teamwork within the institution and across departments to increase faculty productivity (Gabriel, 2017; Maslach, 2011).
- Scholars should collaborate to improve their careers; it is surprising that there are no universally agreed-upon guidelines for scholars looking to initiate collaboration (Shaikh, 2015).
- Collaborative groups can be formed among people with similar interests, passions, and common goals. Group members can motivate each other and provide encouragement. Collaborative relationships include high levels of engagement, innovation, creativity, and pursuit of the greater good (Logan, King, & Fischer-Wright, 2011).

We value collaborative scholarship in many forms, including but not limited to working in small groups to disseminate a teaching strategy or develop curricular innovations, conducting studies on experiential learning activities that cross multiple levels of nursing education, involving staff and administrators in scholarship that promotes program development, and engaging multidisciplinary teams in projects that influence health outcomes. Our most successful collaborations have demonstrated such rich integration that we often forget what each team member contributed to the scholarly endeavor. Some examples of collaborative scholarship are shared in **Table 13-11**.

Table 13-11 Examples of Collaborative Scholarship

Scholarly Activity	Considerations/Details
Collaborative online course development: Trauma-Informed Care	■ Combined clinical and professional expertise from each faculty member ■ Designed to attract students from a variety of disciplines (not limited to nursing) across the institution ■ Enhanced online course offerings across the institution
Policy development, online teaching: Online course expectations Best practices for online teaching Peer Appraisal for online teaching	■ Collaborative development of departmental policies that support online teaching and learning ■ Policies support the application of scholarly evidence to the practice of online teaching. ■ Led to the development of formal quality assurance for online teaching and learning
Grant activity: Coauthored a grant that was funded to perform an evaluation research study on experiential learning in the online program	■ Research conducted with online students and community partnerships as participants ■ Findings informed curriculum development, experiential learning strategies, and evaluation of the online program. ■ Collaboration involved coauthoring the grant and conducting the study (design of study, data collection, data analysis). ■ Led to dissemination of findings in a scholarly nursing education journal ■ Review the study in Chapter 16.
Collaborative research study: Service learning and conceptual learning	■ Primary research study designed to assess conceptual learning in an online program ■ Data collection included assessment of teaching and learning in the online classroom. ■ Led to dissemination of findings at an interdisciplinary public health conference ■ Led to dissemination of an article published in a scholarly nursing education journal
Program development: Development of an interprofessional holistic model for successful academic progression	■ Collaborated with an interprofessional team, including an admission counselor, outreach coordinator, academic advisor, and faculty director, to develop a holistic model for academic progression ■ The model focused on current student success strategies and online program development.

(continues)

Table 13-11 Examples of Collaborative Scholarship *(continued)*

Scholarly Activity	Considerations/Details
	■ The project contributed to ongoing quality assurance in the online program, including partnership development, student satisfaction and perseverance, and program evaluation. ■ Led to dissemination at an annual University Professional and Continuing Education Association (UPCEA) conference, the leading interdisciplinary association for professional, continuing, and online education ■ Led to an article for dissemination in a national community and public health journal ■ *Review the interprofessional module in Chapter 4.*

Summary

We believe that strong preparation and deep, continual engagement in best practices can support faculty members who are making the transition to online teaching. We have spent over a decade engaging in formal study, certification courses, professional development activities, and scholarship in online education to develop our own teaching practices that have been personally and professionally rewarding. As a specialty practice in nursing education, online teaching is ideally suited for the development of scholarly practice. Online faculty *can* fit into traditional academic institutions and meet the same expectations for scholarship as faculty teaching in face-to-face classrooms.

Best-Practice Recommendations for Online Programs

- Nursing education is an area of advanced nursing practice, and online teaching is a specialty practice in nursing education.
- Faculty members need training and support when transitioning to online teaching in order to demonstrate readiness and competence.
- Ongoing professional development and certification for online teaching enhance the quality and credibility of online education.
- Online adjunct faculty benefit from supportive teaching models that provide leadership for orientation and ongoing mentorship for online teaching.
- Full-time faculty benefit from formal mentorship programs designed to help them develop a successful path toward the scholarship of teaching.
- Conducting collaborative scholarship is an effective way to promote faculty development, enhance scholarly productivity, improve faculty satisfaction, and reduce faculty burnout.

References

American Association of Colleges of Nursing. (2016). *Advancing Healthcare Transformation: A New Era for Academic Nursing.* https://www.aacnnursing.org/portals/42/publications/aacn-new-era-report.pdf

American Association of Colleges of Nursing. (2018). *Defining scholarship for academic nursing: Task Force Consensus Position Statement.* https://www.aacnnursing.org/Portals/42/News/Position-Statements/Defining-Scholarship.pdf

American Association of Colleges of Nursing. (2019). *Fact sheet: Nursing faculty shortage.* https://www.aacnnursing.org/Portals/42/News/Factsheets/Faculty-Shortage-Factsheet.pdf

Aspden, L., & Helm, P. (2004). Making the connection in a blended learning environment. *Educational Media International, 41*(3), 245. http://www.anitacrawley.net/Resources/Articles/Making%20the%20Connection%20in%20a%20Blended%20Learning.pdf

Bernstein, J. L., & Ginsburg, S. M. (2009). Toward an integrated model of the scholarship of teaching and learning and faculty development. *Journal on Centers for Teaching and Learning, 1,* 57–72.

Bland, C. J., Taylor, A. L., Shollen, S. L., Weber-Main, A. M., & Mulcahy, P. A. (2009). *Faculty success through mentoring.* Rowman & Littlefield.

Blodgett, M. C. (2008). Adjunct faculty perceptions of needs in preparation to teach online. *Dissertation Abstracts International Section: Humanities and Social Sciences, 69*(6), 2163.

Boyer, E. (1990). *Scholarship reconsidered: Priorities for the professoriate.* Carnegie Foundation for the Advancement of Teaching.

Brookfield, S. D. (1995). *Becoming a critically reflective teacher.* Jossey-Bass.

Dietrich, D. (2015). Why instructor satisfaction cannot be ignored. *eLearn Magazine.* https://elearnmag.acm.org/archive.cfm?aid=2735931

Ellis, P. (2016). Systematic program evaluation. In D. Billings & J. Halstead (Eds.), *Teaching in Nursing: A guide for faculty* (pp. 463–507). Saunders.

Fisher, M. (2016). Teaching in nursing: The faculty role. In D. Billings & J. Halstead (Eds.), *Teaching in Nursing: A guide for faculty* (pp. 1-14). Saunders.

Forbes, M. O., Hickey, M. T., & White, J. (2010). Adjunct faculty development: Reported needs and innovative solutions. *Journal of Professional Nursing, 26*(2),116–124. doi:10.1016/j.profnurs.2009.08.001

Gabriel, S. (2017). Moving from silos and burnout to community and engagement. *Faculty Focus.* Higher Ed Teaching Strategies from Magna Publications. https://www.facultyfocus.com/articles/teaching-careers/moving-silos-burnout-community-engagement/

Grant, M. R., & Thornton, H. R. (2007). Best practices in undergraduate, adult-centered online learning: Mechanisms for course design and delivery. *Journal of Online Learning and Teaching, 3*(4), 346–356. https://jolt.merlot.org/documents/grant.pdf

Hampton, D., Culp-Roche, A., Hensley A., Wilson, J., Otts, J., Thaxton-Wiggins, A.,... Moser, D. K. (2020). Self-efficacy and satisfaction with teaching in online courses. *Nurse Educator.* Advance online article. http://doi.org/10.1097/NNE.0000000000000805

Hanna, D. E., Glowacki-Dudka, M., & Conceicao-Runlee, S. (2000). *147 practical tips for teaching online groups: Essentials of web-based education.* Atwood.

Horvitz, B., Beach, A., Anderson, M., & Xia, J. (2015). Examination of faculty self-efficacy related to online teaching. *Innovative Higher Education, 40*(4), 305–316. http://doi.org/10.1007/s10755-014-9316-1

Hunt, H. D., Davies, K., Richardson, D., Hammock, G., Akins, M., & Russ, L. (2014). It is (more) about the students. Faculty motivations and concerns regarding teaching online. *Online Journal of Distance Learning Administration, 17*(2). http://www.westga.edu/~distance/ojdla/summer172/Hunt_Davies_Richardson_Hammock_Akins_Russ172.html

Igbo, I., Landson, M., & Straker, K. (2019). *Collaboration: A way to promote faculty development and reduce burnout.* https://www.facultyfocus.com/articles/faculty-development/collaboration-promote-faculty-development-and-reduce-burnout-2/

Johnson, A. (2013). *Excellent online teaching: Effective strategies for a successful semester online.* Aaron Johnson.

Johnson, A. E., & Meehan, N. K. (2013). Faculty preparation for teaching online. In K. H. Frith & D. J. Clark (Eds.), *Distance education in nursing* (pp. 33–52). Springer.

Kerka, S. (1998). Competency-based education and training: Myths and realities. *ERIC Digest.* http://eric.ed.gov/?id=ED415430

Koehler, M. J., Mishra, P., Hershey, K., & Peruski, L. (2004). With a little help from your students: A new model for faculty development and online course design. *Journal of Technology and Teacher Education, 12*(1), 25–55.

LERN. (2020). *Certified Online Instructor.* https://lern.org/events-education/faculty-training/certified -online-instructor-coi/

Lin, H., Dyer, K., & Guo, Y. (2012). Exploring online teaching: A three-year composite journal of concerns and strategies from online instructors. *Online Journal of Distance Learning Administrators, 15*(3). http://www.westga.edu/~distance/ojdla/fall153/lin_dyer_guo153.html

Logan, D., King, J., & Fischer-Wright, H. (2011). *Tribal leadership: Leveraging natural groups to build a thriving organization.* Harper Business.

Maslach, C. (2011). Burnout and engagement in the workplace: New perspectives. *European Health Psychologist, 13*(3), 44–47.

McAlpine, L., Weston, C. B., Beauchamp, J., Wiseman, C., & Beauchamp, C. (1999). Building a metacognitive model of reflection. *Higher Education, 37*, 105–131. https://doi.org/10.1023 /A:1003548425626

Mowrer-Reynolds, E. (2008). Pre-service educator's perceptions of exemplary teachers. *College Student Journal, 42*(1), 214–224.

National League for Nursing. (2020). *Certification for nurse educators.* http://www.nln.org/Certification -for-Nurse-Educators

Nilson, L. B., & Goodson, L. A. (2018). *Online teaching at its best: Merging instructional design with teaching and learning research.* Jossey-Bass.

Oermann, M. H. (2018). Becoming a scholar in nursing education. In M. H. Oermann, J. C. DeGagne, & B. Cusatis Phillips (Eds.), *Teaching in nursing and role of the educator: The Complete guide to best practice in teaching, evaluation, and curriculum development* (2nd ed., pp. 379–398). Springer.

Oermann, M. H., DeGagne, J. C., & Cusatis Phillips, B. (2018). *Teaching in nursing and role of the educator: The complete guide to best practice in teaching, evaluation, and curriculum development* (2nd ed.). Springer.

Palloff, R. M., & Pratt, K. (2007). *Building online learning communities: Effective strategies for the virtual classroom.* Jossey-Bass.

Quality Matters. (2020). Why QM? https://www.qualitymatters.org/

Riley, J. M., Beal, J., Levi, P., & McCausland, M. P. (2002). Revising nursing scholarship. *Journal of Nursing Scholarship, 34*(4), 383–389.

Robina, K. A., & Anderson, M. L. (2010). Online teaching efficacy of nurse faculty. *Journal of Professional Nursing, 26*(3), 168–175. http://doi.org/10.1016/j.profnurs.2010.02.006

Shaikh, A. (2015). *A brief guide to research collaboration for the young scholar: Working with other scholars can boost your profile, but some arrangements are more likely to lead to publication.* https:// www.elsevier.com/connect/a-brief-guide-to-research-collaboration-for-the-young-scholar

Stavredes, T. (2011). *Effective online teaching: Foundations and strategies for student success.* Jossey-Bass.

Weston, C. B., & McAlpine, L. (2001). Making explicit the development toward the scholarship of teaching. *New Directions for Teaching and Learning, 86*, 89–97. https://onlinelibrary.wiley.com /doi/abs/10.1002/tl.19

Appendix A

Faculty Mentor Position Summary

Position Summary: The mentor develops a professional relationship with the assigned new faculty member (mentee) for the purpose of assisting the mentee in developing a successful and satisfying career within the School of Nursing.

Responsibilities:

1. Meet with the new faculty member within 2 weeks of being assigned for introductions, welcome, and a review of how they will work together. Begin discussing goals that the mentee would like to accomplish in the first month.
2. Work with the new faculty member to ensure the items found in the Orientation Checklist, as appropriate, are completed within the first semester. Provide information to the mentee regarding the "who, where, and how" of completing the items.
3. Meet with the mentee on an agreed-upon regular basis depending on the mentee's needs—at a minimum, weekly for the first semester to review questions, concerns, and goals and assist with problem solving. Meeting may be in person, by phone, or via Zoom.
4. Ensure the meetings are documented and include the date, agenda for the meeting, outcomes, and plan for time between meetings.
5. Documentation is submitted to nursing administration by the mentor after each meeting. Ask the associate dean for the template.
6. Orient the new faculty member to the overall curriculum and the semesters.
7. Coordinate with other faculty as needed regarding the courses the mentee is or will be teaching. This information is available through the associate dean.
8. The course mentor (preferably will be the mentor if possible) is responsible for thoroughly reviewing the course syllabus, calendar, and assignments.
9. Ensure the mentee is oriented to needed technology, such as Blackboard, Kaplan, and Shadow Health, and has the contact information of the person to go to if questions arise.
10. Orient the mentee to the role of faculty advisor.
11. Assist the mentee in arranging to observe different classes taught by different faculty members.

12. Introduce the mentee to the requirements of the faculty role, such as the three requirements for tenure-track faculty: teaching, professional development, and service.
13. Orient the mentee to the committee structure within the college and the School of Nursing (SON), and explain which meetings all faculty members attend.
14. Coordinate with the associate dean regarding committee observation for the first semester and membership for the subsequent semester.

Qualifications:

1. Excellent interpersonal and communication skills; ability to facilitate conflict resolution
2. Excellent teaching and organizational skills
3. Tenure-track mentees: preferable to be mentored by a tenured faculty member
4. Clinical mentees: preferable to be mentored by an experienced clinical faculty member

Appendix B

Faculty Orientation and Mentorship Checklist

What	Who/Where/How	Date Completed and Initials
Administrative Items		
Workload contracts		
Role and responsibilities of		
■ Dean		
■ Associate dean		
■ Tenure track (TT)		
■ Visiting professor (VP)		
■ Semester coordinators		
■ Integrated Experiential Learning coordinators		
■ Director of clinical education		
■ Experiential Learning Center staff		
■ RN-to-BSN program		
Blackboard		
Payroll, reimbursement procedures, travel authorization		
Health requirements		
Family Educational Rights and Privacy Act (FERPA)		

(continues)

What	Who/Where/How	Date Completed and Initials
Academic integrity		
Americans With Disabilities Act (ADA) plans		
Off campus/vacation notification		
SON Campus Operations		
Peterson Hall/Loveridge—offices		
Keys, office supplies, name badge, business cards		
Ordering supplies		
Mail		
Parking		
Inclement weather policy		
Online text access		
Voice mail		
Help desk		
Curriculum		
Student-based learning Concept-based teaching		
Curriculum progression		
Grade submission		
Textbook resources		
Kaplan		
NCLEX plan		
Shadow Health		
Online Dosage Calculation Program		
Learning assistance plans		
Test-bank question access		
Theory vs. clinical courses		
Syllabus requirements—contract		

What	Who/Where/How	Date Completed and Initials
Clinical		
Experiential Learning Center		
Calculation of clinical hours		
Calculation of simulation hours		
Hi-Fidelity Simulation		
Lab standards		
Electronic Health Record Tutor		
Clinical and lab dress codes		
Records and registration		
Site requirements		
Health passport		
Incident reports		
Clinical reasoning model		
College		
Linfield website		
Mission/values of college		
Discuss two campuses		
Linfield curriculum (general education) credits (LCs)		
Faculty governance		
Faculty assembly		
College committees		
Faculty Handbook		
Professional development—Funds		
School of Nursing		
SON credits		
Mission/values of SON		
SON committees		

(continues)

What	Who/Where/How	Date Completed and Initials
Library/librarian		
SON Faculty Manual		
Faculty Resources/Responsibilities		
Committee responsibilities		
Graduation and pinning ceremonies		
Email communication		
Represent Linfield		
Academic advising		
Annual faculty evaluation process		
Faculty–student collaboration		
Work expectations between semesters		
Working collaboratively or in consultation with other faculty		
Academic freedom		
Student concern/care reports		
Faculty resources on Blackboard		
Faculty development opportunities		
Scantron and item Analysis		
Student		
Student Handbook		
Nursing Student Manual		
Academic alerts		
Counseling resources		
Student Life		
Learning Support Services		
Other		
Recommended articles		
Other resources		

The Influence of Generational Differences on Learning in the Online Classroom: Research Exemplar

Melissa Robinson

Overview

The purpose of this chapter is to share findings from a qualitative dissertation research study conducted by the author to assess the influence of generational differences on student learning in an online registered nurse–bachelor of science in nursing (RN-to-BSN) program. Six major findings emerged from the study: (1) increased nursing knowledge, (2) expanded perspectives, (3) leadership development, (4) enhanced communication skills, (5) personal growth, and (6) improved technology skills. Each of the findings is supported by narratives that describe the perspectives that participants shared following their experiences with learning in the online classroom. The findings contribute to a deeper understanding of the value of generational diversity in online nursing programs and inform the recommendations for best practices in online education presented at the end of this chapter.

Generational Diversity in Nursing Education

Multiple generations of learners are represented in today's university and college classrooms. This is even more common in online classrooms, which tend to attract working adults, especially nurses who are advancing their education. Multiple generations are represented in the nursing workforce, including the millennial, Generation X, baby boomer, and veteran cohorts (Stanley, 2010). Each generational cohort has a common set of values, ideas, ethics, communication styles, worldviews, and cultural influences, which affects how cohort members interact with each other in the classroom (Bednarz, Schim, & Doorenbos, 2010; Lipscomb, 2010). The differences have added to the complexity of the learning needs of a diverse student population while also creating an opportunity to increase awareness of generational issues in the classroom that enhance learning.

Although the nursing education literature indicates that student learning styles and preferences have been studied, the evidence related to generational differences and their effects on teaching and learning is limited (Earle & Myrick, 2009; Walker et al., 2006). An ongoing need exists to examine intergenerational diversity in the classroom in order to understand the impact on teaching and learning (Earle & Myrick, 2009). As the diversity of students in higher education expands to include multiple generations, an understanding of the learning needs of students who are generationally diverse can assist faculty members in developing effective teaching practices (Bednarz et al., 2010). This study addressed a gap in the literature regarding student perceptions of how generational differences influence learning in the online classroom. Recommendations for further research and teaching strategies are suggested based on the findings of this research.

Study Methodology

A social constructivist approach to the qualitative descriptive research was used to place an emphasis on the perspectives of the participants and the meaning that they ascribed to their experiences with learning in the online classroom (Creswell, 2009). Qualitative description (QD) is an approach to research studies that is descriptive and particularly useful for examining experiences related to health care and nursing (Kim, Sefcik, & Bradway, 2017; Polit & Beck, 2014).

The study took place in a small liberal arts college with a population of 16 registered nurses who had completed an online RN-to-BSN program within the last 2 years after Institutional Review Board (IRB) approval was obtained. The population was ethnically and generationally diverse. The participants ranged in age from 26 to 57 and had varied experiences in nursing practice that spanned between 3 and 36 years, thus representing generational groupings from millennials to baby boomers.

Data were collected using open-ended conversational interviews conducted in synchronous electronic chat sessions with the participants. An interview guide was used to ensure that the questions were asked consistently. Participants were asked to share their age, describe their nursing experience, and identify and describe their generation. Participants were also asked to reflect back on experiences in the online classroom that they had with students from different generations (younger or older), describe their experience, and discuss the impact on their learning.

Six major findings were revealed through thematic analysis of the data collected in this study: (1) 75% of participants reported increased nursing knowledge, (2) 63% of participants described expanded perspectives, (3) 63% of participants reported leadership development, (4) 50% of participants reported enhanced communication skills, (5) 44% of participants described personal growth, and (6) 31% of participants reported improved technology skills. Each of the findings is supported by narrative descriptions of the perspectives of the participants.

Finding 1: Increased Nursing Knowledge

Participants reported they benefited from increased nursing knowledge in the online classroom. They reported developing skills that allowed them to build on their existing knowledge, which can be described simply as *informational learning* (Kegan,

---

Table 14-1 Increased Nursing Knowledge

Student Narratives: Informational Learning

"Sometimes it is easy to judge someone of a different generation. I felt that after my interaction with the older generation nurse[,] we both realized that we could share some information and practices to increase both of our knowledge in our own nursing careers."

"These types of interactions with the younger generation allowed me to share experiences and knowledge; while at the same time they may have had a very different interpretation of a situation which introduced me to new ideas and broadened my learning experience."

"The older nurses have tons of nursing knowledge and experience which they share with younger nurses; these may be classified in nursing as 'ways of knowing' I guess; the blend of their expertise and our generation X exposure to EBP can be merged."

"As 'ways of knowing' are shared, we can further bring in research work on such topics so that the two can be merged where the benefit of both translates into patient care."

2000). Participants recognized the value in learning practice information from each other and understood that their learning experiences could be mutually beneficial among older and younger generations. One participant reported learning "different protocols that other nurses use in their hospitals" and recognized that she appreciated learning "changes in nursing practice, medications, nursing education, technology in the workplace, etc.... from newer nurses. I learned from their more recent and up-to-date education." Participants described learning that "merged" various levels of experience in nursing with new knowledge that could be applied to practice. **Table 14-1** includes narratives that demonstrate the value of informational learning.

Finding 2: Expanded Perspectives

Participants described learning experiences that expanded their perspectives. Themes revealed in the narratives included (a) alternative points of view, (b) diversity, and (c) tolerance. Exposure to different experiences and alternative points of view were reported as positive and providing a broader perspective. One participant stated, "I definitely have a broader view of how people see things ... it became a discussion with lots of opinions ... and seemed like everyone got something positive out of the interaction." The same nurse recognized that she gained a broader perspective and "learned to look at things through the eyes of others." Another participant who identified herself as a baby boomer made a connection to the development of the nurse's individual practice: "I have other creators or collaborators who have different experiences and points of view that I can consider and, perhaps, weave into my own practice." She also identified a specific experience with a younger male nurse that led her to see new possibilities based on what the students were learning from each other:

> In the Global Forum classes we all were learning new exciting and depressing ideas about globalization. There were a few people in the classes

that I resonated with, really well. One was a young father, nurse, in the nursing program as well. Our "threads" were quite wonderful as we discovered hidden "gems" of ideas in each other through which the other could develop early ideas of our own. This led to amazing personal satisfaction and the online learning experience of providing deep and meaningful encouragement for the other person.

Generational differences and the years of practice experiences were recognized by students as a component of diversity in the online classroom. Participants identified being intentional with their efforts to learn more about their peers in the classroom, even as the course progressed throughout the semester.

Each class began with an introductory biography[,] which offered a glimpse into a cohort's life and professional experiences. I realize that the majority of on-line students were recent graduates from traditional nursing programs. I would often look back at the bios to see the approximate age of a student, and would adapt my conversations to relate to that person. Points of reference to generation were seen in their life and work experience shared in group discussions.

The theme of tolerance emerged from the participants' descriptions of their growth and learning experiences. An experienced nurse (baby boomer) provided vivid details as she discussed working with a younger student on a group assignment. She described how they worked together to overcome the challenges of the online format in order to achieve a successful outcome. In addition to developing new communication and leadership skills, she identified gaining different perspectives from the younger student, which led her to grow in tolerance and understanding:

I remember working with another student who was younger than me (she shared her age with me) on an assignment. Starting out on the project, I believe we both were frustrated a little trying to find a common ground where we both could work together based on very different personalities and work ethics. While this is challenging in a classroom setting, it can be even more challenging in an online format[;] however, through online education you gain new communication skills that become invaluable, even when communicating face to face. Being organized is extremely important[,] so I took a leading role to create a timeline[,] and we discussed our strengths and weaknesses so we could apply our talents where they would fit best. This experience was great as I was able to gain different perspectives on issues from my project partner that I probably would not have thought about on my own and helped me grow in tolerance and understanding.

Several participants reported growing more aware of barriers to embracing the diversity they encountered in nursing practice. **Table 14-2** includes additional narratives that demonstrate growth in online students' understanding of alternative points of view, diversity, and tolerance.

Table 14-2 **Expanded Perspectives**

Student Narratives: Alternative Points of View, Diversity, and Tolerance

"I discovered that I loved the challenge of formal education, and the interaction with my virtual classmates ... the nature of education it affords the learner the opportunity to find new perspectives and develop new outlooks. The on-line learning experience allowed for the development of a new perspective and positive attitude toward change in the midst of familiar experiences in my personal and professional life." (alternative points of view)

"In an online program, discussion boards are a major part of learning, sharing experiences and knowledge as well as learning from other cultures that may not be so prevalent in a classroom setting that is located in one specific geographical location. Sharing experiences and learning from my peers has truly helped me understand and appreciate different perspectives." (alternative points of view)

"The diversity in opinion and perspective from varying [sic] generations was challenging and fun. It allows the student to free themselves [sic] from pre-conceived notions and biases that we all possess. Maybe just the awareness of our bias and prejudgment frees us and breaks down the barriers that restricts [sic] us from truly embracing the diversity we experience with our patients. (impact on patient care)." (diversity)

"The acceptance of diversity of opinions and perspectives allowed for my personal growth and awareness of the differences in the patients I encounter in my everyday nursing practice. This was a great practice in patience and acceptance, and allowed me to be less quick to judge people in my personal and professional life." (alternative points of view, diversity, tolerance)

"The exposure to multi-generations in the learning environment is a microcosm of the diversity of all the generations that I care for in my nursing practice. I welcome the diversity of opinion that can certainly differ from my personal philosophy. Through the diversity of opinion and perspective, I learn tolerance, and can reflect on new perspectives and outlooks. This can also extend into tolerance and understanding of the cultural diversity encountered in the healthcare environment." (alternative points of view, diversity, tolerance)

"When I interact with different nurses with different background expand my perspective [sic] ... we are more respectful to each other. I remember one time we were discussing ethical issues; I think if it was outside classroom it probably argument [sic]; because of their generation, the interactions online are different." (alternative points of view, tolerance)

Finding 3: Leadership Development

Participants described experiences that demonstrated leadership development as a result of the generational differences in the online classroom. Themes that were re-vealed in the descriptions of their learning included (a) leadership, (b) mentorship, and (c) education.

The baccalaureate-prepared nurse is expected to apply leadership concepts, skills, and decision making to the delivery of high-quality nursing care and team coordination (American Association of Colleges of Nursing, 2008). Several of the nurses recognized that they developed leadership qualities as a result of generational differences in the online classroom. One of the nurses stated, "Many of the older nurses were wonderful leaders and were able to show me how to be a better leader by their examples, and even their responses to my own discussions." Another nurse attributed her growth as a leader to becoming more sensitive to the views of others during her learning experiences:

> This experience has helped me as a leader to be more sensitive and appreciative of others['] views. I might not always agree with anothers [sic] view but this experience has taught me how important it is to respect all views. In recognizing that, I find professional relationships take on a different meaning and you learn to appreciate each person. In working with patients, this is priceless because you don't create preconceptions about a patient, you approach with an open mind so you hear so much more.

One of the younger nurses who identified herself as a member of the millennial generation spoke very specifically about her professional and personal growth:

> Professionally, I began to help out in projects around the hospital and push myself to look at all the aspects of being a nurse and bettering our work environment for our patient. Personally, learning what it takes to be a leader, practicing these things, getting rid of bad habits purposefully and being a more effective communicator (even just as a person in my relationships).

Three of the participants described developing relationships and making connections with younger peers through sharing experiences and engaging in valuable dialogue. At the same time, they believed that they had contributed to the learning experiences of the younger nurses by improving their critical thinking skills and making a positive impact:

> In my Modern Philosophy class I had relationships like this with several of the younger people. I can say that I feel pretty sure that I helped improve the creativity in their critical thinking skills about philosophy and they improved mine. So vast was the breadth of opinions I found it amazing that I could, actually, collaborate within a philosophical discussion! I can say in that class that I really learned the art, as well, of acceptance with grace of others opposing ideas while still remaining open to them as individuals. In these online forums where identity becomes more about what one thinks and believes instead of how old you are or what generation you are from people just discuss the ideas. It's really wonderful. I will never forget how satisfying, poignant, funny or brilliant some of those classroom dialogues were.
>
> Specifically, I found myself connecting with people of the younger generation in really positive ways and feeling like my shared nursing experiences added to overall learning for people. In other words, I feel that I might have made a positive impact at times. Another way is that by watching the younger nurses[,] I learned how to feel comfortable, to navigate sucessfully [sic] in what was really a "younger person" dominated nursing world. I found I like younger nurses and could see their wisdom also.

While she had quite a jump on me in terms of the longevity she will have within the nursing profession, I found that my life experiences both in and out of the healthcare field brought a certain depth to our discussions. These types of interactions with the younger generation allowed me to share experiences and knowledge; while at the same time they may have had a very different interpretation of a situation[,] which introduced me to new ideas and broadened my learning experience.

Mentorship

Mentorship emerged as a consistent theme when the participants described experiences they had with nurses from different generations. Mentorship in nursing has been recognized as an informal process that occurs between an expert nurse and a novice nurse or a more formal assigned role, such as a preceptor in the work setting (Ruthman & Erickson, 2012). The mentoring relationship in nursing has focused on supporting the professional aspects of the nurse's development through listening, encouraging, affirming, coaching, and counseling (Ruthman & Erickson, 2012; Vitale, 2019). The mentoring relationship can be a mutually beneficial experience for both nurses. Three participants in this study described interactions with their peers that demonstrated an awareness of the importance of relationships that are mutually beneficial between nurses. The nurses described experiencing positive mentoring relationships in the online classroom that were encouraging and uplifting. They described the value of nurse mentors and the importance of providing support and encouragement to each other in the following narratives:

> I had one that I remember clearly. She was quite young and a fairly new nurse and mother. Work and family pressures were evident. She felt she wasn't really processing the content of the class and wanted to just talk about it and study with me. We had 2 or 3 sessions that were really helpful to her and me, both. I was touched to see the insecurity she had about this class and her courage in reaching out to me for help and encouragement. It makes me really see the value in nurse mentors for all nurses at all times, not just new hires.
>
> It helps me to realize that if I find myself in a position that is similar to her [*sic*] that I can reach out to someone I consider "helpful" and get support, encouragement, and even instruction that will help me be more effective. This fosters a sense that I will be able to cope with difficulties that arise and engenders resilience because I know that I am not alone in my nursing practice.
>
> "Newer nurses do not seem jaded. When they share their experiences it has more to do with the "warm and & fuzzy" aspect of nursing. They are out there and ready to save the world so to speak. While this seems naive and can leave older nurses shaking their heads and saying "oh, just you wait", their innocence is refreshing and I found myself going back to a time when I was a new nurse. I felt it provided positive affirmations that I can take to my practice.

"Nurses eat their young" is a metaphor for a common practice in professional nursing (King-Jones, 2011)—it has been used in nursing to describe experiences with bullying among peers, nurses in clinical practice, and nursing faculty (Baker, 2012). Research has suggested that the nurse's first exposure to bullying, or horizontal violence, often occurs in nursing school and can have a devastating effect on the self-confidence and self-image of the nursing student (King-Jones, 2011; Meires, 2018). Nurse bullying has been described as behaviors that include ignoring, gossiping, disrespect, sabotage, and verbal attacks (Baker, 2012). Three of the participants used this term, but in every case, it was used in contrast to what they experienced in the online classroom. The nurses shared examples of feeling encouraged and supported by their peers in the online classroom as opposed to experiences in the clinical environment where they may have experienced a sense of separateness among their colleagues. They described the online classroom as a safe environment that supported their growth, which, in turn, inspired them to want to create healthy, supportive relationships and a sense of community among nurses. In the following narratives, the nurses recognize the experiences of newer, younger nurses as well as the experiences of older nurses that helped them achieve additional awareness and insight:

> I guess if nothing else I was around other nurses who did not "eat their young" and believed in growth and change. It was encouraging for me to want to continue to grow and also how [sic] to influence others at my work to improve without telling them "you need to improve". It also gave me some insight into how someone might feel who has been a nurse for a long time and suddenly or even gradually had to change a lot of what they were used to. That would be difficult too and it gave me a little more compassion towards the older nurses at my work.
>
> Many times I could sense the fear, frustration, and lack of support from newer nurses when they shared their experiences in their practice. Many times I or other seasoned nurses could offer advice, support, or refer that new nurse to information that could help them grow and succeed. The old saying "nurses eat their young" was not evident in the online classroom setting.
>
> I would be more willing to listen to others['] wisdom in an open and friendly way. It would make me want to be .... co-creators of solutions that one individual could not have come up with and help create more of a sense of community among nurses (something that can be lacking). I am thinking about the phrase that was used in my last nursing class to describe older nurses in their treatment of younger nurses as, "eating their young". I would want to, now, be a nurse that was humble, inclusive of other nurses, helpful and nonjudgemental [sic]. I would want to create an atmosphere of safety and have resources for myself, first, and then for others in which open, easy collaboration could take place. I think patient outcomes could be significantly improved if they were able to see harmony amongst their caregivers instead of separateness as sometimes happens.

Another participant linked her perspectives on the importance of a safe work atmosphere directly to improving patient outcomes when she recognized the importance of harmony and professionalism among her colleagues in the clinical practice environment. Based on their descriptions, participants recognized the importance of creating healthy peer relationships with nurses of all ages in order to influence the quality of the work environment and patient outcomes.

Education emerged as a common theme in the descriptions of the participants' learning experiences. Nurses have important roles in education, both as learners and as teachers. Nurses have been responsible for teaching individuals and families, teaching groups in the community, and teaching other healthcare professionals and caregivers (Blais & Hayes, 2016). In addition, they teach other nurses in their roles as leaders, preceptors, and educators. Nurses are also required to maintain a commitment to lifelong learning in an effort to maintain the skills and competence needed to perform in multiple professional capacities (American Nurses Association, 2008).

Two of the participants referred to experiences that made a difference in the way they had viewed the orientation of new coworkers and when they had served as a preceptor to students who were learning their roles. One nurse, who identified herself as a millennial, commented on how a healthy learning environment that included generationally diverse students influenced her ability to orient new co-workers and provide feedback to students:

> I was taking a Mexican history class & we had a nice mix of different generations. We often had chat nights & it was refreshing to hear different opinions about the same subject; there was no bickering or arguing... but just listening & discussing; it made me want to have a healthy learning environment where there isn't really a wrong answer & a person is encouraged to ask questions; it made me change how I orient new co-workers & when I have students following me; it definitely changed my views when dealing with different people. I can't just do it the same way every time; now I take time to figure what's the best way for them to learn (vs what they say is the best way for them) & give them feedback as much as I can.

Another participant, who identified herself as a member of Generation X, acknowledged the importance of lifelong learning, mentoring, and serving as a preceptor to younger nurses:

> Being able to interact within a multi-generational environment reminded me that in life there are times to be a teacher and times to be a student. How many times do we hear, that a good nurse is a lifelong learner and a good nurse is a mentor. This experience taught me that I really enjoy "teaching". As a staff nurse on a busy surgical floor, I am now the experienced one and often have nursing students under my tutelage for a shift; I believe my recent opportunities to interact across the generations has strengthened my ability to precept the younger nurses.

One participant, who identified herself as a member of the millennial generation, recognized that she learned about the value of nurses from older nurses and changed her views on education as a result of her learning experiences:

> I think I learn a lot more from older nurses not just because of the experiences that they tell me but the value of nurses; value of the nurses—it's not just about getting by day by day; it's more about the care; One older nurse told me "it is about the relationship with other than [sic] matter, not money"; but throughout the program I learned that education is very important; after my BSN program I changed my view of education.

Table 14-3 Leadership Development

Student Narratives: Leadership, Mentorship, and Education

"It seems to be that the nurses that have 20+ years of nursing experience over me can feel slightly intimidated by a 'younger' nurse coming in to take their jobs ... I think that older generation nurses or more experienced nurses do have a lot to offer us 'younger' nurses but that we have just as much to give to them as well." (mentorship)

"This experience of learning with multi-generations influenced my nursing practice to make sure that I learn everything I can from the more experienced/older generation nurses before they retire. I have learned a lot of job skills and helpful tips from the more experienced nurses that I intend to pass down through my years as [a] nurse." (mentorship, education)

"I feel more prepared to educate patients across generations in the clinical setting since I have had this experience; I feel more qualified." (education)

"I have noticed that many of my opinions on leadership and continuing education have been greatly influenced by what I learned in the RN to BSN program." (leadership, education)

"I have a better understanding of what educational materials to supply for my patients. I don't remember the exact incident but I do remember coming away from one online experience realizing that my younger patients would likely want only website names or an actual computer to use to search their diagnosis, while those about 35 and older would more appreciate printed materials. Now I offer both options to my patients." (education)

"It has led me in the direction of nursing education. I feel it is my role to help educate the nurses of the future; In general, I think there are not as many mentorship programs for new nurses in healthcare these days (identified as Generation X nurse)." (mentorship, education)

Participants consistently commented on the value of learning from more experienced nurses and passing on that knowledge to others. One participant shared her motivation for teaching and learning when she stated, "I think this experience has just fueled me to learn as much as I can so I can provide peer nurses insight on what I've learned." Several commented that age was not a barrier in how they felt they could influence the nursing practice of others, including one participant who stated, "I think I have also learned that it is ok to 'coach' a peer, even if they are older." **Table 14-3** includes additional narratives that demonstrate growth in online students' development in leadership, mentorship, and education.

Finding 4: Enhanced Communication Skills

Participants described experiences that demonstrated they had enhanced their communication skills, which were revealed as communication skills and stories. Effective communication skills have allowed nurses to develop therapeutic relationships with patients and demonstrate professionalism among their colleagues.

Because of advances in technology, nurses have also been required to utilize technology to communicate with clients and other healthcare professionals throughout the healthcare system (Arnold & Boggs, 2019). Two of the study participants described how their experiences in the online classroom contributed to learning new communication skills. They described the nature of the learning environment and shared specific examples of what helped them to develop skills in coordination and professional communication:

> This experience has taught me invaluable skills that I don't believe I would have gained so easily in a classroom setting. When you learn and communicate in an environment where there is no ability to smell, touch, see or feel, it is completely different. You have to learn new skills to be able to communicate and learn effectively[,] which for me, has been amazing. I consider myself an introvert so being able to express myself in an environment that does not lend to "pre judgment" based on physical appearances or body language, facilitates a greater learning experience.

> I learned a lot on how to communicate online and how to coordinate efforts online … Each experience was a learning curve. Being able to communicate online is very different to [sic] communicating in person. I think that having the opportunity to learn online has created opportunities to practice communication. I think that in the end this impacts my overall personal and professional communication. And that is a priceless outcome.

Stories were discovered as an influential component of communication that occurred across generations in the classroom, which participants described as affecting their learning experiences. Stories, particularly stories about health and illness, have long been a part of nursing. Telling and hearing stories can honor and share human experiences and also facilitate the integration of knowledge that is crucial to understanding nursing care (Hunter & Krantz, 2008). As a teaching strategy, stories have been used to assist students in building knowledge, developing listening skills, and developing interpretive thinking skills through verbalizing lived experiences (Darbyshire, 1995; Hunter & Krantz, 2008). One participant, who identified herself as a member of the millennial cohort, described very specific differences in the communication style of students from different generations. Her belief was that older-generation students communicated by telling a story and utilizing a relational approach to communication:

> Maybe the way we convey our information speechwise [sic]. For example, when I were [sic] to present the information I want …. it may come out shorter, conciser [sic] and with certain verbage [sic] when I do my postings versus an older generation student telling more of a story, wanting to be more relational, go beyond the surface; I think my initial thoughts when this would happen were more of "just answer the question"…(that may sound harsh). Rather than wanting to take the time to explore thoughts and go deeper. Just my comment – I have found this as well just by observation. Task focused in education and practice.

> I felt like sometimes projects became more cumbersome and drawn out than they needed to be. This sometimes led to frustration in just

wanting to complete an assignment and be done with it; I think I learned that I need to slow down my pace. Go in depth more. Be ok with ex- plorimg [sic] areas beyond the initial topic; it definitely taught me to go beyond the surface in my nursing practice. Before, I just wanted the quick answer and to do it. But through this experience, I realized its [sic] better to know the background and reasoning in order to more effectively deliver care and understand what I am doing and why.

Three of the participants, members of Generation X and the millennial gen- eration, also stated that stories told by older nurses provided valuable insights for patient care and nursing practices:

Stories from long-time nurses definitely provide a new picture to younger nurses and may allow them to understand their patients better. And the opposite may be true where understanding a younger nurse may allow older nurses to better understand their patients.

I have realized that someday I will be part of that group who have [sic] been working for 10-15 years. And the young nurses who are listen- ing to my stories will have a whole different/new set of standards, morals, practices to think about.

I think when the online interactions became more personal, and stu- dents shared stories from their lives and allowed us to see where they were coming from. This all adds to a better understanding not just of the person but of their generation.

One of the millennial participants added that by sharing personal stories, she had gained a better understanding of generational issues. Her statements indicated that the participants who discussed the stories and the relational approach to com- munication valued this type of modeling by older nurses. A participant who identi- fied herself as a baby boomer characterized the communication style of the younger generation as effective in helping her to learn how to communicate across genera- tion gaps:

I would say the different perspectives I gained were related to our genera- tional differences. From my own experiences, the younger generation has different filters than I do[,] so while they sometimes "shock" me, when I question further why they feel or think a certain way, I find they show me a different way to look at something. Even if I don't agree, it helps me be able to better communicate across generation gaps.

Finding 5: Personal Growth

Participants in this study described personal growth as a meaningful outcome of their learning experiences. Confidence was the most common theme that was re- vealed in the participants' descriptions of their personal growth. Nurses return to higher education to earn a baccalaureate degree based on a variety of personal and professional reasons. Many nurses have been motivated to advance their education for personal achievement and satisfaction related to their educational goals. The confidence of the nurse is highly individualized and often reflected in the nurse's sense of self, self-esteem, sense of self-efficacy, and perspective (Perry, 2011). The narratives of the participants reflected support for the development of confidence. One participant stated, "It has given me a measure of self-esteem." Two of the nurses specifically identified developing confidence as a result of sharing opinions and views with peers in the online classroom:

> I think I became more confident in sharing my views and opinions, and also in questioning those of others. When it is mediated in the right ways, online learning environments can help an individual to thrive and improve on skills such as writing, expressing complex ideas, and organization.
>
> From a professional level, I have so much more confidence in my role as a nurse and am able to take all the knowledge I have gained into the workplace and apply it to create positive change.

Participants described personal and career satisfaction as a result of their diverse online learning experiences, which reflected their confidence and personal growth:

> We definitely shared alot [*sic*] of experiences with the entire class. There were quite a few nurses in my cohort who had been RNs for 10-15 years, sans BSN. They had some wonderful experiences to share that enriched my ideas of what an RN is capable of, even without a BSN. They also made me realize that I am fortunate to be getting my BSN early in my career so I can hopefully stay on top of things.

Finding 6: Improved Technology Skills

Participants in this study described improved technology skills as a result of their learning experiences in the online classroom. *Change* and *groups* were discovered as common themes in their perspectives. The participants considered technology to be an important factor affecting their nursing practice across all settings, including the online classroom.

Change refers to the observable things that happen or are done differently than they were done previously (Austin & Currie, 2003; McLean, 2011). Changing work practices requires people to make an extra effort; therefore, resistance to change and innovation should be expected (Hewitt-Taylor, 2013). Rapid changes in technology have affected health care, and nurses have experienced significant change and innovation in the workplace. One participant, who identified herself as a member of Generation X, reflected on an interaction with a younger nurse who voiced some of the challenges of using technology in the clinical environment:

> One that stands out, however, was a young nurse, newly graduated with ADN and immediately went for a BSN. She expressed frustration with "older" nurses and how they don't understand technology and complain about it; technology is change and, no matter what age the person is, change is hard.

Working in groups was identified as a consistent theme when students described the use of technology and their learning. Working effectively in groups has been a consistent expectation in professional nursing. As providers of care, nurses have been in the position of assisting clients in adapting to the changes they experience in their health or illness state (Otten & Chen, 2011). To meet the needs of the clients they care for, nurses are expected to work cohesively with other nurses as well as other members of the healthcare team. Working successfully in groups has been described as including predictable work patterns, support to maintain competencies, defined roles and expectations, and a strong and effective communication system (Porter-O'Grady & Malloch, 2010). As coordinators of care in many healthcare environments, nurses often lead groups and facilitate group processes. Challenges emerged for the participants when working with online group projects:

> There is a certain level of technological aptitude that is required in order to participate in group projects. This became clear from the start, when a "wiki page" was supposed to be used. No matter how much instruction was given, there were a couple who just couldn't get it right.

Positive experiences with technology also led to them to assist others in improving their technology skills or achieve a particular goal. One participant, who identified herself as a member of the millennial generation, described an experience that she had with assisting an older student: "she had difficulty with finding things online and will ask me questions about it; like how to get to download this, where to find that, but eventually it became easier."

Another credited her experiences with the development of stronger writing skills and confidence. And yet another felt more prepared to access information online: "I am much more savvy and confident online. I feel I can 'treat' people with greater courtesy online because my writing skills are better... I guess as an older nurse I feel more integrated with the modern hi-tech society... I think online learning skills have prepared me to access information online. It also improved my ability to help others with online applications."

Implications for Nursing Education Practice and Research

The findings of this study have direct implications for nursing education practice and research. Capitalizing on the value of a generationally diverse student population can enhance learning in nursing education. The integration of teaching and learning strategies that highlight generational diversity and increase awareness of diverse perspectives has the potential to influence the quality of the learning experience and the knowledge and skills necessary for professional nursing practice (Earle & Myrick, 2009; Wellman, 2009). Additionally, nurses who possess an awareness of diversity and insight into generational differences have the opportunity to contribute to a dynamic work culture that values diverse perspectives and experiences (Earle & Myrick, 2009).

Faculty members in nursing education are in a key position to assist nurses in developing as leaders, educators, and mentors in professional practice. In RN-to-BSN programs, faculty members welcome nurses into academia and assist in their transition to professional practice by recognizing the nurse's life and work experiences and designing course plans that accommodate working students (Megginson, 2008; Wros, Wheeler, & Jones, 2011). Given the findings of this study, recruiting nurses from all generational groups and different levels of experience, from new graduates to those with years of experience, would enhance the educational experience well beyond what can be accomplished by a homogeneous group.

This study reinforces our philosophy, as discussed in Chapter 2. A constructivist approach to teaching that shifts the role of the educator from content expert to that of facilitator of learning can result in a learner-centered classroom where learner support is essential (Legg, Adelman, Mueller, & Levitt, 2009). Constructivist strategies that support technological challenges, provide consistent student feedback, require ongoing peer interaction and dialogue, and guide student learning are recommended to decrease learner isolation and enhance learning (Billings & Halstead, 2009; Legg et al., 2009).

In addition to emphasizing peer interaction in the online classroom, encouraging interaction and communication with faculty members is a strategy supported by the findings of this study. When students have positive experiences with faculty interactions, they are more likely to be involved and engaged in their own learning (Davis, 2013). Given that nurses who return to higher education to obtain a baccalaureate degree need to acquire both academic and discipline-specific knowledge, skills, and identity, simultaneously, modeling by faculty members might provide a valuable teaching and learning strategy in the online classroom (Andrew, McGuiness, Reid, & Corcoran, 2009; Davis, 2013). The development of learning activities that support faculty and peer role modeling and mentoring in the online classroom can assist RN-to-BSN students in developing confidence in their leadership abilities, particularly related to mentorship and education.

Recommendations for Future Research

The findings from this study provide a wealth of information on how students perceive the impact on their learning of interacting with different generations. Further studies that address the generational differences between students and faculty in online nursing education and the effects of those differences could reveal additional perspectives on learning in the online classroom (Bednarz et al., 2010; Earle & Myrick, 2009). Additionally, studies conducted with different student populations, such as traditional undergraduate baccalaureate students, and different settings, such as the face-to-face classrooms or hybrid classrooms, would extend the knowledge base relative to generational differences in nursing education. However, most importantly for online teaching, research that specifically addresses teaching and learning strategies that take full advantage of the generationally diverse online classroom would add to identifying best practices for online teaching. Strategies that support the unique needs of generationally diverse students in the online classroom may increase the opportunity for student success and enhance learning.

Strategies That Support a Generationally Diverse Online Classroom

- Require students to utilize their previous life and work experiences as they build new knowledge.
- Develop interactive activities that capitalize on the generational diversity in the online classroom.
- Build in opportunities for peer mentoring and leadership development; consider having students work collaboratively in pairs or small groups.
- Create learning experiences that enhance interaction between students and faculty to promote faculty members' ability to demonstrate and model the concept of leadership in a multigenerational class.
- Provide meaningful and consistent feedback to guide student learning, decrease student isolation, and develop student confidence in working with nurses of various generations and work experiences.

References

American Association of Colleges of Nursing. (2008). *The essentials of baccalaureate education for professional nursing practice*. http://www.aacn.nche.edu/Education/bacessn.htm

American Nurses Association. (2008). *Professional role competence*. http://www.nursingworld.org/MainMenuCategories/ThePracticeofProfessionalNursing/NursingStandards/Professional-Role-Competence.html

Andrew, N., McGuiness, C., Reid, G., & Corcoran, T. (2009). Greater than the sum of its parts: Transition into the first year of undergraduate nursing. *Nursing Education in Practice*, 9(1), 13–21. http://doi.org/10.1016/j.nepr.2008.03.009

Arnold, E., & Boggs, K. (2019). *Interpersonal relationships: Professional communication skills for nursing*. Saunders.

Austin, J., & Currie, B. (2003). Changing organizations for a knowledge economy: The theory and practice of change management. *Journal of Facilities Management*, 2(3), 229–243. http://doi.org/10.1108/14725960410808221

Baker, C. (2012). Evidence-based practice: A basis challenge for nurse educators? *Oklahoma Nurse*, 57(2), 9.

Bednarz, H., Schim, S., & Doorenbos, A. (2010). Cultural diversity in nursing education: Perils, pitfalls, and pearls. *Journal of Nursing Education*, 49(5), 253–260. http://doi.org/10.3928/01484834-20100115-02

Billings, D., & Halstead, J. (2009). *Teaching in nursing: A guide for faculty*. Saunders.

Blais, K., & Hayes, J. (2016). *Professional nursing practice: Concepts and perspectives*. Pearson.

Creswell, J. (2009). *Research design: Qualitative, quantitative, and mixed methods approaches*. Sage.

Darbyshire, P. (1995). Lessons from literature: Caring, interpretation, and dialogue. *Journal of Nursing Education*, 34(5), 211–216.

Davis, J. (2013). Modeling as a strategy for learning and teaching in nursing education. *Singapore Nursing Journal*, 40(3), 5–10.

Earle, V., & Myrick, F. (2009). Nursing pedagogy and the intergenerational discourse. *Journal of Nursing Education*, 48(11), 624–630. http://doi.org/10.3928/01484834-20090716-08

Hewitt-Taylor, J. (2012). Identifying, analyzing, and solving problems in practice. *Nursing Standard*, 26(40), 35–41.

Hunter, J., & Krantz, S. (2010). Constructivism in cultural competence education. *Journal of Nursing Education*, 49(4), 207–214. http://doi.org/10.3928/01484834-20100115-06

Kegan, R. (2000). What transforms? A constructive-developmental approach to transformative learning. In J. Mezirow & Associates (Eds.), *Learning as transformation* (pp. 35–69). Jossey-Bass.

Kim, H., Sefcik, J. S., & Bradway, C. (2017). Characteristics of qualitative descriptive studies: A systematic review. *Research in Nursing & Health*, *40*(1), 23–42. http://doi.org/10.1002/nur .21768

King-Jones, M. (2011). Horizontal violence and the socialization of new nurses. *Creative Nursing*, *17*(2). http://doi.org/10.1891/1078-4535.17.2.80

Legg, T. J., Adelman, D., Mueller, D., & Levitt, C. (2009). Constructivist strategies in online distance education in nursing. *Journal of Nursing Education*, *48*(2), 64–69. http://doi.org/10.3928 /01484834-20090201-08

Lipscomb, V. (2010). Intergenerational issues in nursing: Learning from each generation. *Clinical Journal of Oncology Nursing*, *14*(3), 267–269. http://doi.org/10.1188/10.CJON.267-269

McLean, C. (2011). Change and transition: What is the difference? *British Journal of School Nursing*, *6*(2), 78–81.

Megginson, L. (2008). RN-BSN education: 21st century barriers and incentives. *Journal of Nursing Management*, *16*, 47–55. http://doi.org/10.1111/j.1365-2934.2007.00784.x

Meires, J. (2018). The essentials: Here's what you need to know about bullying in nursing. *Urologic Nursing*, *38*(2), 95–97, 102. http://doi.org/10.7257/1053-816X.2018.38.2.95

Otten, R., & Chen, T. (2011). Change, chaos, adaptation: The effects of leadership on a work group. *Creative Nursing*, *17*(1), 30–35. http://doi.org/10.1891/1078-4535.17.1.30

Perry, P. (2011). Concept analysis: Confidence/self-confidence. *Nursing Forum*, *46*(4), 218–230. http://doi.org/10.1111/j.1744-6198.2011.00230.x

Polit, D. F., & Beck, C. T. (2014). *Essentials of nursing research: Appraising evidence for nursing practice*. Lippincott Williams & Wilkins.

Porter-O'Grady, T., & Malloch, K. (2003). *Quantum leadership*. Jones & Bartlett Learning.

Ruthman, J., & Erickson, D. (2012). Personal and interdisciplinary communication. In P. Kelly (Ed.), *Nursing Leadership & Management* (pp. 198–221). Cengage.

Stanley, D. (2010). Multigenerational workforce issues and their implications for leadership in nursing. *Journal of Nursing Management*, *18*, 846–852.

Vitale, T. R. (2019). The impact of a mentorship program on leadership practices and job satisfaction. *Nursing Management*, *50*(2), 12–14. http://doi.org/10.1097/01.NUMA.0000552745.94695.81

Walker, J., Martin, T., White, J., Elliott, R., Norwood, A., Mangum, C., & Haynie, L. (2006). Generational (age) differences in nursing students' preferences for teaching methods. *Journal of Nursing Education*, *45*(9), 371–374.

Wellman, D. (2009). The diverse learning needs of students. In D. Billings & J. Halstead (Eds.), *Teaching in nursing: A guide for faculty* (pp. 18-32). Saunders.

Wros, P., Wheeler, P., & Jones, M. (2011). Curriculum planning for baccalaureate nursing programs. In S. Keating (Ed.), *Curriculum development and evaluation in nursing* (pp. 209–240). Springer.

CHAPTER 15

Assessing Online Collaborative Discourse

Henny Breen*

Overview

This study was conducted to examine Harasim's (2007) online collaborative learning theory as a framework for assessing online collaborative discourse in a registered nurse–bachelor of science in nursing (RN-to-BSN) program.

Collaborative Learning

Collaborative learning is a pedagogical approach that is congruent with the curriculum reform that is taking place within nursing education today. This curriculum reform involves a paradigm shift from a content-driven to a concept-driven curriculum to better prepare nursing students for today's healthcare environment. This shift involves faculty becoming facilitators of learning in which collaborative learning is emphasized, rather than deliverers of content in which students are passive learners (Billings & Halstead, 2009; Giddens et al., 2008). Collaborative learning advances active and reflective learning and encourages teamwork, which provides opportunities for students to become accountable for their own and others' work (Billings & Halstead, 2009). These attributes are required of practicing nurses because nurses must be able to collaborate with other nurses and healthcare professionals.

According to the American Nurses Association *Scope and Standards of Practice*, collaboration is defined as "a professional healthcare partnership grounded in reciprocal and respectful recognition and acceptance of: each partner's unique expertise, power, and sphere of influence and responsibilities . . ." (American Nurses Association, 2010, p. 64). Gardner (2005) makes the point that true collaboration is seldom practiced because of its complexity and the level of skills required. Collaboration is conceptualized as a dynamic process in which the group moves through

---

*Breen, H. (2015, October). Assessing online collaborative discourse. *Nursing Forum, 50*(4), 218–227.

different developmental stages. At the same time, collaboration is also seen as an outcome in which there is a merging of different perspectives to understand complex problems for the purpose of coming to a solution (Gardner, 2005).

There is a renewed emphasis on collaboration in all healthcare disciplines, requiring nurse educators to ensure collaboration is addressed in the curriculum. In the document that defines the essentials of baccalaureate education for professional nursing practice, the American Association of Colleges of Nursing (2008) identified intra- and interprofessional collaborative skills as critical to providing safe, evidence-based patient care. Collaborative skills are essential to nursing practice, and their development begins during nursing education.

To maximize the impact of the learning experience, it is important for nursing faculty to be able to differentiate between cooperation and collaboration. *Collaboration* and *cooperation* are most often used interchangeably. However, Tutty and Klein (2008) placed collaboration and cooperation on either end of a continuum, whereas Harasim (2012) identified cooperative learning as a division of labor and collaboration as co-labor. Breen (2013) defined virtual collaboration as "an interdependent and democratic online group process grounded in constructivist pedagogy in which students debate and reflect on shared knowledge, to construct new understanding of relevant information" (p. 267). The design of an online collaborative course is structured to provide opportunities for the students to construct or build knowledge as a group toward a common goal. This is in contrast to cooperative group learning, in which students work independently on a part of a project to contribute to the final product rather than building knowledge together. When collaborating, they are working together so that the final product is better than any one person could do on his or her own (Harasim, 2012).

Literature Review

In a literature review, very little research was found on the actual process of collaboration in online higher education, and no research was found in online nursing education. There have been a number of studies that examined the outcomes of online collaborative learning, such as learner completion rates; learner satisfaction; differences between online and face-to-face learning; cognitive, social, and teaching presence; interactivity; and, more recently, learning outcomes (De Wever, Schellens, Valcke, & Van Keer, 2006; Dennen, 2008; Oncu & Cakir, 2011). Menchaca and Bekele (2008), in their study of success factors of both learners and instructors, recommended that "the quality and nature of online collaboration . . . be further examined" (p. 249). Enhancing learner engagement and collaboration has been identified as a priority for research in online learning environments. In order to meet this goal, one area of study is investigating the patterns that enhance effective collaboration among online learners (Oncu & Cakir, 2011). Given the proliferation of online learning within nursing education, it is imperative that this modality of learning be closely examined to ensure that the outcomes for nursing education are met.

There have been a number of studies done using different instruments in an effort to conduct a quantitative content analysis of online asynchronous discussion groups in a number of different undergraduate- and graduate-level online courses outside of nursing. These instruments differed in their theoretical orientation, level of detail, and type of analytical categories used. As a result, there is a weak empirical base for the validity of the instruments developed to date because of a lack of coherence between the theoretical base and the operational translation of the theory in the instruments (De Wever et al., 2006; Dennen, 2008). A review of 15 content analysis schemes to analyze transcripts of online asynchronous discussion groups found that standards had not yet been established in spite of this technique being frequently used (De Wever et al., 2006). Given this finding, a qualitative study using transcript analysis to examine Harasim's online collaborative learning theory was undertaken for the purpose of understanding the usefulness of this theory for the assessment of collaborative discussions in nursing education.

Online Collaborative Learning Theory

Harasim's online collaborative learning theory was developed from a grounded study and has three processes or phases, which describe a path from divergent to convergent thinking (Harasim, 2007). These three phases are idea generating, idea organizing, and intellectual convergence.

Phase One: Idea Generating

This phase refers to divergent thinking within a group. It may involve brainstorming, talking, or writing it out. Ideas are shared, and information is generated. It is a democratic process; different perspectives are shared from group members' personal observations and experiences.

Phase Two: Idea Organizing

As group members share different ideas, they begin to seek clarification. In comparing and contrasting the different ideas, the ideas are organized according to their similarities to one another. It involves selecting the strongest ideas and weeding out the weaker ones. This phase is the beginning of group members acknowledging and recognizing different perspectives. They begin to identify how the different perspectives relate or do not relate to one another and the topic. In this phase, there is a beginning movement toward convergence.

Phase Three: Intellectual Convergence

Convergent thinking requires the ability to narrow down the options based on the information available and the analysis of that information so that the best ones are applied. During this phase, there is shared understanding as intellectual synthesis occurs. Group members in the discussion either agree to disagree or coproduce a product, which could be anything from a solution to a problem to a design, an assignment, a theory, a publication, or a work of art.

Method and Design

This qualitative study investigated the collaborative process by identifying empirical evidence of collaboration in an online class in which RN-to-BSN students were working on a virtual case study in a learning module on disaster management.

Transcript analysis was the qualitative method used for this study because it is a valuable methodology to study asynchronous online educational discourse (Garrison, Cleveland-Innes, Koole, & Kappelman, 2006). *Transcript analysis* refers to a system for making replicable and valid inferences from texts to the contexts of their use. The three phases of Harasim's online collaborative learning theory provided the basis for the analytical constructs for the study. The transcripts were from a 2-week discussion about nursing following a disaster in a virtual community.

The Neighborhood, which features the unfolding stories of several characters representing community and nurse members, was used as the virtual community. The stories are enhanced with pictures, video clips, medical records, and newspaper clippings (Giddens, 2010). Students were required to become familiar with several members of the community in the weeks preceding an announcement in the course management system, Blackboard Learn, that an earthquake had struck the Neighborhood. Videos and articles about earthquakes were added to the module. During that first week, each student produced a nursing action plan as he or she role-played being a community health nurse in the community. For the second week, the class was divided into four smaller groups in which the members developed a more comprehensive nursing action plan together.

Setting and Participants

The setting for the study was a fully online RN-to-BSN program offered through the School of Nursing and Adult Education Program in a small northwest liberal arts college in the United States. Participants for the study were 19 RNs enrolled in their final nursing course during the summer of 2012. This student group represented different generations and came from a variety of nursing backgrounds, with varying years of experience. This diversity provided a rich community of learners for baccalaureate nursing education built on a philosophy of constructivism.

This sample was also chosen because these students had experience working collaboratively from their work in earlier courses. In the studied RN-to-BSN program, the curriculum is carefully scaffolded to move the students toward meeting the program outcomes, which include communicating effectively and collaboratively in professional practice as well as providing effective nursing care that incorporates diverse values. In their first-level courses, students were required to work in groups in which collaboration and cooperation were introduced as different concepts. The expectation is that students are able to move from cooperative to collaborative work as they progress in the program. Given that collaboration is not easily achieved, it was decided that using transcripts of asynchronous discourse from students who had developed some skill in collaboration would provide an appropriate sample to study the collaborative process.

Data Collection, Coding, and Analysis

The college used Blackboard Learn as the platform for online courses, from which the data were extracted and placed into an Excel spreadsheet for coding. Data for the study consisted of discussion-board transcripts over a 2-week period from five different discussion forums. The first week involved all 19 students collaborating together in one forum consisting of two discussion threads. One discussion thread was for role-playing being community nurses, and the other discussion thread was for posting their individual case studies and providing feedback to each other. For the second week, the class was divided into four smaller groups of four or five students to make up the remaining four forums. Each of these forums had a discussion thread to collaborate on and a file exchange in which they could develop their final group nursing action plan.

Each discussion post was used as a unit of analysis and was coded into the most relevant category of Harasim's (2012) three phases of collaboration. It was also recognized that there was a possibility that a single post might display characteristics or indicators of more than one of the analytical constructs. Anderson, Rourke, Garrison, and Archer (2001) found that this procedure had the advantage of being more efficient and provided more meaningful information because the percentage of total posts contained in each of the categories was reported. This method for determining the unit of analysis was used for this study because it was considered to be a valuable method, given that the chosen theoretical framework had defined indicators. Furthermore, Harasim (2012) noted that it is the nature and quality of the posts that are the key indicators, and these indicators can be customized according to the assignment.

The number of posts in these discussions allowed for a rich database, which was used for the analysis guided by the online collaborative learning theory indicators. **Table 15-1** presents how the data were analyzed using the theory. The use

Table 15-1 The Coding Tool

Idea generating	<ul><li>Divergent thinking</li><li>Individual points of view presented, leading to multiple perspectives</li><li>New ideas generated</li><li>Participants are engaged and contribute</li><li>Democratic participation</li><li>Number of initial postings</li><li>Personal understanding</li><li>Providing examples</li><li>Use of "I" and "my"</li></ul>
Idea organizing	<ul><li>Idea linking</li><li>Identifying associations between ideas</li><li>Ideas become clarified and grouped into various positions</li><li>Movement from individual comments to building on previous comments</li><li>Early form of convergence as participants contribute to shared ideas</li><li>Increased number of references to previous messages</li><li>Increased number of references to other participants by name</li><li>Number of agreement and disagreement statements; shared understanding; weaving ideas together</li><li>Shared understanding</li></ul>
Intellectual convergence	<ul><li>Synthesis of ideas</li><li>Co-construction of knowledge based on shared understanding</li><li>Discussions leading to conclusion on plans or ideas for action</li><li>Increased number of substantive contributions (messages that compare, structure, extend, and synthesize ideas)</li><li>Number of conclusive position statements</li><li>Development toward shared understanding</li><li>Working toward closure</li><li>Use of "we" and "our"</li></ul>

Note: The online collaborative learning theory guided the analysis of the data. These characteristics and indicators are based on Harasim's theory and customized based on the case study in the course module (Harasim, 2012).

of a theoretical framework situates the analysis and does not exclude inductively derived insights gained through the transcript analysis (Garrison et al., 2006). A constant comparative analysis method was used in the analysis of the data. This involved taking one unit of analysis and comparing it with all other units of analysis to see what made it different or similar. An Excel database was created to support the coding process. The message texts (posts) were numbered and individually placed in a comment folder in a cell identified by a letter code representing a student name. In addition, separate columns were created for the date and time of the post, the three phases of the theory, and comments. The comments field was used to capture the coder's notes about the posts and potential inductively derived inferences.

Reliability and validity issues are related to the rigor of the theoretical frameworks, models, and coding schemes designed to guide the analysis of transcripts (Garrison et al., 2006; Krippendorff, 2013). The sound theoretical framework of the online collaborative learning theory addressed potential validity issues. Harasim has been focusing on online education since the late 1980s, and the three phases of collaboration came from a grounded theory study she conducted. Reliability was addressed by checking the coding at two intervals with 3 weeks separating them, and the 80% code–recode reliability according to Miles and Huberman (1994) was reached. A colleague was also asked to code 25% of the data. Areas of disagreement were discussed, and a 100% agreement was reached.

Ethical Considerations

Informed consent had been obtained by email as directed by the Institutional Review Board of the university where the students were enrolled. Using student numbers in the coding program and substituting names for any quoted postings protected anonymity. One area of concern may be related to the participants having been students of the researcher. This concern was alleviated by the fact that at the time of the analysis, the researcher was no longer their faculty member because the students had completed the final nursing course for the RN-to-BSN program.

Findings

The transcripts that were studied represented five different forums related to the disaster case study over a 2-week period. The first week involved all 19 students collaborating together in one forum. There was a total of 154 posts coded during the first week, in which students role-played being nurses in the community following an earthquake. In addition, they each developed a nursing action plan and provided feedback to each other. For the second week, the class was divided into four smaller groups to make up the remaining four forums. There was an average of 75 posts in each small group forum as they worked together to develop one nursing action plan to respond to the needs of agreed-upon members of the virtual community. All five forums had evidence of moving through the three phases of Harasim's (2012) online collaborative learning theory.

Week One (Entire Class)

The students placed themselves as community health nurses in the virtual community experiencing the disaster. Throughout this forum, they provided their

Table 15-2 Percentage Distribution of Online Collaborative Learning Phases During Week One

Day	Posts	Posts With Phase One Indicators	Posts With Phase Two Indicators	Posts With Phase Three Indicators
Day 1	8 posts	50%	75%	25%
Day 2	28 posts	39%	71%	21%
Day 3	26 posts	15%	81%	31%
Day 4	21 posts	0%	81%	19%
Day 5	25 posts	16%	92%	8%
Day 6	35 posts	11%	57%	43%
Day 7	11 posts	27%	64%	45%

assessment of their client needs, what the priority issues were for their clients and the community, the available resources, methods of communication, means of transportation and their location, and what they were doing to help. One student identified herself as a team leader of a triage center. **Table 15-2** shows the percentage of messages in each of the three phases.

Phase One

Indicators that were coded as idea generating included participants being engaged and contributing, divergent thinking with new ideas generated, personal understanding, and providing examples. Students presented new evidence based on personal experience, the virtual community information, and information from the literature. Citations from the literature and examples to illustrate their points reflected personal understanding. An example of divergent thinking that was not linked to another member's contribution is "What are our lab capabilities? Are we able to run labs on Yvonne to assess renal status?" Another example is a lengthy post by a student who provided information comparing Hurricane Katrina to the Japanese tsunami in terms of looting and cautioned the team to be aware of this, expressing safety concerns.

Phase Two

Indicators of idea organizing include idea linking, identifying associations between ideas, ideas becoming clarified and grouped into various positions, and movement from individual comments to collaboration. Phase Two indicators are noted in the following post:

> Tyler's whereabouts are definitely a priority [agreement with previous posts] considering the mental well[-]being of Mark as well as Randall for Yvonne. Both of these individuals are under a lot of stress prior to the earthquake [information from the virtual community][,] and that has

substantially increased with this event. In an article written by Margaret Cole Marshall[,] there are 5 lessons learned from Hurricane Katrina and Rita . . .

The student goes on to provide information from the article reflecting personal understanding, which is a Phase One indicator. Phase One and Phase Two indicators were often seen in the same message.

Phase Three

Intellectual convergence is characterized by the synthesis of ideas and the co-construction of knowledge based on shared understanding and ideas for action. This was noted when a student posted a comment that was identified as going out to all disaster team members:

> There seems to be a general consensus that community members are searching for missing family members. The Neighborhood High School has been designated as a safe shelter. If you are looking for missing family members, please refer all community members to this location. There is a Healthcare Disaster Team member that will be logging who has arrived at this location. [Student name] RN

In summary, idea generating and then moving on to idea organizing included indicators in which the students shared ideas by adding new information to build on the role-play, linking similar ideas and statements of agreement. Movement to intellectual convergence was noted when students provided an update bringing together the information that had been shared and plans for action that would be needed to provide care. The three phases did not occur in a circular process but tended to be one of continual movement advancing based on a feedback spiral. For example, the phase of idea organizing may move directly to intellectual convergence, or it may trigger further idea generating (Harasim, 2012). Several themes or topics came up in the discussion that students built on using their imagination, the literature, and the data from the Neighborhood. Some of the topics included the following:

1. Communication included comments about who had cell phones, cell phone batteries dying, having access to ham radios, loss of Internet access, and asking others to contact the hospital.
2. Missing persons from the community were designated as a priority because of the need to alleviate the stress experienced by family members. This was agreed upon.
3. Resources, such as the role of the Red Cross, Federal Emergency Management Agency, and Coast Guard, were researched and discussed.
4. Triage and transportation—a student researched and provided information about simple triage and rapid transport (START). There was a discussion about how to transport Mark, and the students agreed he needed transport by helicopter because of his declining condition.
5. Treatment—issues related to supplies; oxygen for Jimmy Bley; electricity and generators; lessons learned from other disasters; and whether people needed a safe shelter (they set up the high school to be the safe shelter), triage (assisted

living center was set up for this), or hospitalization (discussion about what the hospital could do and which patients they could accept) were discussed.

6. Loss—some members of the community died, including one of the volunteer nurse's family members. She was Jewish, and there was a discussion about Jewish cultural practices when there is a death. There was also a discussion about debriefing, supporting each other and their clients, and self-care.

Week Two: Group Forums

All four groups had evidence of moving through all three phases of the online collaborative learning theory. Examples are taken from different groups to illustrate this evidence.

Phase One

Idea generating included posts that referred to the work students did on their individual care plans, reflecting individual points of view with some new ideas. For example, "Tracie was in college. . . . This would be another place for shelter as colleges are usually prepared for disasters and have stadiums or large structures to house people."

Phase Two

Once students had shared information from their individual care plans, students moved quickly into the phase of idea organizing. They demonstrated early forms of convergence as they contributed to shared ideas, had agreement and disagreement statements, weaved ideas together, and increasingly referred to each other by name. Some examples include the following: "Hi [student name]. . . . Is there any need to mention immunizations?" "[group member names], I was thinking for the assessment, while we are assessing for anxiety, we should also assess Mark's depression. I also agree about the immunization as Tyler was behind."

Phase Three

Intellectual convergence was evident in the following post in which the student synthesized several posts: "I was thinking of using a combination of our initial openings and then follow the family details. Here is what I got from our posts." Shared understanding was exemplified in the following post:

> I agree with [student name] assessment that the Bleys are vulnerable due to their age and Jimmy's chronic respiratory condition . . . without adequate medications, food, and water, the health conditions can deteriorate rapidly. As [other student name] had indicated, the Bley's strong family ties are [a] strength and rejoining them will decrease their vulnerability.

Group Structure

Groups One and Two set up a separate thread for each part of the nursing action plan, which lent itself to a very similar pattern for each thread. Examples of subject headings for these threads included community resources, references, prioritization of physical and psychological needs, short- and long-term goals, and assessment data. Each thread started with Phase One, then moved to Phase Two, followed by

Phase Three, as they took the information provided by the group members and made final decisions for each part of the nursing action plan, finally resulting in closure of the discussion. The final care plan was developed with no more than three drafts.

By contrast, Groups Three and Four did not separate parts of the nursing action plan into separate threads. They had more drafts of the nursing action plan synthesizing the information gained (Phase Three), which led to more idea generating before they settled on their final nursing action plan. One can posit that the pattern of moving through the phases of the theory may be related to how the discussion threads were set up by the group members and did not influence the ability to move through the phases.

Group Process

In coding the group discussions, it was noted that several of the posts did not have any of the indicators that are foundational to Harasim's (2012) online collaborative learning theory. The three phases of the online collaborative learning theory relate to the process of collaborative learning and building knowledge through discourse (Harasim, 2012). The posts that were not coded as one of the three phases were coded as group process. *Group process* was narrowly defined to include posts that discuss how to set up the group, directions, availability, expressions of support or frustration, and social comments such as "thank you" and "good job."

Three of the groups worked well together, with no apparent conflict. One group did face some challenges in working together, as reflected in the following post: "We are all busy but this is a group assignment. I managed to squeeze in time and log on several times in between my busy day as well and stayed up until 1 am after working a morning shift." Even with these group-process challenges, they were still able to move through all the phases of the online collaborative learning theory and produce a good final product.

Table 15-3 shows the total percentage of group-process indicators and messages in each of the three phases for the four small groups. The total percentage of messages in the three phases for the class as a whole is also included for comparison purposes.

Discussion

The main purpose of this study was to examine Harasim's (2012) online collaborative learning theory as a framework for assessing online collaborative discourse. The transcript analysis provided empirical evidence of moving through all three phases of the theory in both the class and small-group discussions. The most striking difference between the class and small-group forums was the number of process indicators. These indicators were only present in the small groups. This is probably related to the fact that there was no group project or outcome required for the class discussion as there was in the small groups. Collaborating for the purpose of producing a group assignment requires decisions to be made about how students will work together. There was no need to discuss these issues when working on an individual assignment. These findings suggest that group-process indicators may not be required for collaboration to occur and reinforce the chosen

Table 15-3 Percentage Distribution Comparing Entire Class and Small-Group Discussion

Day	Posts	Posts With Phase One Indicators	Posts With Phase Two Indicators	Posts With Phase Three Indicators	Group-Process Indicators
Class	154 posts	19%	74%	27%	0%
Group One	80 posts	18%	25%	26%	34%
Group Two	56 posts	11%	41%	21%	30%
Group Three	84 posts	17%	27%	15%	57%
Group Four	73 posts	10%	40%	14%	40%

theory. This finding is contrary to the findings of the concept analysis of virtual collaboration, which found that group process was an antecedent to collaboration (Breen, 2013).

Harasim's (2012) online collaborative learning theory differs from other theoretical models that place collaboration on a continuum from social presence to production, such as Murphy's (2004) model. Many of the indicators of social presence found in Murphy's study were similar to those labeled as group-process indicators in this study. For example, references to working together as a group, expressions of appreciation for contributions made, and expressing emotions such as feeling overwhelmed were found in this study as well as in Murphy's study. Given that these process indicators were not found in the class discussion, it is suggested that they should not be included in a theoretical model of collaboration. Furthermore, there does not seem to be any relationship between the number of group-process indicators and reaching intellectual convergence. Groups Three and Four had the most group-process indicators, and Group Two had the most intellectual convergence indictors. In comparing the way the groups set up their forums, Groups One and Two set up specific threads addressing the different parts of the nursing action plan, whereas Groups Three and Four had one thread to address the nursing action plan. Again, this did not affect the number of indicators of intellectual convergence.

The class discussion had the most Phase Two (idea organizing) indicators. This was probably related to the fact that there was no dependency on each other to develop their final product, leaving more time to contribute to each other's ideas without having to come to any group decisions on the final assignment. Intellectual convergence was mostly noted in their individual nursing action plans. Co-construction of knowledge was evident in that their individual action plans were different from what they could have done on their own. Their action plans reflected the synthesis of ideas from their discussion in the role-play.

No other indicators that reflect collaboration were inductively derived from analysis of the transcripts, suggesting that the theory provides a good framework for evaluating collaboration if the group-process indicators are seen as separate from collaboration. Three relevant findings to suggest separating group process from the collaborative process are as follows: (a) Group-process indicators were not required to move through the phases of the online collaborative learning theory if an individual outcome was required, (b) the number of group-process indicators did not seem to affect the movement through the phases, and (c) conflict and unequal participation did not prevent a group from moving through the three phases of the theory.

It is recommended that group process and collaboration be assessed separately. Doing so would facilitate the purposeful assessment of cognitive and affective domains of learning to enable targeted areas for student development, depending on the outcome of the evaluation. Harasim (2007) recommends that a grading rubric address the quality of posts by including such elements as citations, adding new insights, posing new ideas and questions, and building knowledge, measured by moving through the three phases of the theory. Including citations and adding new insights from reading the course content, research outside the course content, and personal experience are common features of discussion grading rubrics. Using a grading rubric that incorporates the theory would enhance the evaluation of the student's ability to meaningfully contribute to the collaborative process. It would provide the instructor with the ability to assess the student's skill and growth. For example, a student may be strong in generating new ideas but needs to develop skills in identifying associations between ideas. This would also have the potential of furthering the understanding of how collaboration is different from cooperation.

Conclusion/Recommendations

This qualitative study examining the collaborative process using Harasim's (2012) online collaborative learning theory may be the first to use it in nursing because no other nursing studies were found that used this theory. This study offers a way to evaluate students' collaborative skills. The following recommendations are based on the findings and analysis of this study and are related to the use of online collaborative learning theory in RN-to-BSN education. These recommendations are followed by suggestions for further research.

Online Instruction

The following recommendations for online instruction are offered:

1. For some individual assignments, a class discussion regarding the assignment could be set up prior to the students submitting the assignment. This is related to the finding that the students moved through all three phases only if an outcome was required. This would be appropriate for assignments in which input and feedback from classmates in addition to personal research would facilitate the development of being able to merge different perspectives.
2. Although not a direct finding of this study, it is recommended that faculty consider how they scaffold their programs and courses to facilitate students' ability

to learn how to collaborate. This would dictate how prescriptive the faculty member needs to be in setting up the collaborative activities and how involved he or she needs to be in the discussion. For example, students new to collaborative learning need help in understanding how collaboration is different from working together cooperatively. They may also need help in structuring their discussion forums.

3. When groups are brought together to develop a group outcome, the instructor needs to keep an eye on the group process and may need to provide assistance if the group dynamics are interfering with their ability to work together. Knowing when to step in and when to leave the group to work through conflict on their own needs to be carefully considered. The instructor needs to take into consideration the learning objectives of the group assignment and the experience of the students with online learning and group work.

4. Consider the use of role-playing as a different approach to learning. Although not the focus of this study, it was found to be an engaging strategy for immersing the students in collaborative work.

5. The virtual community was found to be an interesting avenue for engaging students in the collaborative process and is recommended for use in exploring complex concepts.

Evaluation

In evaluating a group's ability to collaborate, it is recommended that the phases of the online collaborative learning theory be used to evaluate the group's and/or individual students' ability to collaborate. Group-process skills should be evaluated separately. Group process has more to do with interpersonal skills, whereas collaborative learning has more to do with cognitive skills. Both are required for practicing nurses. When evaluated separately, the students' learning needs would be more clearly delineated.

Further Research

Given the findings of this study, it is recommended that further studies be done that investigate the relationship between group development and the collaborative process. Other recommendations include the following:

1. Further research to closely examine the role of the instructor in facilitating the collaborative process to facilitate understanding best practices for instruction in the online environment as related to collaborative learning with nursing students is recommended.

2. To further enhance the understanding of the value of this theory for nursing education, it is recommended that a study be conducted to investigate how the students' understanding of a concept changes as they progress through the phases of the theory. This is particularly important in light of the change from content- to concept-driven curriculums in nursing.

3. Given that nursing is a practice discipline, it is recommended that a study be conducted investigating how engaging in collaboration online affects the nurse's ability to collaborate in practice.

References

American Association of Colleges of Nursing. (2008). *The essentials of baccalaureate education for professional nursing practice.* http://www.aacn.nche.edu/education-resources/baccessentials08.pdf

American Nurses Association. (2010). *Nursing: Scope and standards of practice* (2nd ed.). Author.

Anderson, T., Rourke, L., Garrison, D. R., & Archer, W. (2001). Assessing teaching in a computer conferencing context. *Journal of Asynchronous Learning Networks, 5*(2). http://sloanconsortium.org/publications/jaln_main

Billings, D. M., & Halstead, J. A. (2009). *Teaching in nursing: A guide for faculty* (3rd ed.). Saunders/Elsevier.

Breen, H. (2013). Virtual collaboration in the online educational setting: A concept analysis. *Nursing Forum, 48*(4), 262–270. http://doi.org/10.1111/nuf.12034

De Wever, B., Schellens, T., Valcke, M., & Van Keer, H. (2006). Content analysis schemes to analyze transcripts of online asynchronous discussion groups: A review. *Computers &Education, 46*(1), 6–28. http://doi.org/110.1016/j.compedu.2005.04.005

Dennen, V. P. (2008). Looking for evidence of learning: Assessment and analysis methods for online discourse. *Computers in Human Behavior, 24*(2), 205–219. http://doi.org/110.1016/j.chb.2007.01.010

Gardner, D. (2005). Ten lessons in collaboration. *Online Journal of Issues in Nursing, 10*(1). http//:www.nursingworld.org:MainMenuCategories:ANAMarketplace:ANAPeriodicals:OJIN:TableofContents:Volume102005:No1Jan05:tpc26_116008.html

Garrison, D. R., Cleveland-Innes, M., Koole, M., & Kappelman, J. (2006). Revisiting methodological issues in transcript analysis: Negotiated coding and reliability. *Internet & Higher Education, 9*(1), 1–8. http://doi.org/110. 1016/j.iheduc.2005.11.001

Giddens, J. (2010). *The neighborhood: Instructor's navigation guide.* Pearson.

Giddens, J., Brady, D., Brown, P., Wright, M., Smith, D., & Harris, J. (2008). A new curriculum for a new era of nursing education. *Nursing Education Perspectives, 29*(4), 200–204.

Harasim, L. (2007). Assessing online collaborative learning: A theory, methodology, and toolset. In B. H. Khan (Ed.), *Flexible learning in an information society* (pp. 282–293). Information Science Publishing.

Harasim, L. (2012). *Learning theory and online technologies.* Routledge.

Krippendorff, K. (2013). *Content analysis: An introduction to its methodology* (3rd ed.). Sage.

Menchaca, M. P., & Bekele, T. A. (2008). Learner and instructor identified success factors in distance education. *Distance Education, 29*(3), 231–252. http://doi.org/110.1080/01587910802395771

Miles, M. B., & Huberman, A. M. (1994). *Qualitative data analysis* (2nd ed.). Sage.

Murphy, E. (2004). Recognising and promoting collaboration in an online asynchronous discussion. *British Journal of Educational Technology, 35*(4), 421–431. http://doi.org/110.1111/ j.0007-1013.2004.00401.x

Oncu, S., & Cakir, H. (2011). Research in online learning environments: Priorities and methodologies. *Computers & Education, 57*(1), 1098–1108. http://doi.org/110.1016/j.compedu.2010.12.009

Tutty, J., & Klein, J. (2008). Computer-mediated instruction: A comparison of online and face-to-face collaboration. *Educational Technology Research & Development, 56*(2), 101–124. http://doi.org/110.1007/s11423-007-9050-9

Academic Partnerships: Social Determinants of Health Addressed Through Service Learning

Henny Breen and Melissa Robinson*

Overview

The purpose of this study was to evaluate the impact of service learning through academic partnerships. Although there is an abundance of literature regarding service learning as a pedagogical strategy for teaching prelicensure students, there is a gap in the literature regarding associate degree nurses returning to school to earn a bachelor's degree. A qualitative study that included student assignments and interviews, written feedback, and focus groups with staff from community organizations was used to evaluate the service-learning program. Five primary themes emerged from the data: a deeper understanding of vulnerable populations, increased knowledge of challenges in access to care, improved leadership skills, improved awareness of community resources, and impact on nursing practice. Community organizations recognized the expertise of the registered nurse–bachelor of science in nursing (RN-to-BSN) students and benefited from their work, and at the same time, students recognized their expertise and leadership in ways they had not done before. This chapter describes the findings from a qualitative research study conducted to evaluate experiential learning in an online RN-to-BSN program that utilizes service learning with community organizations.

Background

Nursing in the United States is unique in that there are multiple educational pathways for nurses to enter the profession as registered nurses. Nursing students can qualify to take the licensure exam after completing a diploma in nursing, an associate degree in nursing, or a baccalaureate degree in nursing. However, many

---

*Breen, H., & Robinson, M. (2019). Academic Partnerships: Social Determinants of Health Addressed though Service Learning. *International Journal of Nursing Education Scholarship, 16*(1).

healthcare settings in several parts of the country are now requiring nurses to have a bachelor's degree at a minimum.

Online RN-to-BSN programs have the opportunity to support expanded roles for nurses in health promotion, population health, and leadership by providing a variety of experiences in the community (Wros, Wheeler, & Jones, 2014). A stronger curricular focus on population health with an emphasis on the social determinants of health (SDOH) is critical to helping nurses provide care that recognizes culture, social context, and specific needs in partnering with their clients to make decisions about their care (American Association of Colleges of Nursing [AACN], 2013).

A community-based philosophy that prioritizes learner-centered education, health promotion, awareness of vulnerable populations, and social justice guides the design of the online RN-to-BSN program. In the first course, students conduct an in-depth, epidemiological assessment of their community that includes a wind-shield survey and key informant interviews. The assessment is designed to increase the students' awareness of SDOH and build on their knowledge of the individual- or illness-focused perspective, moving them toward a perspective that recognizes the importance of health promotion and disease prevention while caring for the community. As students move through the program, the World Health Organization (2018) definition of SDOH, "the conditions, in which people are born, grow, work, live, and age, and the wider set of forces and systems shaping the conditions of daily life," provides context for knowledge development.

In the RN-to-BSN leadership course, students engage in activities that are focused on how social and economic conditions affect health as students study healthcare finance, economics, policy, and the need for care coordination using a complex systems perspective. The population health course is organized using an SDOH framework that includes (1) economic stability, (2) education, (3) health and health care, (4) neighborhood and built environment, and (5) social and community context. During the capstone course, students engage in a less traditional care setting in the community through service learning. Simply stated, service learning is learning through serving. Service learning is defined as an experiential learning approach where students work to meet the needs of the community while addressing academic requirements. It is more than volunteerism because of the connection to academic coursework (Trail Ross, 2012).

Students gain hands-on experience in serving vulnerable members of the community, and the goal is that service learning will help them integrate the theory they have learned in the classroom into real-life situations and nursing practice (Bassi, 2011). A unique feature built into the experience is that students have a primary role in developing their experience in consultation with the service-learning coordinator, the faculty member, and the community organization. It is through that experience that students have the opportunity to develop their leadership skills in autonomy and collaboration while establishing a mutually beneficial relationship between the college, student, and community organization.

Literature Review

An abundance of literature supports the value of service learning as a pedagogical strategy in nursing education, particularly in BSN programs. However, less is known about the impact of service learning on RN-to-BSN students' learning and the organizations they work with. Examples of service learning discussed in the literature address caring for vulnerable populations, such as elders, culturally diverse groups, immigrants, homeless individuals and families, women, and at-risk youth (August-Brady & Adamshick, 2013; Gillis & MacLellan, 2010; Kolomer, Quinn, & Steele, 2010; Riner, 2013; Spurr, Bally, Ogenchuk, & Walker, 2012). The focus of service learning is on providing health promotion and education. Students have gained insight into health care, social justice issues, and the value of civic engagement. Further, they developed skills in group collaboration, team building, leadership, and advocacy. Service learning integrates meaningful community service with instruction and reflection to enrich the learning experience, meet academic course requirements, teach civic responsibility, and strengthen communities (Trail Ross, 2012; Voss, Mathews, Cohn, Scott, & Schaffer, 2015).

In a phenomenological study that explored the lived experiences of 14 BSN and RN-to-BSN students, five themes emerged from their service-learning experiences with homeless families (Hunt, 2007): eye-opening experience; feeling intense emotions; homeless families are both different from and similar to families who have housing; challenging and transforming assumptions, perceptions, and stereotypes; and reflection in action. A sixth theme emerged for the RN-to-BSN students. They were forced to consider nursing in a different light, and they began to feel a sense of futility as their understanding of how these families faced issues related to broader social and political forces grew. At the same time, they began to appreciate how their role required advocacy, citizenship, and political action (Hunt, 2007).

In a previous qualitative study of our own, we examined the effectiveness of service learning for enhancing conceptual learning in the RN-to-BSN curriculum. We found that students demonstrated higher-level thinking by linking concepts, such as vulnerable populations, and critical reflection that could be applied to nursing practice. This knowledge enhanced their leadership, teamwork, and collaboration through a greater appreciation of community, vulnerable populations, and health promotion (Breen & Robinson, 2016). Although it was not a specific aim of that study to examine the impact of SDOH, we did find that service learning affected students' understanding of the ways that SDOH influence the health of populations.

Effective academic–practice partnerships are important for creating systems that support nurses in achieving educational and career advancement and preparing nurses to practice, lead, and develop as lifelong learners (AACN, 2012). However, there is limited research on the impact of service learning on the organizations that students work with because the focus has been on student learning. This is a new area of research (Smith Budhai & Lewis Grant, 2018). A study that looked at the relationship between students and host organizations identified four tensions that resonate with our experience, although not part of our study. They included a student emphasis on hours, learning, and flexibility versus an agency emphasis on commitment, efficiency, and dependability (Mills, 2012). Mills also identified idealism versus reality, which was not part of our RN-to-BSN students' experience. Within nursing, Beal (2012) found numerous articles that describe academic–service partnerships but, again, few studies that address outcomes. No studies were found that evaluated the impact of RN-to-BSN student service on the organizations.

Methodology

The purpose of this qualitative evaluation study was to evaluate the RN-to-BSN service-learning experience. Our aim was to evaluate the impact that service learning had on student learning and how the service of the RN-to-BSN student affected the organization. Given how little research has been conducted in this area, a qualitative evaluation methodology was chosen. When little is known about a certain subject area or social phenomenon, qualitative designs are particularly valuable and are used to discover knowledge directly from the participants' perspective of their experience (Cheek, Onslow, & Cream, 2004; Fain, 2004). Further, an evaluation study can provide the opportunity to examine the effectiveness of service learning and at the same time work to build relationships with partner organizations and improve the program (Lodico, Spaulding, & Voegtle, 2010). Institutional Review Board (IRB) approval was secured, and consent for participation was obtained from the volunteers who participated in the study.

The limitations of this study include the lack of generalizability and the potential for researcher bias. A rigorous process of identifying and controlling potential sources of bias was implemented by ongoing reflection to examine personal beliefs, experiences, and feelings, and the two researchers engaged in regular debriefing to assist with challenging assumptions and considering different ways of challenging assumptions (Lodico et al., 2010). The transcripts of the student interviews were also compared to the written assignments.

Data Sources and Analysis

The research study included 49 RN-to-BSN students from two different semesters who volunteered to share their input on service learning in two written course reflection assignments. The assignments were developed specifically for the study and completed in the online classroom. The students were also invited to participate in a face-to-face focused interview to share their experiences with service learning. The interviews were limited because only two students volunteered to participate. The student interviews took place after the course ended and the grades were submitted. The focus groups took place after the students had completed their service-learning experience at the organization. This was to reinforce that participation would not affect the student's grade, as was stated in their consent to participate.

Data sources from the community organizations included written feedback from 55 organizations. Some examples included an immigrant and refugee senior center, community clinics, schools, an organization offering housing for the homeless, drop-in centers, and Adult Protective Services. As part of the service-learning program, organizations were asked to comment on their experience in having an RN-to-BSN student work with them and if they would welcome students in the future. Additionally, a focus group was held with six participants from a day shelter for women and eight participants from a homeowners' association (HOA) for a senior housing complex, and an interview was conducted with a nurse manager and staff member in two different residential facilities. **Table 16-1** provides a list of data sources and the community organizations.

Interview protocols were developed and adapted from an assessment model developed by Gelmon, Holland, Driscoll, Spring, and Kerrigan (2001) for the student interviews and focus groups with the organizations. A field test was conducted to allow us to become comfortable with the interview process and establish the validity of the protocols (Creswell, 2009). Two doctorally prepared nurse researchers experienced in qualitative design were asked to participate in an expert review of the protocols. They were asked to evaluate the appropriateness of the questions

Table 16-1 Data Sources

Data Source	Number	Community Organization
Reflective assignments	49 RN-to-BSN students	Students were involved in 55 different organizations within their local communities (some students worked with more than one organization).
Written feedback	55 organizations	Organization representatives provided feedback about the students when validating their hours and also indicated if they would welcome another RN-to-BSN student the following semester.
Focus-group interviews	Six participants (director and staff); two students	Participants were from a nonprofit day shelter and community center for women and children located in an urban neighborhood of a metropolitan community that serves between 60 and 90 guests per day. Services include the provision of immediate needs (clothing, food, hygiene, computer access), advocacy (housing, emotional support, financial assistance, medical and health support), education and socialization (health education, spirituality, support groups), and community (relationship building, safety, respect).
Focus group	Eight participants	Participants were from a homeowners' association for residents over the age of 55, located in a suburban community. The association is managed entirely by volunteers and governed by a board of directors who participate in governance and decision making.
Interview	Manager and one staff member	Participants were from a residential home for young, single women who are pregnant and need a safe place for themselves and their unborn baby, located in an urban community. The staff members focus on supporting women locally, in their own communities and close to the resources that they need to complete their education and find employment. The focus is on creating a safe community for young mothers and their children by addressing their physical, emotional, and spiritual needs.

(continues)

Table 16-1 Data Sources   *(continued)*

Data Source	Number	Community Organization
Interview	Manager and one staff member	Participants were from a residential facility in the metropolitan community that serves the healthcare and housing needs of low-income persons living with HIV. The team works with individuals to help them manage the complexities of HIV and also the challenges of managing independent living. In addition to 24-hour residential care, the clinical team provides home visits in the community for clients experiencing similar challenges.

for the population and to assess alignment with the overall purpose of the study. No changes were made as a result of these strategies to ensure the validity of the protocols.

During the interview and focus groups, casual conversations put the participants at ease and allowed them to openly discuss their experiences (Lodico et al., 2010). The interviews were conducted by the investigators and were taped and transcribed for data analysis. The transcripts obtained from the course included a reflective assignment that had the same questions that were asked of the two students during the interviews and a discussion question that specifically addressed what they learned regarding the SDOH and how the experience would affect their practice. All the transcripts were analyzed by each researcher throughout the data-collection process using thematic analysis, which is a method for identifying, analyzing, and reporting patterns (themes) within data (Braun & Clarke, 2006). Following individual analysis, the researchers worked collaboratively to make comparisons. In this way, reliability was addressed. Having two researchers check the data for themes individually at different intervals, followed by discussing differences until at least 80% agreement is met, is the recommendation (Merriam, 2009). In this case, 100% agreement was met.

Findings: Students

Analysis of the data written by the students and confirmed in the two interviews revealed that reflecting on their experiences enabled them to appreciate how SDOH were a major factor in population health. Many students also reported that they felt very anxious about collaborating with an organization in the community to organize their own experience. However, being successful was empowering, and they began to appreciate how much they were respected as nurses. This helped them learn and develop their leadership skills in the community setting because they often had to work independently in assessing the learning needs of the clients they worked with. They planned and provided education and nursing care to the clients they worked with. Further, some students ended up in organizations that also had BSN nursing students from other programs with their faculty member. In an interview, an RN-to-BSN student discussed how she ended up taking a leadership role with the BSN students, who felt insecure and wanted an RN to double-check things like blood pressure, for example, and also provided feedback on their teaching when their own teacher was absent. She said the students' attitude was "I am a sponge—give it to me please." The students appreciated working closely with the RN-to-BSN student.

During a student interview, the affective impact of the service-learning experience was captured when the student said, "This, the service learning experience itself, helped me get out of my head in this program because this is a very cerebral thing, if you're doing it all on the computer and it's all what you read and it's all these ... (pause, sigh) articles that are so deep that sometimes they just wanna make you walk away ... What I really liked about it was that it got me out of head."

The primary themes that emerged from the assignments and interviews included (1) deeper understanding of the needs and struggles of vulnerable and marginalized populations specifically through social and economic disadvantages; (2) increased knowledge of challenges in access to care; (3) improved leadership skills involving communication, collaboration, and advocacy skills; (4) improved awareness of community resources; and (5) impact on nursing practice. Student quotes related to each of the themes are found in **Table 16-2**.

Table 16-2 Primary Themes—Student Quotes

Themes	Student Quotes
Vulnerable populations	"Opened my eyes, less judgmental when I know nothing about their stories, made me more aware of my own biases and how that can affect the care I provide." "Anyone who essentially lives paycheck to paycheck or with minimal savings can become part of a vulnerable population just by losing their job."
Access to care	"I worked with a vulnerable population that needs more advocacy and activism to support it. I think a lot of people are unaware of the extent of poverty, and mental health ... and the resulting living situations[,] and as nurses[,] we can help educate. There are obviously nonprofits working for change and improved quality of life. Within each organization there are defined goals and leadership, but what they lack is overarching leadership to tie them together. As a nurse, I see an opening for bringing these resources together to work in collaboration instead of in tandem. Perhaps a coalition is in order here, and now I have the skills, knowledge and connections to make that happen."
Leadership skills	"I worked as a volunteer RN... [at] a Day Shelter ... for women and their children. Part of my responsibilities included spending time assessing patient's medical needs such as wound care with dressing changes, checking blood pressures when requested, referring women to seek health care at local clinics or emergency rooms and participating in active listening, that helped me to be an advocate working with other staff."

(continues)

Table 16-2 Primary Themes—Student Quotes *(continued)*

Themes	Student Quotes
	"Being able to communicate and collaborating with the staff while working with the guest helped with finding the right services they needed. ... Working with a vulnerable population allowed me to help out my community and discover new ways I can contribute to a much-needed cause."
Community resources	"It was eye opening to volunteer at the annual community education day[,] and I plan to be a volunteer again next year. I learned about many fantastic resources available to people with cancer that I did not know about before, such as the numerous support groups and events that are free to people going through cancer. I made connections with the Cancer Resource Center and the Project Coordinator. I feel like with these connections I may have bridged a small gap for some of the disadvantaged coastal patients."
	"I also learned that advocacy for this group can come from a variety of sources. For example, I learned about many different foundations and groups working around Sarcoma research. Some focused on the families themselves by offering a support network, some offered fund raising support for individual families, some were disease specific and worked on fundraising for research in this area, all advocating for this vulnerable population but in different ways. It was amazing to see how they did not work against each other but filled different niches and supported each other when they were able to."
	"I enjoyed the diabetic clinic evening group meetings. It was amazing to see physicians, dieticians, physical therapists, nurses, prayer leaders, and interpreters all come together, all volunteering, just to help those patients. The patients were always so grateful for those evening meetings. The local food bank always donated a large bag of healthy groceries to each patient at the meetings, too. Seeing the generosity of the community and the knowledge that we were improving our patients' lives was the most rewarding part to me."
Nursing practice	"Nursing is so much more than meeting the clinical needs of patients and their families. It really hit me hard at the shelter, that nursing really needs to be more involved in the self-sufficiency of individuals, families and communities—brought me back to the reason I wanted to practice nursing—the care coordination and support for the vulnerable."

Vulnerable Populations

As a primary finding in this study, service learning enhanced student understanding of how social determinants affect health. Economic instability stood out as a major barrier to achieving positive health outcomes. Many students demonstrated a deeper appreciation and compassion for those who suffer from poverty and homelessness as they challenged their own preconceptions and judgments. They identified many factors that lead to vulnerability, including homelessness; discrimination related to mental illness and being transgender; physical illness leading to job loss and depleted savings; unemployment; lack of job skills; inadequate pay, transportation, education, childcare, and health insurance; no support system; and undocumented immigrant status. Further, they identified high levels of stress related to transgender status and being in an unsafe or abusive environment at home or on the streets (including young mothers with young children trying to escape abuse). They identified that being with vulnerable clients made them more aware of the need to provide holistic care and compassion to promote health.

One student wrote about how gratifying it was to help a single mother with two children get back on track after losing her job because of her children being sick and then losing her apartment. The student had cancer herself and was not able to work. The experience had her wondering if she could hold on to her home if she could not go back to work. The student came to a deeper realization that anyone could become homeless as a result of economic circumstances. The service-learning experience provided an opportunity to experience firsthand, through their engagement with vulnerable and marginalized people, what it is like to live in poverty.

Challenges in Access to Care

Access to care was a common theme; students recognized that not only was it difficult to find resources but also that accessing care related to childcare issues, lack of transportation, and feeling judged were barriers. They also recognized a lack of coordination. A student reported that she became aware that many nonprofit organizations are "literally next door to each other and have no clear knowledge of exactly what the other does or what resources they offer." She mentioned the importance of working together to optimize client outcomes and identified her interest in becoming involved, following her educational experience, in a way that would connect resources in the community. She also identified goals related to lobbying on behalf of organizations and possibly developing a coalition for organizations to come together.

Leadership Skills—Communication, Collaboration, and Advocacy

Multiple students reflected on their communication skills, including their ability to collaborate and advocate. Their skills were enhanced by the service-learning experience as well as the appreciation they experienced related to their expertise in having advanced communication skills. For example, when working in a day shelter for women, several students found that they were able to communicate with the women to ensure they followed up with local clinics and providers in ways other staff could not because of their role as an RN and their therapeutic communication skills.

Improved Awareness of Community Resources

Students reported learning about the resources available in the community to assist those who are marginalized and suffering. They learned that people were grateful rather than manipulative, as is often the prevailing belief: "even the smallest things mean a great deal[,] such as time spent with people." Some expressed shock to learn how many local restaurants and food chains donate food, and another student expressed that she felt better sending babies home with moms who live in a shelter as a result of her experience working in a shelter.

Impact on Nursing Practice

For some students, the experience led to serving as a change agent within their organizations. For example, one student shared with her peers that she learned a lot about social discrimination related to homelessness and challenged the assumption that individuals are homeless due to drug or alcohol use or other lifestyle choices. Another student reported that in her community hospital (the only hospital in town), staff would not collaborate with case managers or other shelter staff to meet the needs of the homeless community members. They would send patients back to the shelter from the hospital in taxis with no communication to the shelter staff regarding a discharge plan, and often no paperwork was sent. As a result, the RN-to-BSN student offered in-services at her place of employment about the importance of collaboration with community organizations. She stated that she learned that the need was great and that nurses have the power to make a difference.

Findings: Community Organizations

Each of the community organizations reported positive outcomes associated with having RN-to-BSN students placed in their organizations. When describing their experiences, staff members recognized differences in supporting students who were already licensed nurses compared with BSN students, who require more orientation, closer supervision, and more investment of staff time and resources. Terms that were used to describe the RN-to-BSN students included *mature, systems-oriented, efficient, skilled, organized, experienced, professional, knowledgeable, compassionate,* and *nonjudgmental*, among others.

The primary themes that reflected the impact that service learning had on the community organization included (1) increased access to health support and education for the population, (2) improved involvement of the community members in health activities as a result of the credibility and qualifications of the student, (3) higher quality of care and services based on the expertise of the students, and (4) increased trust and confidence in the organization based on effective and therapeutic communication with clients. Quotes from managers and staff in the organizations are provided in **Table 16-3**.

Access to Health Education

Increased access to health education and support was a primary theme identified by participants in the focus groups from the community organizations. These organizations do not have nurses as part of their organizations. Having an RN-to-BSN student available regularly made it possible to provide regular access to health promotion, which was perceived as "immediate access to health care" and a way to "eliminate barriers" for clients accessing care. Participants identified that it made a difference to be able to offer follow-up and consistent access by stating, "Come back tomorrow—there will be a nurse here."

Table 16-3 Primary Themes—Community Organization Quotes

Themes	Community Organization Participant Quotes
Access to health education	"A client divulged that she normally goes somewhere else [to have wound cleaning and assistance bandaging up her wounds] but they were shut down for services that day, so the fact that we were able to provide that service meant that she actually received care."
Involvement of clients in health-promotion activities	"Building trust [building that trust is a big part of how we operate] and knowing that nurses are held at such high stature in any community but especially vulnerable populations ... so they would want that professional support and opinion and help." "It is clear they need to go to the emergency room and seek medical attention for many reasons some of them, I'm unsure why they won't seek medical attention somewhere else, I think it's been comfortable here ...there's the level of respect they may not receive at the hospital when you have um, abscess or drug inflicted wounds or, you know, those things that you may not be treated that way um ... when to an emergency room or another medical facility. That's the feedback I seem to hear from our [clients]." "The home visits and educational events made the efforts visible to a larger number of residents than the committee could have done on their own. Each term the students presented their accomplishments at a board meeting. This assisted the Emergency Preparedness committee in successfully obtaining a budget line, however small, in the HOA annual budget. With this heightened profile residents became aware of the grass roots efforts and gave donations of medical equipment, supplies and some cash donations that can be used by the Medical Aid and CERT team members to provide care if needed."
Increased quality of care and services	"Our model is very holistic, we're wanting to help the women and their children, attend to the things they are the most concerned about ... if you are experiencing illness or injury, that hierarchy of needs, our ability to address some peoples very basic needs right away is important to our model and achieving our mission." "One of the common things that we hear from women who come who are experiencing poverty and homelessness and abuse ... there's the frustration in the trauma sometimes of just trying to access service ... it really does fit into our mission and I think it's a significant ... having nurses here to further their learning, but with this degree of competency and experience allows us to, allows us to really ... realize our mission more fully." "It is significant for us to be able to share with our community partner agencies, funding agencies, or foundations that we have [volunteer] nurses available during

(continues)

Table 16-3 **Primary Themes—Community Organization Quotes** *(continued)*

Themes	Community Organization Participant Quotes
	our service hours ... we work with such vulnerable population ... it enhances our position as a day shelter and community center for women and children in terms of our perceived role in the community and ability to serve."
	"The student was self-directed and had a macro understanding of healthcare systems ... her strengths were system level[,] which helped to develop a formal system for what we were doing to address medication errors ... this allowed her to serve us, and our clients, on a whole other level."
	"She had the ability to 'zoom out' on a clinical problem to think about the system, rather than just the individual problem (i.e. medication error, impact on client). She came with skills ... that would be sustainable in its effect on client outcomes. She also interacted with clients and staff to understand the level of care and day-to-day operations of our program[,] which informed her understanding of the factors involved in medication errors."
	"She was more independent and serving in a way that served us ... she was a resource that we would not have had ... we believe she also benefited from the experience."
	"We appreciated the student's ability to look at our program and our system ... then to address the issue without any judgment. She was professional and understanding about the reality of the delivery of clinical care. She asked questions in the process that made us think deeply about the issues; she looked at things from a different perspective. The work she did was sustained and the program has been implemented. We learned more about our program from her assessment."
Increased trust and confidence in the organization	"[It is] reassuring to guests when we say 'we have a nurse here'[;] it is true that the nurses we have here are continuing their education[,] but they are already working and experienced in their field. [My] observation is that there is ... more effective communication with the population we serve[,] and it's not a criticism of our student nurses who are working toward their nursing licensure[,] it's just the experience level ... and that is ... great support for staff because we deal with people who have many, many different concerns and, and helping them address their physical health ... it's a real enhancement for us and our service model."
	"It's not just the basic first aid ... a lot of it is therapeutic communication and active listening and empowering them ... how to get to the places that they need to get resources. Truly what I found beneficial was that the [nurses] allowed them to open up and feel better ... they are so thankful to have that person to be able to effectively, you know listen and communicate and empower. I found that to be a blessing."

During an outreach event in a local park, a client had a seizure. The nurse was able to triage the client's urgent needs and ensure her safety in the community setting. A participant reported that the student "was able to put that person aside and take care of her; we were able to continue on ... this was in the middle of a major event for us with over 100 of our clients there at the park." The participant valued that the nurse could assess her condition quickly, obtain a medical history, and access 911 appropriately.

Involvement of Clients in Health-Promotion Activities

Participants from a day shelter identified that clients expressed increased interest and involvement in promoting their own health by seeking interaction with the students. Further, clients, based on nurse recommendations, would seek health care within systems they normally avoided. They attributed this to the level of trust that nurses have within the community. Within the HOA, students assisted in emergency preparedness, and their work with the committee helped successfully obtain a budget line in their annual budget for emergency preparedness and facilitated the donation of supplies.

Increased Quality of Care and Services

Participants identified that service learning increased the quality of the care and services that the organization could provide to the community. They shared that students provided "expertise" and "advanced skills," which resulted in a "higher-quality experience" for not only the clients they serve but also for staff and volunteers who benefited from the role modeling and services provided. One participant described a "certain power dynamic that comes with being a Registered Nurse ... they are more of a resource and an expert ... they look at things differently; they are honest and mature." As nurses, they felt the students came prepared and were "vocal in recognizing an issue" and bringing it to their attention.

In a residential facility, participants reported being able to "capitalize" on the expertise and knowledge of the RN-to-BSN student, especially in the area of quality assurance, while also providing a unique experience. Having the student's expertise made it possible to implement a state-sponsored program aimed at increasing quality and safety.

At times, issues were identified by students in which the service-learning coordinator had to get involved. For example, students questioned the availability of over-the-counter (OTC) medications at a shelter that were donated to the organization and that they were asked to administer without having the appropriate policies and procedures in place. This concern was expressed to the administrator and her faculty member. The faculty member contacted the administrator, and they agreed that an RN-to-BSN student would work on researching what was needed to ensure the appropriate regulations and policies were in place. Given the challenges, during a subsequent meeting between the service-learning coordinator and the director of the shelter, it was decided that OTC medications would no longer be available within the shelter and that appropriate referrals would be made. Students continued to educate clients on the use of OTC medications. This kind of experience is also an indication of increased awareness of professionalism and leadership as students gained insights into the regulations regarding community organizations.

Increased Trust and Confidence in the Organization

Participants described that service learning increased the trust and confidence that the community had in the organization as a result of the higher level of effective and therapeutic communication skills demonstrated by the RN-to-BSN students. A participant shared that having student volunteers "blends comfort and credibility to what we are doing to have licensed nurses here[,] which also gives our volunteers a level of comfort too." Another participant described the students' ability to provide compassionate listening, which she believed affected clients' self-worth because of "the fact that you deserve a licensed nurse to be here[,] and this is really important to your well-being."

Discussion

In the online classroom, there is a great deal of emphasis on the cognitive level of learning, with some affective learning through case studies and reflective exercises. However, the service-learning experiences augmented the cognitive learning of RN-to-BSN students with affective learning, as described by the students. Students described feeling a deeper level of empathy as their assumptions and judgments about poverty and homelessness were challenged. This is not unlike the findings of Hunt (2007), in which the themes of eye-opening experience; feeling intense emotions; homeless families are both different from and similar to families who have housing; challenging and transforming assumptions, perceptions, and stereotypes; and reflection in action were identified. Our study also found, as Hunt did, that RN-to-BSN students began to appreciate how their role required advocacy, citizenship, and political action. On the other hand, our students did not begin to feel a sense of futility as their understanding of how these families faced issues related to broader social and political forces progressed.

As nurse educators, we have a responsibility to help students gain a broader understanding of health that includes the SDOH in order for nurses to connect people to the resources that are essential to their recovery (Zangerle, 2016). This became very clear following our study that examined the effectiveness of service learning for enhancing conceptual learning in the RN-to-BSN program. It was this study that led us to look more closely at how service learning affected the students' understanding of how SDOH influences population health, in addition to looking at the impact of having RN-to-BSN students serve in community organizations.

Organization participants recognized the expertise of the RN-to-BSN students and benefited from their work, and, at the same time, students recognized their expertise and leadership in ways they had not done before, which was professionally empowering for them. Students recognized that they were influencing change when their contributions were valued through building relationships with staff in the organizations (Grossman & Valiga, 2017). Ultimately, nurses began to realize that they had skills that could be translated into practice in the community. As they grew in their role as a professional within the community, they also began to recognize the gaps that exist, particularly related to unmet health needs and risks directly affected by SDOH. Nurses are uniquely suited to leverage this knowledge by integrating knowledge of SDOH into their practice. They can demonstrate leadership when it comes to interprofessional collaboration with various community agencies and sectors and advocate for supportive interventions that integrate knowledge of the individual's SDOH (Zangerle, 2016).

Through service experiences for RN-to-BSN students, we have been able to develop and strengthen the collaborative relationships with our academic–practice partners that have proven to be mutually beneficial (AACN, 2012). This is a step in demonstrating that effective academic–practice partnerships are important for creating systems that support nurses in achieving educational and career advancement and prepare nurses to practice, lead, and develop as lifelong learners (AACN, 2012). The number of partnerships has grown dramatically, which allows us to sustain the placement of students in organizations where health promotion can be provided regularly. We have expanded our outreach and service to a variety of organizations, including community clinics, tutoring programs for teens, mental health organizations for youth, maternal/child programs, specialized summer youth camps, housing associations, parish nursing programs, and more. Several students developed a strong commitment to continue their service long after their service-learning experience concluded, and several organizations now regularly request RN-to-BSN students.

To expand on the findings in this study and the value of academic–practice partnerships, a future study that examines the impact on clients served by the organization within the framework of service learning is recommended. Once a study that examines the impact on clients is completed, a theoretical framework could be developed for RN-to-BSN service learning in the community, with SDOH as a major construct that could lend itself to further qualitative and potentially quantitative research to examine the theory for generalization.

Acknowledgments

This publication/project was made possible through a cooperative agreement between the American Association of Colleges of Nursing (AACN) and the Centers for Disease Control and Prevention (CDC), Grant U360E000003-05; its contents are the responsibility of the authors and do not necessarily reflect the official views of the AACN or CDC.

Funding

This work was supported by the AACN and CDC, Grant U360E000003-05.

References

American Association of Colleges of Nursing. (2012). *AACN-AONE Task Force on Academic Practice Partnerships.* http://www.aacn.nche.edu/leading-initiatives/academic-practice-partnerships/Guiding Principles.pdf

American Association of Colleges of Nursing. (2013). *Public health: Recommended baccalaureate competencies and curriculum guides for public health nursing.* http://www.aacnnursing.org/Portals/42 /Population%20Health/BSN-Curriculum-Guide.pdf

August-Brady, M., & Adamshick, P. (2013). Oh, the things you will learn: Taking undergraduate research to the homeless shelter. *Journal of Nursing Education, 52*(6), 342–345. http://doi .org/10.3928/01484834-20130515-02

Bassi, S. (2011). Undergraduate nursing student's perceptions of service learning through a school-based community project. *Nursing Education Perspectives, 32*(3), 162–167. http://doi.org/10 .5480/1536-5026-32.3.162

Beal, A. (2012). Academic-service partnerships in nursing: An integrative review. *Nursing Research and Practice,* Article ID 501564. http://doi.org/10.1155/2012/501564

Braun, V., & Clarke, V. (2006). Using thematic analysis in pscychology. *Qualitative Research in Psychology, 3*(2), 77–101. http://dx.doi.org/10.1191/1478088706qp063oa

Breen, H., & Robinson, M. (2016). Service learning enhances conceptual learning in a RN to BSN program. *International Journal for Innovation Education and Research, 4*, 10. https://iiier.net/index .php/ijier/article/view/609

Cheek, J., Onslow, M., & Cream, A. (2004). Beyond the divide: Comparing and contrasting aspects of qualitative and quantitative research approaches. *Advances in Speech Language Pathology, 6*(3), 147–152. http://doi.org/10.1080/14417040412331282995

Creswell, J. (2009). *Research design: Qualitative, quantitative, and mixed methods approaches.* Sage.

Fain, J. (2004). *Reading, understanding, and applying nursing research.* F.A. Davis.

Gelmon, S., Holland, B., Driscoll, A., Spring, A., & Kerrigan, S. (2001). *Assessing service-learning and civic engagement: Principles and techniques.* Campus Compact.

Gillis, A., & MacLellan, M. (2010). Service learning with vulnerable populations: Review of the literature. *International Journal of Nursing Education Scholarship, 7*(1). https://doi.org/10.2202 /1548-923X.2041

Grossman, S. C., & Valiga, T. M. (2017). *The new leadership challenge: Creating the future of nursing* (5th ed.). F.A. Davis.

Hunt, R. (2007). Service-learning: An eye-opening experience that provokes emotion and challenges stereotypes. *Journal of Nursing Education, 46*(6), 277–281. https://www.healio.com /nursing/journals/jne

Kolomer, S., Quinn, M., & Steele, K. (2010). Interdisciplinary health fairs for older adults and the value of interprofessional service learning. *Journal of Community Practice, 18*(2–3), 267–279. http://doi.org/10.1080/10705422.2010.485863

Lodico, M., Spaulding, D., & Voegtle, K. (2010). *Methods in educational research: From theory to practice.* Jossey-Bass.

Merriam, S. B. (2009). *Qualitative research: A guide to design and implementation.* Jossey-Bass.

Mills, S. D. (2012). The four furies: Primary tension between service-learners and host agencies. *Michigan Journal of Community Service Learning, 19*(1), 33–43. https://its.fsu.edu/sites/g/files /imported/storage/original/application/86f4384df876eb969db799807a8ea758.pdf

Riner, M. E. (2013). Globally engaged nursing education with local immigrant populations. *Public Health Nursing, 30*(3), 246–253. http://doi.org/10.1111/phn.12026

Smith Budhai, S., & Lewis Grant, K. S. (2018). First encounters, service experience, parting impressions: Examining the dynamics of service-learning relationships. *Journal of Higher Education Outreach and Engagement, 22*(3), 69. https://files.eric.ed.gov/fulltext/EJ1193371.pdf

Spurr, S., Bally, J., Ogenchuk, M., & Walker, K. (2012). A framework for exploring adolescent wellness. *Pediatric Nursing, 38*(6), 320–326. http://www.aii.com/services/pblshng/pnj/default .htm

Trail Ross, M. E. (2012). Linking classroom learning to the community through service learning. *Journal of Community Health Nursing, 1*, 53–50. http://doi.org/10.1080/07370016.2012.645746

Voss, H., Mathews, L. R., Cohn, T. F., Scott, G., & Schaffer, M. (2015). Community-academic partnerships: Developing a service-learning framework. *Journal of Professional Nursing, 31*(5), 395–401. http://doi.org/10.1016/j.profnurs.2015.03.008

World Health Organization. (2018). *Social health determinants.* http://www.who.int/social_determinants /sdh_definition/en/

Wros, P., Wheeler, P., & Jones, M. (2014). Curriculum planning for baccalaureate nursing programs. In S. Keating (Ed.), *Curriculum development and evaluation in nursing* (3rd ed., pp. 245–284). Springer.

Zangerle, S. M. (2016). Population health: The importance of social determinants. *Nursing Management, 47*(2), 17–18. http://doi.org/10.1097/01.NUMA.000047944475643.e5

Index

A

AACN. *See* American Association of Colleges of Nursing
ACA. *See* Affordable Care Act
academia, faculty role
  CNE, 218–219
  COI, 219–220
  collaborative scholarship, 230–232, 231–232*t*
  demand for faculty, 212
  exchanging knowledge about teaching and learning, 227
  faculty promotion and tenure, 222–223, 222–223*t*
  formal mentorship program, 227–229, 228*t*
  mentorship, 214–215, 215*t*, 216*t*
  nurses in, 211
  online adjunct faculty, 213–214
  online teaching
    competence, 213
    preparation and competency, 212–213
    readiness for, 212
  orientation, 214
  professional development, 215–218, 217*t*, 218–219*t*
  QM, 220
  scholarship
    application, 221
    Boyer's Model of, 221
    discovery, 221
    integration, 221–222
    nursing education in, 220
    teaching/learning, 221, 224
  teaching
    growth, 224
    growth in the scholarship of, 229, 229*t*
    philosophy, 225–227
    reflection, 224–225
academia, nurses in, 211
academic advising, feedback from students, 54–56
academic advisor, 49–50, 51*t*
academic integrity, online nursing, learning through writing, 156–158, 158*t*
Academic Nurse Educator Certification Program, 4
academic partnerships, service learning
  access to care, challenges in, 281
  community organizations, 282, 283–284*t*
  community resources, 281–282
  data sources and analysis, 276–278, 277–278*t*
  discussion, 286–287
  health education, access to, 282, 285
  health-promotion activities, clients involvement in, 285
  leadership skills, 281
  literature review, 274–275
  methodology, 275–276
  nursing practice, impact on, 282
  quality of care and services, 285
  students, 278–279, 279–280*t*
  trust and confidence in organization, 286
  vulnerable populations, 280–281
academic program review, 76
acceptance, of online education, 62–63
access to care, challenges in, 281
ACEs. *See* Adverse Childhood Experiences
active learning and teaching, online teaching strategies, 130–132, 131–132*t*
adapting model, online nursing education, experiential learning, 170–172, 171*f*, 173–175*t*
ADDIE process, 103, 104*t*
admissions counselor, 48–49, 49*t*
adult learning theory, 15, 17*t*, 134
Advancing Healthcare Transformation: A New Era for Academic Nursing, 220
Adverse Childhood Experiences (ACEs), 123
advocacy, leadership skill, 281
Affordable Care Act (ACA), 178
alignment, curriculum development, 88–90, 90–91*t*
  design, 95

American Association of Colleges of Nursing
(AACN), 4, 106, 127, 152, 187, 212,
220, 222, 224, 260
American Nurses Association (ANA), 3, 24,
129, 259
ANA. *See* American Nurses Association
andragogy, defined, 15
APA style, 155, 156, 159
appraisal, peer, 79, 80–81*t*
art forms: literature, cinema, podcasts, music,
198–201, 199–201*t*
arts and literature activity, online nursing
education, experiential learning,
172–176, 176*t*
assessment
and grading rubrics, 114–120, 115–120*t*
and learning activities, 111–114,
111*t*, 113*t*
online course design, 108–111, 109*t*, 110*t*
asynchronous discussions, online teaching
strategies, 138–139, 140*t*
audio- and video-conferencing tools, 150
automated-response software programs, 143

B

baby boomers, 28, 241
bachelor of science in nursing (BSN), 2,
43, 150, 152
behaviorist approach, 193
blackboard learn, 262
Bloom's/Fink's taxonomy, 138
Boyer's model, 221–222, 224, 229
BSN. *See* bachelor of science in nursing
bullying, 248

C

caring, definition of, 33
CDC. *See* Centers for Disease Control and
Prevention
Centers for Disease Control and Prevention
(CDC), 143
certified nurse educator (CNE), 4–5,
127–128, 218–219
certified online instructor (COI), 219–220
change, defined, 253
CINAHL, 151
clear/consistent structure, online course
design, 102
clients, involvement in health-promotion
activities, 285
clinical reasoning, 184–185, 188–189
CNE. *See* certified nurse educator

coalition building, 187–188, 190–191
cognitive constructivism, 10, 11, 13, 14,
16*t*, 101
cognitive presence, online teaching
strategies, 134
COI. *See* certified online instructor
CoI model. *See* community of inquiry model
collaboration
defined, 3, 259–260
leadership skill, 281
collaborative
and individual reflection, 103
design and development process, 105, 106*f*
leadership model, 63–64, 65*t*
learning, 183, 259–260
online course design, 102
online course design, 103
model, for online nursing education,
1–6, 4*f*
scholarship, 230–232, 231–232*t*
work, 177
collaborativist learning theory, 12–13, 17*t*,
134, 138
communication, leadership skill, 281,
250–252
community
-based philosophy, 274
concepts of, 189–190
of learners, 132, 194, 195
organizations, 282
quotes, 283–284*t*
partner survey, 56, 57*t*
partnerships, 52–53
resources, awareness of, 281–282
community of inquiry (CoI) model, 132, 133,
133*f*, 135–136, 138, 141
concept-based and competency-based
teaching, online teaching
strategies, 129
concept-based curriculum, 91
in postlicensure programs, 92–95, 93–94*t*
confidence, service learning, 286
constructivist learning theory, 10–12, 101,
102, 183, 255
cognitive constructivism, 10, 11
social constructivism, 10, 11–12
cooperative work, 177
coordinator, of online programs, 64, 66, 66*t*
service-learning, 67, 68*t*
course evaluation, online learning, 74–75, 75*t*
course lead, 67, 69*t*
course learning outcomes, online course
design, 105–106
crisis, student support during, 37, 37–38*t*
cultural constructivism. *See* social
constructivism

culture, online nursing students, 24–26
curriculum development
    concept-based, 91–92
        in postlicensure programs, 92–95,
            93–94t
    design, 91–95
        alignment, 88–90, 90–91t, 95
        integrated, 95
    learning
        assessment of, 96
        through semesters, progression of, 96, 98
    in nursing education, 9
    RN-to-BSN, integration of models, 96, 97t

D

Dee Fink's taxonomy language, 95–96, 98
Defining Scholarship for Academic Nursing,
    221–222
Defining Scholarship for Academic Nursing:
    Task Force Consensus Position
    Statement, 222
demonstrate presence and engagement, online
    teaching strategies, 136–137, 137t
design and development, online course
    design, 105
design, curriculum, 91–95
    alignment, 95
    concept-based curriculum, 91–92
        in postlicensure programs, 92–95, 93–94t
    integrated, 95
dialectic poles, online nursing education,
    experiential learning, 170
disaster nursing, 185–187, 189–190
discipline, online nursing, learning through
    writing, 154–155
diversity
    gender, 24–26, 25t, 27t
    generational, 28–29, 30t
        enhanced communication skills,
            250–252
        expanded perspectives, 243–244, 245t
        improved technology skills, 253–254
        in nursing education, 241–242
        increased nursing knowledge,
            242–243, 243t
        leadership development, 245–247, 250t
        mentorship, 247–250, 250t
        online classroom strategies, 256
        personal growth, 252–253
        practice and research, 254–255
        study methodology, 242
DNP. See doctor of nursing practice
doctor of nursing practice (DNP), 22
documentary: the invisible war, 201

E

embedded librarians, online nursing, learning
    through writing, 150–151
emergency remote teaching, 5
English as a second language (ESL), 26–28
enrollment trends, in higher education, 21–22
epistemology, 10
ESL. See English as a second language
ethnicity, online nursing students, 24–26
evaluation, online course design, 125
Evolution of Nursing course, 143
exchanging knowledge about teaching
    and learning, 227
expectations, online course, 79, 81–82t
experiential learning theory, 13–14, 17t
experiential storytelling, 204–205, 204–205t
extroverted students, 30

F

facilitating reflective, critical, and analytical
    thinking, online teaching strategies,
    139–141, 140t
facilitation challenges, online teaching
    strategies, 142
faculty preparation, online teaching strategies,
    127–128, 128t
faculty promotion and tenure, 222–223,
    222–223t
faculty role, online teaching strategies, 129
faculty storytelling, 205–208, 206t, 207–208t
Federal Emergency Management Agency
    (FEMA), 123, 143
feedback banks, online teaching
    strategies, 143
FEMA. See Federal Emergency Management
    Agency
formal mentorship program, 227–229, 228t
Future of Nursing report, 23, 43–44, 87

G

gathering: welcoming and calling forth,
    195–196
gender diversity, online nursing students,
    24–26, 25t, 27t
generation X, 28, 241, 249, 252
generational diversity, 28–29, 30t. See also
    diversity, generational
Gibbs's model, 205
Google Scholar, 151
grading and feedback, online teaching
    strategies, 142

grading and timeliness, online teaching
strategies, 145–146, 146t
group feedback, online teaching strategies,
143, 144t
group process, defined, 268
group work, online teaching strategies,
138, 254

H

health care issues, affecting nursing
education, 87–88
health education, access to, 282, 285
health-promotion activities, clients
involvement in, 285
higher education, enrollment trends, 21–22
higher-level thinking, 177
horizontal violence. *See* bullying
humanistic education, 32–34

I

ICN. *See* International Council of Nursing
IEL. *See* Integrated Experiential Learning
The IEL course, 184
*I'm Here: Compassionate Communication in
Patient*, 201–202
information literacy, online nursing, learning
through writing, 150
informational learning, 242–243, 243t
informed consent, 264
institutional-level policies, online nursing,
learning through writing, 154
Institutional Review Board (IRB), 242
institutional support, for quality online
education, 72–73
instructional designers, 103
instructional resources, online teaching
strategies, 142–143
integrated design, curriculum
development, 95
Integrated Experiential Learning (IEL),
184, 185
International Council of Nursing (ICN), 186
internet, 156
interpretative approach, 194–195
interpreting: unlearning and becoming, 196
interprofessional model, 45–46, 46f
program evaluation, 53–54
interprofessional team, 47
academic advisor, 49–50, 51t
admissions counselor, 48–49, 49t
community partnerships, 52–53
online faculty, 50–51, 53t

outreach coordinator, 48, 49t
program director, 50–51, 53t
interviews, online nursing education,
experiential learning, 177
introverted students, 30
inviting: waiting and letting be, 196–197
IRB. *See* Institutional Review Board

J

jing, 151
Journal of Community & Public Health Nursing,
46
Journal of Continuing Education, 165

K

kolb and kolb, online nursing education,
experiential learning, 166, 167f

L

leadership
dedicated program, 63
development, 245–247, 250t
for online programs, 61–69
acceptance of education, 62–63
collaborative model, 63–64, 65t
coordinator, 64, 66, 66t
course lead, 67, 69t
dedicated, 63
service-learning, 67, 68t
skills, 281
learner-centered teaching
online teaching strategies, 128–129
learner presence, 135
learning, 166–170, 167–168t, 169f
assessment of, 96
domains of, 164
materials, 122–124, 123f
modules, 121–122, 122–123f
online course design, 102
and practicing interpretative
thinking, 196
-style preference, 29–30
taxonomy of, 106–108, 107–108t
through semesters, progression of, 96, 98
learning management systems (LMSs), 111,
114, 121, 125, 150, 152
Learning Resources Network (LERN), 219
LERN. *See* Learning Resources Network
leveling and scaffolding, online course design,
124–125, 124–125t

librarians and nursing faculty, collaboration, online nursing, learning through writing, 150

Likert scale, 56

Linfield-Good Samaritan School of Nursing, 187

listening: knowing and connecting, 197

literature review
  collaborative learning, 260–261
  service learning, 274–275

LMSs. *See* learning management systems

M

mechanics, online nursing, learning through writing, 155–156, 155–156*t*, 157*t*

mentorship, 214–215, 215*t*, 216*t*, 247–250, 250*t*

millennials, 28–29, 241, 249, 252

motivation
  for higher levels of nursing education, 44
  student, 31–32, 32*t*

N

narrative pedagogy, 15–16, 18*t*
  art forms: literature, cinema, podcasts, music, 198–201, 199–201*t*
  documentary: the invisible war, 201
  experiential storytelling, 204–205, 204–205*t*
  faculty storytelling, 205–208, 206*t*, 207–208*t*
  gathering: welcoming and calling forth, 195–196
  I'm Here: Compassionate Communication in Patient, 201–202
  interpretative approach, 194–195
  interpreting: unlearning and becoming, 196
  inviting: waiting and letting be, 196–197
  listening: knowing and connecting, 197
  schooling learning teaching, concernful practices of, 195
  strengths of, 194*f*
  use of, 197
  virtual community, 198
  When Breath Becomes Air, 202–203

National Academy of Medicine, 23, 43, 87

National Center for Education Statistics (NCES), 22, 45

National League for Nursing (NLN), 4, 24, 127

national licensing exam (NCLEX), 89

NCES. *See* National Center for Education Statistics

NCLEX. *See* national licensing exam

Neighborhood™, 165, 184, 185, 186, 187

NLN. *See* National League of Nursing

nurses
  barriers to degree advancement, 44
  bullying, 248
  holistic academic progression for, 45–46, 46*f*
  motivation, for higher education, 44

nursing education
  advanced practice, 4–5
  curriculum
    online nursing, learning through writing, 152–154, 153*t*
  demand for faculty, 212
  demand for higher levels of, 23
  educational pathways, 22
  generational diversity. *See* diversity, generational
  health care and societal issues affecting, 87–88
  online. *See* online nursing education
  practice and research, implications for, 254–255

nursing practice, impact on, 282

O

online adjunct faculty, 213–214

online collaborative activities, online teaching strategies, 137–138

online collaborative learning theory, 261
  data collection, coding, and analysis, 262–264, 263*t*
  discussion, 268–270
  ethical considerations, 264
  findings
    week one (entire class), 264–267, 265*t*
    week two (group forums), 267–268
  method and design, 261–262
  phases, 261
  setting and participants, 262

online collaborative theory. *See* collaborativist learning theory

online course design
  assessment, 108–110, 109*t*
    and grading rubrics, 114–120, 115–120*t*
    and learning activities, 111–114, 111*t*, 113*t*
    online assessments, types of, 110–111, 110*t*
  best practices, 101–102, 125–126

online course design (*Continued*)
 clear/consistent structure, 102
 collaborative and individual reflection, 103
 collaborative design and development
  process, 105, 106*f*
 collaborative learning, 102
 course learning outcomes, 105–106
  learning, taxonomy of, 106–108,
  107–108*t*
 design and development, 105
 evaluation, 125
 learning, 102
  materials, 122–124, 123*f*
  modules, 121–122, 122–123*f*
 leveling and scaffolding, 124–125,
  124–125*t*
 process of, 103–105
 structure and sequencing of, 121
online course expectations, 79, 81–82*t*
online faculty, 50–51
online learning
 academic program review, 76
 assessment and evaluation, 74–76
 course evaluation, 74–75, 75*t*
 student persistence rates, 75
online nursing education
 collaborative model for, 1–6, 4*f*
 experiential learning
  arts and literature activity,
   172–176, 176*t*
  dialectic poles, 170
  interviews, 177
  by kolb and kolb, 166, 167*f*
  learning, 166–170
  model for, 170–172, 171*f*, 173–175*t*
  service learning, 178–179
  simulation, 164–165, 165*t*
  small-group work, 177–178
  strategies, 172
  synchronous versus asynchronous
   simulation, 166
 guiding principles, 4
 integrated within institution, 5–6
 philosophical and theoretical
  approaches, 9–18
  adult learning theory, 15, 17*t*
  collaborativist learning theory,
   12–13, 17*t*
  constructivist learning theory, 10–12
  experiential learning theory, 13–14, 17*t*
  narrative pedagogy, 15–16, 18*t*
  transformative learning theory, 14, 17*t*
 subspecialty of, 5
online nursing, learning through writing
 academic integrity, 156–158, 158*t*
 discipline, 154–155

 embedded librarians, 150–151
 information literacy, 150
 institutional-level policies, 154
 librarians and nursing faculty,
  collaboration, 150
 mechanics, 155–156, 155–156*t*, 157*t*
 nursing education, curriculum,
  152–154, 153*t*
 research guides and tutorials, 151
 student-centered learning, 151–152, 152*t*
 writing students, types of, 159
online nursing programs
 leadership. *See* leadership, for online
  programs
 quality assurance. *See* quality assurance
online nursing students
 characteristics of
  cultural, ethnic, and gender diversity,
   24–26, 25*t*, 27*t*
  English as a second language, 26–28
  generational diversity, 28–29, 30*t*
  learning styles and preferences, 29–30
  personality traits, 30
  student motivation, 31–32, 32*t*
 demand for higher levels of education, 23
 educational pathways, 22
 enrollment trends, in higher
  education, 21–22
 humanistic education, 32–34
 respect, 35
 sense of belonging, 35
 social presence, 35–36
  individual phone calls, 36
  student support during crisis, 37,
   37–38*t*
  synchronous meeting times, 36
 student–faculty relationships, 34, 34*t*
 successful academic progression, 43–58
  barriers to degree advancement, 44
  community partner survey, 56, 57*t*
  interprofessional model. *See*
   interprofessional model
  interprofessional team. *See*
   interprofessional team
  motivation, for higher education, 44
  program evaluation, outcomes of, 56–57
  RN-to-BSN program, 47, 47*t*
  student persistence. *See* student
   persistence
  student survey, 54–56
 teacher immediacy, 35–36
online teaching
 best practices for, 76, 77–79*t*
 competence, 213
 peer appraisal, 79, 80–81*t*
 preparation and competency, 212–213

preparation for, 76, 77*t*
readiness, 212
online teaching strategies
active learning and teaching, 130–132,
131–132*t*
asynchronous discussions, 138–139, 140*t*
cognitive presence, 134
community
of inquiry model, 132, 134, 135–136
of learners, 132, 133
concept-based and competency-based
teaching, 129
demonstrate presence and engagement,
136–137, 137*t*
facilitating reflective, critical, and analytical
thinking, 139–141, 140*t*
facilitation challenges, 142
faculty preparation, 127–128, 128*t*
faculty role, 129
feedback banks, 143
grading and feedback, 142
grading and timeliness, 145–146, 146*t*
group feedback, 143, 144*t*
group work, 138
instructional resources, 142–143
learner-centered teaching, 128–129
online collaborative activities, 137–138
personalization, 143–145, 145*t*
scaffolded learning, 129–130
social presence, 133–134
Socratic method, 141–142, 141*t*
teaching presence, 134–135
ontology, 10
OPT model. *See* Outcome-Present State Test
model
organization, trust and confidence in, 286
orientation, 214
Outcome-Present State Test (OPT)
model, 184
outreach coordinator, 48, 49*t*

P

PBL approach. *See* problem-based learning
approach
pedagogical preparation, 128
pedagogical principles, 101, 102
peer appraisal, 79, 80–81*t*
personalization, online teaching strategies,
143–145, 145*t*
philosophical approach, 10
phone, 150
phone call, with students, 36
Planning Document for a Community
Coalition Activity, 188

postlicensure programs, concept-based
curriculum in, 92–95, 93–94*t*
PowerPoint presentations, 130
pragmatic approach, 193
problem-based learning (PBL)
approach, 185
process, online course design, 103–105
professional development, 215–218, 217*t*,
218–219*t*
program director, 50–51
psychomotor learning, 164
PubMed, 151

Q

QD. *See* Qualitative description
QM. *See* Quality Matters
QSEN. *See* Quality and Safety Education for
Nurses
qualitative description (QD), 242
Quality and Safety Education for Nurses
(QSEN), 129
quality assurance, in online nursing programs,
71–83
assessment and evaluation, 74–76
academic program review, 76
course evaluation, 74–75, 75*t*
student persistence rates, 75
institutional support, 72–73
online course expectations, 79,
81–82*t*
online teaching
best practices for, 76, 77–79*t*
peer appraisal, 79, 80–81*t*
preparation for, 76, 77*t*
peer appraisal, 79, 80–81*t*
specific, 76
student feedback, 79, 82, 83*t*
quality, in online programs, 73–74, 73*t*
Quality Matters (QM), 73–74, 164, 220
quality of care and services, 285
quotes
community organizations, 283–284*t*
student, 279–280*t*

R

reflective practice, 207
registered nurse–bachelor of science in
nursing (RN-to-BSN) program, 168,
178, 183–184
registered nurses (RNs), 2, 133, 150
regulated learning, 135
remote teaching, 5

research guides and tutorials
online nursing, learning through
writing, 151
respect, practicing and modeling, 35
RN-to-BSN program, 2, 274
curriculum, integration of models,
96, 97t
development, 88
online, key features of, 47, 47t
RNs. *See* registered nurses
Robert Wood Johnson Foundation, 43

S

SBAR. *See* situation, background, assessment,
and recommendation
scaffolded learning, online teaching strategies,
129–130
scholarship
application, 221
Boyer's model of, 221
discovery, 221
integration, 221–222
nursing education in, 220
teaching/learning, 221, 224
schooling learning teaching, concernful
practices of, 195
SDOH. *See* social determinants of health
self-determination, 32
semesters, learning through, 96, 98
sense of belonging (SoB), 35
service learning
academic partnerships. *See* academic
partnerships
defined, 274
online nursing education, experiential
learning, 178–179
service-learning coordinator, 67, 68t
Seven Principles of Good Practice in
Undergraduate Education, 73, 73t
simulation, online nursing education,
experiential learning, 164–165, 165t
situation, background, assessment, and
recommendation (SBAR), 166
Sloan Consortium (Sloan-C), 53
small-group work, online nursing education,
experiential learning, 177–178
SoB. *See* sense of belonging
social constructivism, 10, 11–12, 16t, 132
zone of proximal development, 12, 16–17t
social determinants of health (SDOH), 274
definition of, 274
social presence, 35–36
individual phone calls, 36
online teaching strategies, 133–134

student support during crisis, 37, 37–38t
synchronous meeting times, 36
societal issues, affecting nursing education,
87–88
Socratic method, online teaching strategies,
141–142, 141t
strategies, online nursing education,
experiential learning, 172
structure and sequencing, online course
design, 121
student
feedback, 79, 82, 83t
quotes, 279–280t
student-centered learning, online nursing,
learning through writing,
151–152, 152t
student evaluation, 188
student persistence, 45
measurements of, 54, 54t
rates, online learning, 75
student retention, 45
student–faculty relationships, 34, 34t
students
on academic advising, feedback
from, 54–56
extroverted, 30
introverted, 30
motivation, 31–32, 32t
support during crisis, 37, 37–38t
survey
community partner, 56, 57t
student, 54–56
synchronous meeting times, 36
synchronous versus asynchronous
simulation, online nursing education,
experiential learning, 166
systems thinking, leadership, 64

T

teacher immediacy, 35–36
teaching
growth, 224
scholarship of, 229, 229t
reflection, 224–225
teaching philosophy, 225–227
teaching methods, learning style application
in, 30–31, 31t
teaching presence, online teaching strategies,
134–135
technology, secondary to education theory, 6
technology skills, 253–254
transcript analysis, 261–262
transformative learning theory, 14, 17t
Trauma-Informed Care, 204

trust, service learning, 286
2019 novel coronavirus (COVID-19)
    pandemic, 37

U

understanding, defined, 95

V

veteran cohorts, 241
video or audio-conferencing technology, 138
virtual collaboration, defined, 260
virtual community, 198
vulnerable populations, 280–281
When Breath Becomes Air, 202–203

W

World Health Organization, 274
writing students, types of, online nursing,
    learning through writing, 159

Y

YouTube, 151

Z

zone of proximal development (ZPD), 12,
    16–17*t*, 112, 129–130, 166–167
Zoom, 151
ZPD. *See* Zone of proximal development